Clinician's Guide to

Mental Illness

Clinician's Guide to
Mental Illness

Edited by

Dennis C. Daley, Ph.D.

Associate Professor of Psychiatry
Chief, Drug and Alcohol Services
Director, Center for Psychiatric and Chemical Dependency Services
University of Pittsburgh Medical Center
Western Psychiatric Institute and Clinic
Pittsburgh, Pennsylvania

Ihsan M. Salloum, M.D., M.P.H.

Associate Professor of Psychiatry
Medical Director, Drug and Alcohol Services
Medical Director, Center for Psychiatric
and Chemical Dependency Services
University of Pittsburgh Medical Center
Western Psychiatric Institute and Clinic
Pittsburgh, Pennsylvania

McGraw-Hill
Medical Publishing Division

New York   Chicago   San Francisco   Lisbon   London   Madrid   Mexico City
Milan   New Delhi   San Juan   Seoul   Singapore   Sydney   Toronto

9/2001

McGraw-Hill

A Division of The **McGraw-Hill** Companies

1 2 3 4 5 6 7 8 9 0 DOC DOC 0 9 8 7 6 5 4 3 2 1

ISBN 0-07-134716-X

This book was set in Korinna by Keyword Publishing Services.
The editor was Martin Wonsiewicz.
The production supervisor was Catherine Saggese.
Project management was provided by Keyword Publishing Services.
The cover design was by Aimee Nordin.
R.R. Donnelley & Sons was the printer and binder.

This book is printed on acid-free paper.

Library of Congress Cataloging-in-Publication Data
Daley, Dennis C.
  Clinician's guide to mental illness / editors, Dennis C. Daley, Ihsan M. Salloum.
    p. ; cm.
  Includes bibliographical references and index.
  ISBN 0-07-134716-X
    1. Mental illness.   2. Substance abuse—Patients.   3. Patient compliance.   4. Psychiatry.
  I. Salloum, Ihsan M.   II. Title
    [DNLM: 1. Mental Disorders—diagnosis.   2. Mental Disorders—therapy.   3.
  Substance-Related Disorders—diagnosis.   4. Substance-Related Disorders—therapy.   WM
  140   D141c   2001]
  RC454.D25   2001
  616.89—dc21   00-049623

Contents

ACKNOWLEDGMENTS

We wish to thank our colleagues who spent considerable time and effort writing chapters for this book. Their extensive clinical experience and knowledge of the clinical and empirical literature and ability to write for other medical and health care professionals are evident throughout each chapter. We also wish to thank David J. Kupfer, M.D., Thomas Detre Professor and Chair of the Department of Psychiatry at Western Psychiatric Institute and Clinic (WPIC), and Diane Holder, President of WPIC, for their support of our work. Thanks to Cindy Hurney, administrative coordinator at the Center for Psychiatric and Chemical Dependency Services at WPIC, for her usual excellent help with the many tasks needed to write a book. Finally, we wish to thank Karen Chernyaev, our editor, for help and support throughout this process, and Alan Hunt of Keyword Publishing Services Ltd for his help during the editorial process.

D.C.D.
I.M.S.

Contributors

Dennis C. Daley, Ph.D.
Associate Professor of Psychiatry
Chief, Drug and Alcohol Services
Director, Center for Psychiatric
and Chemical Dependency
Services
Western Psychiatric Institute and
Clinic
University of Pittsburgh Medical
Center

Noreen Fredrick, M.S.N.
Program Administrator,
Comprehensive Care
Services
Western Psychiatric Institute and
Clinic
University of Pittsburgh Medical
Center

Rohan Ganguli, M.D.
Professor of Psychiatry,
Pathology, Health and
Community Systems
Vice Chaiman and Chief of Clinical
Services
Office of Clinical Affairs
Western Psychiatric Institute and
Clinic
University of Pittsburgh Medical
Center

Tad Gorske, Ph.D., C.A.C.
Partial Program Coordinator,
Research Project Clinician
Center for Psychiatric and
Chemical Dependency
Services
Western Psychiatric Institute and
Clinic
University of Pittsburgh Medical
Center

Roger Haskett, M.D.
Professor of Psychiatry
Medical Director, Adult Services
Western Psychiatric Institute and
Clinic
University of Pittsburgh Medical
Center
Chief, Department of Psychiatry
Magee Women's Hospital

Mark Jones, D.C.S.W., L.S.W.
Program Director, Center for
Treatment of Obsessive-
Compulsive Disorders
Western Psychiatric Institute and
Clinic
University of Pittsburgh Medical
Center

Member, Board of the Obsessive-
  Compulsive Foundation of
  Western Pennyslvania

Thomas M. Kelly, Ph.D.
Assistant Professor of Psychiatry
Investigator, Pittsburgh
  Adolescent Alcohol Research
  Center
Western Psychiatric Institute and
  Clinic
University of Pittsburgh Medical
  Center

Maria La Via, M.D.
Assistant Professor of Psychiatry
Medical Director, Eating
  Disorders and Behavioral
  Medicine Program
Western Psychiatric Institute and
  Clinic
University of Pittsburgh Medical
  Center

Oommen Mammen, M.D.
Assistant Professor of Psychiatry
Western Psychiatric Institute and
  Clinic
University of Pittsburgh Medical
  Center

Marsha Marcus, Ph.D.
Associate Professor of Psychiatry
  and Psychology

Chief, Behavioral Medicine and
  Eating Disorders Program
Western Psychiatric Institute and
  Clinic
University of Pittsburgh Medical
  Center

Paul A. Pilkonis, Ph.D.
Professor of Psychiatry and
  Psychology
Western Psychiatric Institute and
  Clinic
University of Pittsburgh Medical
  Center

Jason Rosenstock, M.D.
Assistant Professor of Psychiatry
Chief, Comprehensive Care
  Services
Western Psychiatric Institute and
  Clinic
University of Pittsburgh Medical
  Center

Ihsan M. Salloum, M.D., M.P.H.
Associate Professor of Psychiatry
Medical Director, Drug and
  Alcohol Services and Center for
  Psychiatric and Chemical
  Dependency Services
Western Psychiatric Institute and
  Clinic
University of Pittsburgh Medical
  Center

Preface

This book was written for health care professionals in both behavioral health care settings and primary medical health settings who encounter adult patients with mental health, substance use, or dual disorders (i.e., co-occurring mental health and substance use disorders). We provide a comprehensive and practical review of assessment and treatment of the more common adult mental disorders and substance use disorders. Our aim is to provide information that is easy to read and integrate into clinical practice, especially by busy professionals whose time is limited. This book was written in a style that lends itself for easy use by mental health professionals as well as primary medical care professionals.

The chapters were written by highly experienced teams of researcher-practitioners and clinicians from Western Psychiatric Institute and Clinic (WPIC), the Department of Psychiatry of the University of Pittsburgh Medical Center. WPIC is one of the leading research institutions in the world, and the faculty and staff who have contributed to this current treatment guide have extensive experience in developing and managing treatment programs for patients with psychiatric, substance use, and dual disorders, developing clinical models of treatment, providing direct clinical services in a variety of treatment contexts (hospital, partial hospital, and ambulatory) and formats (individual, group, and family), teaching medical students, psychiatric residents, and professionals from all other disciplines, and conducting clinical trials of psychosocial and/or pharmacological interventions.

Since our contributors are psychiatrists, psychologists, social workers, and nurses, we provide a multidisciplinary perspective on the assessment and treatment of mental and substance use disorders. We believe this book provides an excellent integration of the empirical, clinical, and recovery-oriented literature. Current clinical practice demands that clinicians be aware of current research and ways to translate this to the world of direct treatment.

The introductory chapter summarizes mental disorders and substance use disorders (types, causes, symptoms, common adverse effects on the patient, family, and society) and provides an overview of psychosocial and medication treatments, and the continuum of care. Since a major problem in treating patients with mental health or substance use disorders is poor adherence to treatment, considerable attention is given to clinical and systems strategies that can be used to improve patient adherence to treatment. In addition, strategies are presented that can help the health care professional facilitate a referral for treatment in cases where direct service cannot be provided (e.g., a primary care physician referring a depressed or alcohol-dependent patient to a behavioral health specialist; a mental health therapist facilitating a heroin-addicted patient's entry into a detoxification or rehabilitation program; an addictions therapist helping a patient with a psychotic disorder find the appropriate mental health care). Finally, a framework for "recovery" is presented that is applicable to the various types of disorders discussed throughout this book.

The subsequent chapters provide practical information about assessment and treatment of mood, anxiety, psychotic, substance use, eating, and personality disorders. Family issues, relapse prevention, the use of self-help groups, and comorbidity are also addressed throughout this book since many patients have multiple disorders, their families are often adversely affected, and relapse risk is high. In addition, this book integrates considerable information about treatment adherence, and provides the reader with helpful strategies on ways to enhance patient compliance with pharmacotherapy and psychotherapy, as well as strategies for increasing motivation to change.

1

Chapter One

Helping Patients with Mental Health and Substance Disorders

Dennis C. Daley

Introduction and Overview of Book

Mental health disorders (also referred to as mental disorders or psychiatric disorders) and substance use disorders are common clinical conditions encountered by health professionals in a wide range of medical and behavioral health care settings. Both mental disorders and substance use refer to specific types of psychiatric illnesses as defined by the American Psychiatric Association's *Diagnostic and Statistical Manual of Mental Disorders* (APA, 1994). While mental and substance use disorders are referred to as behavioral disorders and usually treated in mental health or substance abuse treatment systems, individuals with these disorders are often seen in medical settings as well. Mental and substance use disorders, alone or in combination, can create suffering for the patient, impair functioning, create a burden for the family, and impact on the health care delivery system. With this in mind, the primary aims of this book are to help medical and behavioral health care professionals:

- Understand the more common types of mental health and substance use disorders frequently seen in mental health and medical treatment settings.
- Become more knowledgeable and skillful at identifying and assessing these disorders even when the patient does not

specifically acknowledge, or is not primarily seeking treatment for them.

- Increase their ability to educate patients and families about mental health and substance-related disorders, including how they interact with medical disorders or the treatment of medical disorders.
- For mental health practitioners, becoming more comfortable and skillful at addressing substance use disorders among patients (related to assessment, treatment, and/or referral). Substance use disorders are common among mental health patients and clinicians need to be able to address these disorders if patients are to gain the maximum benefit from treatment.
- For substance abuse practitioners, becoming more comfortable and skillful at addressing mental health disorders among patients (related to assessment, treatment and/or referral). Mental health disorders are very common among patients with alcohol or drug abuse or dependence and clinicians need to address these disorders for patients to have the optimum chance of recovery from the substance use disorder.
- For medical health practitioners, becoming more comfortable and skillful at making appropriate recommendations for treatment of mental disorders or substance use disorders by behavioral health professionals such as psychiatrists, psychologists, social workers, therapists, and counselors. Physicians and other health professionals are often the first professionals to encounter patients with mental health and substance use disorders. The more equipped they are to intervene with these patients, the more likely these patients are to benefit from behavioral health care treatments.

Chapters 2–7 in this book are devoted to the more common disorders including substance use (alcohol or drug abuse and dependence), mood (depression and bipolar), anxiety, eating, schizophrenic, and borderline and antisocial personality as these are the common ones encountered by health and mental health care professionals. In these chapters we review the specific symptoms of these disorders as well as assessment and treatment strategies.

Overview of Chapter

This chapter is divided into several sections. In the first section, we review the types and prevalence of mental and substance use disorders; discuss comorbidity, or multiple disorders; and the patterns, causes, and effects of these disorders. The next section covers the process of conducting a comprehensive and thorough assessment of psychiatric and substance use disorders utilizing the Diagnostic and Statistical Manual of Mental Disorders (DSM-IV) multi-axial format (APA, 1994). We also discuss the importance of conveying assessment findings to the patient and/or family. The third section covers the continuum of care, levels of care, treatment approaches, and treatment issues. The importance of therapeutic alliance between caregivers and patient is discussed since this is one of the major variables affecting treatment outcome. The fourth section reviews the process of recovery and relapse. We define the terms, discuss factors mediating recovery, and identify signs of relapse. Next, we review suicide and violence, the family, and involvement in treatment, and self-help groups. Families are grossly affected by disorders and their perspective must be understood and appreciated so that they can be involved in treatment. Self-help programs for family and patients are becoming increasingly important as people recovering from specific disorders have much to offer one another. Finally, we review ways to measure outcome for patients treated for a mental health or substance use disorder. In an age of increasing accountability by administrators and payers, caregivers must have ways of demonstrating that what they do is effective in helping improve patients' clinical conditions, level of functioning, and quality of life.

The material presented in this initial chapter is based on the clinical and empirical literature, our extensive experience providing treatment to psychiatric, substance abuse, and dual diagnosis patients over the past two decades, and research studies we have conducted in our treatment programs. The information provided in this chapter is relevant to a multiplicity of psychiatric and substance use disorders.

■ TYPES OF MENTAL AND SUBSTANCE USE DISORDERS

DSM-IV diagnostic categories for adults include organic mental, psychoactive substance use, schizophrenic, paranoid, and other psychotic, affective, anxiety, somatoform, dissociative, psychosexual, factitious, impulse control, adjustment, and personality disorders (see Table 1-1). While these disorders are discussed more extensively in Chapters 2–8 of this book, following is a brief description of these disorders and some of the associated symptoms (APA, 1994):

TABLE 1-1. DSM-IV MULTI-AXIAL FORMULATION FOR MENTAL AND SUBSTANCE USE DISORDERS

Axis I: Clinical disorders
Substance use, mood, anxiety, somatoform, factitious, dissociative, sexual and gender identity, eating, sleep, impulse control, and adjustment disorders

Axis II: Personality disorders
Prominent maladaptive personality features or defense mechanisms
Mental retardation

Axis III: General medical conditions

Axis IV: Psychosocial and environmental problems
Primary support groups
Social environment
Educational
Occupational
Housing
Economic
Access to health care
Legal
Other problems

Axis V: Global assessment of functioning

1. Affective (mood) disorders. These involve a disturbance of mood or prolonged emotional state that is not caused by a medical or other mental disorder. *Major depression* involves a dysphoric mood or loss of interest or pleasure in the patient's usual activities or pastimes along with other symptoms such as poor appetite, sleep disturbance, fatigue, loss of energy, or suicidality. *Bipolar disorder* involves mania, an elevated, expansive or irritable mood accompanied by other significant symptoms such as an increase in activity, restlessness, or pressured speech. The patient with a bipolar illness may experience a manic episode, depressive episode, or mixed episode. Major depression or bipolar disorders may also include psychotic features. Major depression may be experienced as a single episode, or as a recurrent disorder with multiple episodes of depression over time.

2. Anxiety disorders. This group of disorders involves anxiety as the predominant symptom and includes phobias, panic disorder, generalized anxiety disorder, obsessive–compulsive disorder, and post-traumatic stress disorder. *Phobias* involve persistent and irrational fears of objects, activities, or situations that lead to avoidant behavior. The three major types of phobias are agoraphobia, social phobia, and simple phobia. *Agoraphobia* is the most severe and pervasive form and involves a fear of being alone or in public places from which escape would be difficult. This disorder is sometimes accompanied by *panic attacks*, which involve sudden and intense periods of apprehension or fear along with physical symptoms such as heart palpitations, dizziness, sweating, shaking, or trembling. A *social phobia* involves a persistent and irrational fear of, and a desire to avoid, a situation where the person is worried about being scrutinized by others (e.g., speaking or eating in front of others). The person also is afraid that he or she may act in a way that is humiliating or embarrassing. A *simple phobia* is a persistent or irrational desire to avoid objects (e.g., certain animals) or situations (e.g., closed spaces, heights, or flying in an airplane). A *generalized anxiety disorder* involves persistent anxiety along with symptoms of motor tension (e.g., shakiness, trembling, trouble relaxing), autonomic hyperactivity (e.g., pounding heart, dizziness, upset stomach), apprehension (e.g., anxiety, worry, or fear in antici- pating some misfortune will occur), and vigilance and scanning (e.g., feeling on edge or impatient). An *obsessive–compulsive dis- order* involves obsessions and/or compulsions that are distressful and interfere with the person's ability to function. *Post-traumatic stress disorder* involves the re-experiencing of a psychologically traumatic event (e.g., rape, assault, combat, accident, or natural disaster) through recurrent dreams or recollections of the event along with a numbing of responsiveness or reduced involvement with the world.

3. *Schizophrenia.* This category of mental disorder involves psychotic symptoms (e.g., hallucinations), disturbances in think- ing (e.g., delusions, illogical thinking, loose associations), affect, sense of self, goal directed activity, interpersonal relationships, and psychomotor behavior that contribute to a significant dete- rioration in routine functioning. This disorder represents one of the most chronic and potentially debilitating categories of psy- chiatric illness as many schizophrenics experience a lifelong course of the illness.

4. *Eating disorders (anorexia and bulimia).* These are char- acterized by gross disturbances in eating behavior. In *anorexia*, the person has an intense fear of becoming obese, a disturbed body image, loses a significant amount of weight, and refuses to maintain a normal body weight. *Bulimia* involves recurrent epi- sodes of binge eating followed by depressed mood and self- deprecating thoughts about the binges. Self-induced vomiting, restrictive diets, and diuretics may be used in attempts to lose weight.

5. *Borderline and antisocial personality disorders.* Personality disorders involve a long-term pattern of experience and behavior that deviates from what is normal in the person's culture. This pattern shows in a variety of personal and social situations and causes significant personal distress or impair- ment in functioning. The person has a distorted way of viewing self, others and the world problems with emotional responses; poor impulse control; and/or significant relationship problems.

A *borderline personality disorder (BPD)* involves unstable and intense relationships, impulsiveness, emotional lability, inappropriate and intense anger or problems controlling anger, recurrent suicidal threats, gestures or behaviors or self-mutilating behaviors, identity disturbance, chronic emptiness, and frantic efforts to avoid abandonment. Some individuals with BPD experience psychotic symptoms. This disorder is much more common among women than men and is associated with other types of psychiatric and substance use disorders. An *antisocial personality disorder (ASP)* involves a pattern of antisocial behavior in which the rights of others are violated. The person with ASP often breaks the law, deceives others, lacks remorse for behaviors, and is irresponsible and impulsive. ASP is much more common among men than women, and the majority of individuals with this disorder also have problems with alcohol or drug abuse.

6. *Substance use disorders.* These include a pattern of alcohol or other drug use that leads to personal distress or impairment in functioning. Specific diagnostic categories include substance intoxication, withdrawal, abuse, and dependence or substance-induced mood, anxiety, psychotic or sleep disorders.

■ PREVALENCE OF DISORDERS

The National Institutes of Health conducted the Epidemiologic Catchment Area (ECA) study to determine the prevalence of select adult mental and substance use disorders among individuals (Robins & Regier, 1991). The ECA study involved over 20,000 individuals from across the country. Results showed that 22.5 percent of adults in the United States met lifetime criteria for a non-substance abuse mental disorder, and 16.4 percent met lifetime criteria for an alcohol or drug use disorder. The lifetime prevalence of the more common adult disorders was:

- Alcohol abuse or dependence   13.7 percent
- Phobias   12.6 percent
- Drug abuse or dependence   6.1 percent

- Major depression   5.1 percent
- Antisocial personality disorder   2.5 percent
- Obsessive–compulsive disorder   2.5 percent
- Dysthymia   1.5 percent
- Panic disorder   1.5 percent
- Cognitive dysfunction   1.1 percent
- Schizophrenia   1.0 percent
- Mania   0.4 percent
- Somatization   0.1 percent
- Anorexia   0.1 percent

■ COMORBIDITY OR CO-OCCURRING DISORDERS

The ECA study found high rates of comorbidity, or multiple disorders. Results showed that 29 percent of adults with a mental disorder met lifetime criteria for a substance use disorder. Of these, 53 percent had a drug use and 37 percent had an alcohol use disorder. Numerous studies of clinical populations also show high rates of comorbidity, or multiple disorders, among patients in treatment (Daley, Moss & Campbell, 1993; Ries, 1995; NIAAA, 1997; O'Connell, in press). Many patients with a mood disorder have a comorbid anxiety or substance use disorder; many with schizophrenia have a comorbid mood or substance use disorder; many with an anxiety disorder have a comorbid depressive or substance use disorders; and many with a cocaine use disorder have a comorbid mood, personality, or alcohol use disorder. In one of our recent studies of psychiatric patients, we found an average of 3.13 active DSM-IV diagnoses among patients who had both a mental and substance use disorder, and an average of 1.65 diagnoses among patients with mental disorders and no substance use disorder (Daley, 1999). Also, it is common for patients diagnosed with a specific disorder not to meet full criteria for another disorder, yet experience symptoms of one or more disorders that impact on their recovery.

■ PATTERNS OF MENTAL AND SUBSTANCE USE DISORDERS

Many individuals experience a single episode of a mental disorder and function well when the disorder is in remission, with no residual adverse effects. Others experience occasional episodes over time with little or no serious residual disability between episodes. However, there is a significant group of patients who experience repeated episodes with significant residual disability. These patients have persistent symptoms that are more or less present all of the time and are sometimes referred to as having serious and persistent mental illness (SPMI). Although patients with SPMI can include those from most of the DSM-IV diagnostic categories, many have schizophrenia, recurrent mood or anxiety disorders, or borderline personality disorder. Many SPMI patients also have comorbid substance abuse or dependency (Minkoff & Drake, 1991; Montrose & Daley, 1995; Ryglewicz & Pepper, 1996). These are the patients most likely to need long-term psychiatric or dual diagnosis treatment, inpatient care during periods of symptom exacerbation, and ancillary social services such as case management, housing, community residential programs, vocational training, partial hospital programs, or intensive outpatient programs.

■ CAUSES OF MENTAL OR SUBSTANCE USE DISORDERS

It is widely accepted that mental and substance use disorders are caused by a number of interacting biological, psychological, and social–cultural (environmental) factors (Anthenelli & Schuckit, 1997; Daley & Marlatt, 1997b; Miklowitz & Goldstein, 1997; Sadock & Sadock, 2000; Ott, Tarter & Ammerman, 1999). The biopsychosocial framework is a widely used paradigm for understanding mental and substance use disorders as it considers multiple interacting causal and protective factors in the development of an episode of illness. The degree of influence of each of these major elements depends on the specific type of disorder as some disorders may have more of a genetic vulnerability and biological component than others.

1. *Biological.* These include diseases, genetic vulnerability, dysregulations in dopamine, norepinephrine, serotonin, acetylcholine and gamma-aminobutyric acid systems, and differences in brain structure. Many mood, anxiety, psychotic, and addictive disorders run in families, increasing the risk to offspring or first-degree relatives. The relative risk of acquiring a specific disorder is higher than that of chance.

2. *Psychological.* These include attitudes and beliefs, psychological defenses, coping skills, problem-solving abilities, and personality factors. For example, studies show that there were often early childhood personality indicators (e.g., higher levels of aggressiveness and affective expressiveness) among children of bipolar parents (Miklowitz & Goldstein, 1997).

3. *Social–cultural.* These include early experiences within the family and one's culture, environmental influences, and level of social support. On the other hand, there are also "protective" factors such as a supportive family or social environment that may reduce vulnerability to mental or substance use disorders among some individuals.

■ EFFECTS OF MENTAL AND SUBSTANCE USE DISORDERS

Mental and substance use disorders are associated with a range of problems in all areas of functioning for the affected patient, the family, and society (APA, 1994; Daley, Salloum & Thase, in press). The specific effects on a patient will depend on the type and severity of the disorder(s), personality, personal competencies, coping mechanisms, and behaviors exhibited. Areas of functioning affected include medical or physical, psychological or emotional, family, social or interpersonal, spiritual, occupational, legal, and financial status. Following are examples that illustrate how various areas of functioning can be affected by various psychiatric disorders.

- A patient's life is seriously jeopardized due to severe weight loss and poor nutrition associated with her anorexia.

- A patient with borderline personality disorder makes multiple parasuicide or suicide gestures, creating havoc with the family and significant relationships, leading to family conflict and distress. Her behaviors also lead to feelings of rejection, which in turn contributes to her increased depression.

- A drug-dependent patient with problems with violence suffers physical injuries and causes serious injuries to another due to a violent altercation. His involvement in illegal activities to support an expensive drug habit, increases his risk of being incarcerated.

- A patient in a manic episode is convinced that he has the perfect business idea that will make him rich. He takes out a large loan and uses his family's saving account to finance his idea and subsequently loses all of the money.

- An alcoholic patient misses work due to hangovers, loses a job, and seriously jeopardizes the financial stability of her family. Her erratic and unpredictable behavior when drinking causes her husband and children to worry, and her vulgar verbal attacks upset and bother her family.

- A patient with schizophrenia and poor social skills feels alone and isolated due to her difficulties interacting with others and building interpersonal relationships. She spends much of her time alone and also feels depressed.

- A patient with recurrent depression feels guilty and shameful about being ill and unable to function adequately as a parent. He feels a sense of "emptiness" and that little in life seems meaningful or important to him besides his children. He also feels demoralized due to multiple episodes of depression over time.

- A woman is so anxious and fearful that she can barely leave her home to buy groceries or see a doctor. She feels like a prisoner in her own house and is increasingly despondent as a result. She will not even leave to visit her adult children who live in a nearby town.

Assessment of Mental and Substance Use Disorders

■ DSM-IV MULTI-AXIAL FORMAT FOR ASSESSMENT

Multiple methods are used to gather information during the assessment process in order to determine diagnoses and make treatment recommendations according to five axes. These methods include clinical interviews and observations of the patient, review of previous records (treatment, medical, psychological test results) or laboratory tests, collateral interviews (family, significant others, other caregivers, or social service professionals), and the use of pen and paper questionnaires that elicit information about specific disorders such as depression, social phobia, and substance abuse. While non-behavioral health care professionals usually will not have time to conduct full psychiatric assessments, an understanding of the assessment process can help them become better at determining how to help patients with mental health or substance use disorders. For example, if a physician or nurse suspects a depressive disorder, he or she can have the patient complete a brief written, self-test on depression such as the Beck Depression Inventory. Results of this inventory can then help the physician determine if a more comprehensive psychiatric assessment is needed and then make a referral to a mental health specialist. Or, if a physician or nurse suspects a patient has an alcohol problem, he or she can ask the patient to complete the Michigan Alcoholism Screening Test, the results of which can be used to discuss the need for a more comprehensive substance abuse evaluation or treatment.

The assessment process can be complicated when the patient is psychotic, intoxicated, uncooperative, denies or minimizes problems or symptoms, or has no motivation or interest in being helped. An assessment may take one or more sessions, depending on the patient's condition and the complexity of the situation. A patient may have multiple psychiatric, substance use, personality or medical diagnoses as well as multiple social problems or significant stressors.

Provisional, or "rule-out," diagnoses can be given in cases in which it is not clear if an actual DSM disorder is present and more information is needed. For example, a patient with alcohol dependence may have symptoms of depression. The clinical history may show that this patient never suffered major depression when not drinking, and that he has been drinking heavily during the entire current episode of depression. A provisional diagnosis would be given until it can be determined if clinical depression exists in the absence of active symptoms of alcohol dependence. In the absence of a clear-cut prior history of major depression, this particular case would require that the patient be abstinent from alcohol for a period of time, usually several weeks or longer, before it can be determined if indeed a major depression exists.

The DSM-IV multi-axial format provides a comprehensive approach to assessment of the patient on five axes (APA, 1994, pp. 25–37) (see Table 1-2):

1. *Axis I: Clinical disorders.* These include schizophrenia, other psychotic, mood, anxiety, somatoform, factitious, dissociative, sexual and gender identity, eating, sleep, impulse control, and adjustment disorders. Each specific disorder has a cluster of symptoms (physical, emotional, behavioral, cogni-

TABLE 1-2. DSM-IV DIAGNOSTIC CATEGORIES

Types of disorders	Severity and course specifiers
Psychotic	Mild to severe
Mood	Partial to full remission
Anxiety	Relapse and recurrence
Somatoform	
Factitious	
Dissociative	
Sexual and gender identity	
Eating	
Sleep	
Impulse control	
Adjustment	
Personality	
Substance use	
Other conditions that may be a focus of clinical work	

tive), time requirements, and functioning impairments associated with it.

2. *Axis II: Personality disorders and mental retardation.* These include paranoid, schizoid, schizotypal, antisocial, borderline, histrionic, narcissistic, avoidant, dependent, obsessive-compulsive, and personality disorder not otherwise specified. Even if the patient does not meet full criteria for a personality disorder, the clinician can note significant "traits" on Axis II (e.g., antisocial, narcissistic, paranoid, etc.).

3. *Axis III: General medical conditions and disorders.* These include any condition, disorder, or disease caused by injury, poisoning, or infection, associated with pregnancy, childbirth or the post-partum period; or involving the nervous system, blood, sense organs, skin, or any of the major systems (circulatory, respiratory, digestive, genitourinary, musculoskeletal). These conditions or disorders may be etiologically significant to the primary mental disorder. Or, an Axis III condition may not be etiologically significant but have implications for the management of the mental or substance use disorders.

4. *Axis IV: Psychosocial and environmental problems.* These include problems with the primary support group or social environment, education, occupation, housing, economic status, access to health care, crime, and related to the legal system. These problems may contribute to the exacerbation of the current disorder or result from it. Axis IV is also coded for severity (e.g., none, minimal, mild, moderate, severe, extreme).

5. *Axis V: Global assessment of functioning (current and past year).* This is the clinician's judgment of the patient's current overall level of functioning and highest level of functioning within the past year related to interpersonal relationships, occupation, and use of leisure time. Level of functioning includes superior, very good, good, fair, poor, very poor, and grossly impaired.

As part of the comprehensive psychiatric assessment, the clinician includes current or past suicidal ideation or behavior;

aggressive ideation or behavior; drug or alcohol use; developmental and social history; significant family history of medical, psychiatric, and substance use disorders; level of motivation; impact of disorders on self and others; and patient strengths or personal resources. A mental status examination is also performed to assess orientation, attention and calculation, recall, and language.

Substance use is a significant problem among many psychiatric patients and has major implications for their recovery and for the development of the initial treatment plan. The presence of any type of substance abuse or dependence can complicate psychiatric assessment and recovery in a number of ways. Therefore, a thorough substance use history should be gathered to document current and past substance use, patterns of use, consequences of use, perception of substance use, motivation to address a comorbid substance use disorder, and relapse history. In Chapter 2, we provide more specific details on the assessment and treatment processes for substance use disorders.

Findings of the psychiatric assessment are used to establish diagnoses, including provisional ones, using Axes I–V, determine recommendations for further evaluation, discuss treatment options with the patient, and make an initial agreement on the treatment plan and disposition. In the current climate of managed care, in which treatment services have to be authorized and are subject to review, thorough assessments are all the more important to justify both initial treatment recommendations as well as ongoing treatment.

■ CONVEYING ASSESSMENT FINDINGS TO THE PATIENT AND FAMILY

Once a psychiatric and/or substance abuse evaluation is complete, the clinician can review the findings with the patient in order to present the diagnosis and the clinical information upon which it is based. If the patient meets criteria for a specific DSM-IV disorder, the symptoms and associated behaviors can be reviewed in specific detail to identify the disorder for the patient. This process often leads to discussion of the possible etiology of the disorder, what the patient thinks and feels about the diagnosis, and the recommendations for treatment. Patients who deny or minimize their disorder can be helped to accept it through this process of sharing findings of the assessment. If the family is involved in the assessment process, they can also be involved in this feedback process so that they can share their reactions and ask questions.

In some instances, the patient will have some symptoms of a mental health disorder, but not meet full criteria of the diagnosis. In these cases of "sub-syndromal" disorders, the patient can be referred for mental health treatment if the health care professional believes that such treatment could benefit the patient.

■ ROLE OF MEDICAL HEALTH CARE PROFESSIONALS

A significant number of patients who see physicians, nurses, and other health care professionals for medical problems and treatments have additional mental health and/or substance abuse disorders. Unrecognized and untreated, these "other" disorders can have an adverse impact on the treatment of the medical condition as well as contribute to suffering and impaired functioning in the patient. A major challenge for health care professionals is taking a "holistic" approach to care and considering mental health and substance use issues in their work with patients. Some patients will openly tell their doctor or health care professional about mental health symptoms or problems with alcohol or other drugs, and even ask for help. Many, however, will not spontaneously discuss these problems; in some cases, patients may even be unaware that they suffer from a mental health disorder such as depression or an addictive disorder such as alcohol dependence. Therefore, it is incumbent upon the health care professional to inquire about these other types of disorders and facilitate referrals to mental health or substance abuse treatment professionals as needed. If a patient accepts a referral for a mental health or substance abuse evaluation or treatment, the referring professional can facilitate the process by having a brief telephone discussion with the clinician to whom the patient is being referred. The health care provider can also initiate a discussion with the mental health or substance abuse professional for patients already active in treatment if he or she has any questions or concerns about the patient's current substance abuse, mental health symptoms, an actual or potential relapse, interactions between psychiatric medications and other medicines, interactions between alcohol and medications, or other significant issues that have implications for the patient's health.

■ ROLE OF MENTAL HEALTH CLINICIANS

Since significant numbers of mental health patients have alcohol- or drug-related disorders that complicate their recovery or cause additional problems in their life, mental health clinicians must be able to determine if a substance use disorder exists. While there are different approaches to treatment of mental health patients with co-occurring substance use disorders, the ideal strategy is to provide integrated treatment that addresses issues and problems associated with all of the patient's disorders. However, there may be times in which a given patient needs a specific type of substance abuse treatment such as medical detoxification or residential rehabilitation in order to help stabilize from acute symptoms of more severe types of substance dependency. In such cases, the mental health clinician needs to be conversant with specific types of substance abuse treatment resources in order to facilitate referrals and coordinate treatment efforts.

■ ROLE OF SUBSTANCE ABUSE PROFESSIONALS

Similarly, substance abuse professionals need to be aware that high rates of psychiatric comorbidity are common among patients with alcohol and/or drug-related disorders. While some of these disorders can be treated within the context of substance abuse treatment agencies if staff are adequately trained, others will require that patients be referred to appropriate mental health professionals for evaluation and treatment of specific types of mental disorders. Facilitating referrals may require the clinician to persuade or motivate the patient to accept a mental health treatment referral as well as coordinating care with another professional and/ or treatment system.

■ GETTING THE PATIENT TO ACCEPT HELP

Common Barriers in Seeking Treatment

Some patients willingly accept recommendations to seek treatment for a psychiatric and/or substance use disorder. However, many do not seek treatment despite the serious nature of their problems (Blackwell, 1997; Carroll, 1997). They refuse treatment recommendations, accept them but then fail to follow through with the treatment referral, drop out of treatment prematurely, or comply poorly with the treatment plan. They may, for example, miss treatment sessions, fail to take medications as prescribed, or not follow other specific recommendations made by the treating professional. Resistance is common and caregivers need to understand factors affecting patient motivation to engage in treatment and to determine how to lower resistance so that the patient follows through with the treatment referral.

Table 1-3 summarizes the major factors affecting a patient's adherence to the recommendations of a professional to get help for a mental health, substance use, or dual disorder (Daley & Zuckoff, 1999). These include patient-related factors, illness or symptom-related factors, relationship and social support variables, and treatment systems variables. Usually, a combination of factors adversely impact a patient's willingness to engage in treatment. Awareness of these common internal and external barriers to seeking help can help the professional develop strategies to increase treatment compliance.

How to Facilitate Referrals to Specialized Treatment Programs

There are a number of strategies that the physician or other health care professional can use to increase the odds of a patient following through with specific recommendations for treatment of the problem of depression, alcoholism, or violence. Table 1-4 summarizes clinical strategies and Table 1-5 summarizes systems

TABLE 1-3. FACTORS AFFECTING PATIENT ADHERENCE WITH TREATMENT RECOMMENDATIONS

Patient variables	Illness & symptom related variables	Relationship & social support variables	Treatment & system variables
Motivation	Symptoms of addiction	Negative social supports	Therapeutic alliance
Beliefs	Symptoms of psychiatric	Unstable living situation	Friendliness of treatment
Stigma	illness	Poverty	staff
Expectations	Obsessions or cravings	Homelessness	Competence of staff
Satisfaction with	to use		Demands on counselor
treatment	Social anxiety		Supervision of staff
Personality	Previous history of illness		Access to treatment
Other addictions	and relapse		Characteristics of
(gambling, smoking, etc.)	Failure to catch early		treatment setting
Other life events or	warning signs of relapse		Type of treatment offered
problems	Improvement in		Duration of treatment
	symptoms or problems		Intensity of treatment
			Appropriateness of
			treatment
			recommendations
			Medication problems
			Expense of treatment
			Ineffective treatment
			Continuity of care
			Availability of other
			services

Adapted from Daley and Zuckoff (1999, p. 40).

strategies that can improve the patient's adherence with the treatment referral and ongoing participation.

Treatment of Mental and Substance Use Disorders

■ THE CONTINUUM OF CARE FOR MENTAL HEALTH DISORDERS

Effective intervention with patients who have mental and/or substance use disorders requires that the health care professional be conversant with the continuum of care. Professionals who do not provide direct treatment services or who need specialized services due to the specific nature of a given patient's problems also need strategies to increase patient motivation for treatment in order to facilitate acceptance of, and adherence to, referrals for treatment.

TABLE 1-4. CLINICAL STRATEGIES TO IMPROVE ADHERENCE

Therapeutic relationship
Express empathy and concern
Convey helpfulness in attitudes and behaviors
Encourage discussions of the counseling process
Encourage discussions of patient–counselor relationship

Motivation
Accept ambivalence as normal
Accept and appreciate small changes
Accept varying levels of readiness to change
Anticipate noncompliance at various stages of treatment
Discuss prior history of compliance
Discuss current compliance problems immediately

Treatment preparation
Provide aftercare counseling prior to discharge from residential or inpatient care
Help the patient anticipate roadblocks to change
Explore expectations and hopes for treatment

Treatment plan development
Negotiate rather than dictate change plans
Emphasize responsibility to the patient
Regularly review treatment goals and progress
Discuss pros and cons of treatment
Discuss pros and cons of self-help groups
Discuss pros and cons of abstinence
Provide options regarding treatment

Treatment process and strategies
Provide interventions based on empirical support
Change treatment frequqency and intensity as needed
Provide direct feedback to patient
Discuss patient's reaction to feedback
Provide reinforcement for treatment compliance
Provide reinforcement for compliance with abstinence
Address social anxiety about treatment groups or self-help groups
Provide education to the patient and family
Elicit family support and involvement

Symptom monitoring: psychiatric disorders
Monitor psychiatric symptoms
Address persistent or residual psychiatric symptoms
Monitor psychiatric relapse warning signs

Symptom monitoring: substance use disorders
Monitor substance use recovery issues
Monitor cravings and thoughts of using substances
Monitor people, places and events and close calls
Focus on patient's motivation
Monitor substance use relapse warning signs

TABLE 1-4 (Continued)

Medications
Discuss medication for mental or substance use disorders
Prepare patient for taking medications
Monitor medication compliance
Elicit agreement to not stop medicines without discussing with caregiver
Address adverse side effects of lack of efficacy of medications
Facilitate medication changes for ineffective medicines
Facilitate augmentation therapy
Prepare for negative reactions to medications, of self-help members
Discuss potential interventions between alcohol or illicit drug use, and medicines used for psychiatric or mental disorders

Adapted from Daley and Zuckoff (1999, p 83).

The continuum of care for mental disorders, from the most to the least restrictive level, involves the following treatment settings and services:

1. Long-term psychiatric hospitalization. This is for the more persistently and chronically mentally ill patient who continues to

TABLE 1-5. SYSTEMS STRATEGIES THAT IMPROVE ADHERENCE

Develop a clinic philosophy on compliance
Encourage staff training on motivational and compliance counseling
Provide easy access to treatment
Offer flexible appointment times
Offer consistent appointment times
Call and remind patients of the initial evaluation session
Call patients who fail to show for the initial evaluation
Call patients or family members prior to regularly scheduled treatment sessions
Use prompts to remind patients of scheduled sessions
Use written compliance contracts
Use creative ways of scheduling treatment appointments
Outreach to poorly compliant patients
Encourage treatment dropouts to return for services
Determine the reasons for poor compliance or early treatment drop out
Use case management services
Help the patient access other services
Contact patient to make sure referrals were followed up
Provide assistant with practical problems
Establish clinic and counselor thresholds for acceptable levels of treatment compliance or completion
Conduct regular patient and family satisfaction surveys
Continuously seek quality improvement
Offer integrated treatment for patients with dual disorders

Adapted from Daley and Zuckoff (1999, p.100).

evidence serious psychiatric symptoms, impairment in functioning and an inability to function in the community due to the serious
threat of harm to self or others. Long-term care focuses on treating
symptoms, improving coping skills, and preparing patients for
the community. Length of stay varies from weeks to months or
longer. In recent years, there has been an decrease in the number
of long-term hospital beds with more patients returned to their
community after brief periods of hospitalization.

   2. *Community residential programs.* Some chronically
impaired patients need to live in supervised residential programs
in order to function outside of a hospital setting. Many of these programs have on-site mental health treatment services, but in some
cases patients attend day hospital programs. They receive social
support and supervision in the residential facility and clinical care
at a local mental health treatment program.

   3. *Acute-care psychiatric hospital.* These are short-term programs (days to a few weeks) that aim to establish diagnoses, stabilize acute symptoms of the mental disorder, and develop an
ongoing treatment plan for continued care. Chronic patients may
have episodic admissions during periods of symptom exacerbation. Individual, family, group, and milieu therapies, aftercare
planning, and pharmacotherapy assessment and management
are provided during the acute care stay. In addition, some patients
may receive Electroconvulsive Therapy (ECT).

   4. *Twenty-three-hour bed.* This service allows the treatment
team the opportunity to observe the patient over an extended period of time to determine if an inpatient admission is needed or if
the patient can be better served by referral to an ambulatory program (e.g., partial hospital or outpatient care). Since the acute
effects of substances also affect psychiatric symptoms and behaviors, a 23-hour bed provides time to assess whether current
symptoms may be caused by alcohol or other drug use.

   5. *Ambulatory care: partial hospital or day program.* This program is used to divert a potential inpatient admission, as a "step-
down" program for discharged inpatients, or for patients with
more severe levels of symptoms and impairment who need a
structured program with frequent clinical contact. Acute-care pro-

grams last up to several weeks, and longer-term programs last up to several months. A day in a partial hospital program includes participation in a variety of treatment groups. Individual therapy, medication management, and/or vocational training may also be provided.

6. *Ambulatory care: outpatient or aftercare programs.* These programs are used by higher functioning patients who do not need high levels of care and by chronically impaired patients who need follow-up care after treatment in a hospital or partial hospital program. Intensive outpatient programs may involve several treatment sessions per week. Stable patients in the maintenance phase of care may only be seen every several months. Individual, group, family, and medication management are the main treatments offered in outpatient and aftercare programs. Some patients may also receive ECT as an outpatient.

7. *Other services.* Many psychiatric patients have comorbid substance use disorders and may be detoxified while an inpatient or partial hospital patient. Or, they may participate in "dual diagnosis" programs as part of their psychiatric care. Chronic psychiatric patients also benefit from intensive case management, social work services, vocational assessment and counseling, neuropsychological assessments, chaplain services, leisure counseling, and participation in self-help programs.

■ THE CONTINUUM OF CARE FOR SUBSTANCE USE DISORDERS

Patients with substance use and comorbid mental disorders may utilize the services listed above. Specific substance abuse related services that these dual diagnosis patients, as well as those with primary substance use disorders, may use include the following (ASAM, 1998):

1. *Hospital-based detoxification or rehabilitation.* These are short-term, medically managed services aimed at stabilizing the addiction. They are recommended for more severely dependent patients with significant medical (e.g., seizures, history of delirium tremens) and/or psychiatric (e.g., suicidality) problems that

require close access to physicians and nurses. Detoxification usually last several days, depending on which drugs the patient has been using and is dependent on. Hospital-based rehabilitation programs previously involved 4 weeks of structured, recovery-oriented group treatment to help the patient understand and accept the addiction, to develop skills for sober living, and to prepare an aftercare plan. Managed care has greatly affected length of stay, and patients who attend medically managed programs often stay for less than 2 weeks.

2. *Short-term residential rehabilitation programs.* These are medically monitored programs with goals similar to the ones above. Some last 4 weeks but others are briefer now due to the impact of managed care. Group treatment is the primary approach used in these residential programs.

3. *Longer-term residential programs.* These include therapeutic community (TC) and halfway house programs (HWH) lasting several months or longer. Both TCs and HWHs focus on helping patients make changes in self and lifestyle. TCs usually are more rigorous in terms of the therapy provided. Both TC and HWH programs also focus on the need to develop vocational skills. Following a period of stable adjustment in the TC or HWH, the patient may also attend academic or vocational training programs to prepare them for the job market.

4. *Partial hospital (PH) or intensive outpatient treatment programs (IOP).* These are time-limited, structured treatment programs that aim to help patients stabilize from the addiction and to learn to live without using substances. These programs may serve to divert patients from inpatient programs, as a "step-down" from residential or inpatient addiction treatment, or as a "step-up" from less-intense outpatient care. PH patients may attend daily for several weeks, for up to six to eight hours per day. PH is sometimes also linked to the detoxification process for patients needing help withdrawing safely from substances. IOP involves fewer treatment days and hours per day than the partial program but has similar goals. Both PH and IOP aim to get patients involved in an ongoing recovery process through participation in self-help programs such as A.A. or N.A. Group treatment is the

primary approach used in these programs although patients may also receive individual or family sessions.

5. *Outpatient/aftercare.* Many patients benefit from regular individual and/or group sessions weekly or less often. Outpatient care may be used for the patient who does not need a higher level of treatment, or for the patient who needs continued care following completion of an inpatient, residential, partial hospital, or intensive outpatient program.

6. *Other services.* Many substance abusers benefit from other services such as case management, vocational assessment and counseling, social work services, neuropsychological assessments, chaplain services, leisure counseling, and participation in self-help programs. These services address problems or needs that often interfere with the patient's ability to utilize treatment. However, some of these services such as vocational training may not be offered until the patient demonstrates an ability to remain substance free for a period of time (e.g., 6 months or longer).

■ TREATMENT APPROACHES AND MODELS

Clinicians should become conversant with the empirical literature in order to be informed of the clinical approaches found most effective through randomized clinical trials. There is an increasing body of empirical literature that clearly shows that there are many effective treatments for mental health, substance use, and combined disorders (for reviews see Hester & Miller, 1995; Washton, 1995; Onken, Blaine, Genser & Horton, 1997; Lowinson, Ruiz, Millman & Langrod, 1997; ASAM, 1998; Kendall et al., 1998; Nathan & Gorman, 1998; McCrady & Epstein, 1999; Weissman, Markowitz & Klerman, 2000; Sadock & Sadock, 2000; see also the NIAAA and NIDA references of specific treatment models).

Individual, group, family, and somatic treatments (i.e., pharmacotherapy or ECT) are the treatment approaches used with mental and substance use disorders. Treatment models used depend on the clinician's training and preference, but as mentioned above, should be based on empirical evidence. Several of these treatment models will be discussed in greater detail in the subsequent chapters on specific disorders. Treatment models may vary, depending on the specific type and combination of disorders. Some models such as cognitive behavior therapy (CBT) are used across a range of age groups and psychiatric and substance use disorders. The theoretical underpinnings and intervention techniques of many of the current treatment models are described in mental health clinician manuals. Following is a list of treatment models that have been used with mental- and/or substance-related disorders:

- Behavioral therapy and social skills training (Liberman, DeRisi & Mueser, 1989; Bellack, Mueser, Gingerich & Agresta, 1997; Kadden et al., 1995)
- Cognitive-behavioral therapy (Beck, 1976; Basco & Rush, 1996; Beck, Wright, Newman & Liese, 1993; Layden, Newman, Freeman & Morse, 1993; Foy, 1992; Kozak & Foa, 1997; Beck & Freeman, 1990; Steketee, 1993; NIDA, 1998a)
- Dialectical behavior therapy (Linehan, 1993)
- Family and marital therapies (Anderson & Stewart, 1983; Anderson, Reiss & Hogarty, 1986; Mueser & Glynn, 1999; Miklowitz & Goldstein, 1997; O'Farrell & Fals-Stewart, 1999)
- Interpersonal psychotherapy (Klerman, Weissman, Roussaville & Chevron, 1984; Weissman, Markowitz & Klerman, 2000)
- Interpersonal and social rhythm therapy (Frank, Swartz & Kupfer, 2000)
- Supportive-expressive therapy (Luborsky, 1984).

For substance-related disorders and dual disorders, there are several other treatment models in addition to the ones listed above (these are discussed in Chapter 2):

- Community reinforcement approach (Meyers & Smith, 1995; NIDA, 1998b)
- Cue exposure (NIDA, 1993)
- Dual disorders recovery counseling (Daley & Thase, 2000)

- Group drug counseling (Daley, Mercer & Carpenter, 1998; NIDA, 2001)
- Individual drug counseling (NIDA, 1999)
- Motivational enhancement therapy (NIAAA, 1995b)
- Rational emotive therapy (Ellis, McInerney, DiGiuseppe & Yeager, 1988)
- Relapse prevention (Daley & Marlatt, 1997a–c)
- Skills training (Monti, Abrams, Kadden & Cooney, 1989; NIAAA, 1995c; Roberts, Shaner & Eckman, 1999)
- Social network therapy (Galanter & Kleber, 1999)
- Twelve-Step facilitation therapy (NIAAA, 1995a).

■ FACILITATING TREATMENT ENTRY AND ADHERENCE

Health and mental health caregivers who do not provide direct treatment for mental or substance use disorders can play a major role in helping the patient by facilitating entry into an appropriate treatment program. This requires knowledge of existing treatment programs and resources, an ability to help the patient to overcome barriers to getting help and to increase motivation to change and follow through with treatment referral.

There are a number of clinical strategies that can improve the patient's adherence with a treatment referral. These include the following (Daley, Salloum, Zuckoff, Kirisci & Thase, 1998; Daley & Zuckoff, 1999; Daley et al., in press; Miller & Rollnick, 1991; Meichenbaum & Turk, 1987):

- Being aware of the patient's motivation to enter treatment, accepting ambivalence or resistance to change, and discussing the patient's questions and concerns regarding the referral.
- Providing a rationale for the referral, relating the treatment recommendation to the patient's current problems and concerns.
- Providing an orientation to the service or program to which the patient is being referred (i.e., "role induction" to treatment).
- Providing a motivational session prior to referral.

- Using "prompts" (phone calls or letters) prior to the initial appointment.
- Engaging the family as an ally in treatment to support the patient's entry into treatment.
- Making a follow-up call to the patient to determine if the referral was completed; helping the patient who failed to follow through re-engage in treatment.

In recent years, motivational strategies have been used to improve adherence rates for patients entering treatment or moving from one level of care to another (e.g., inpatient to outpatient care). These strategies have been successful with a variety of mental and substance use disorders. Even a single motivational session can have a positive impact on increasing treatment adherence.

■ THERAPEUTIC ALLIANCE: IMPORTANCE OF THE CAREGIVER–PATIENT RELATIONSHIP

The alliance between caregiver and patient is one of the main therapeutic factors affecting treatment outcome (Frank, Kupfer & Siegel, 1995; Onken, Blaine & Boren, 1997). The relationship is one of the primary vehicles for influencing the patient to change. A positive therapeutic alliance is one in which the patient feels free to self-disclose thoughts, feelings, problems, and conflicts. The patient feels heard, understood, accepted, respected and not judged, and believes that the professional is a helpful ally and "working with" him. The professional contributes to the alliance through acceptance of the patient, sharing empathy, maintaining a sense of trust and confidentiality, supporting the patient's efforts to change, and being optimistic about the patient's chances of success. A good alliance also is one in which therapeutic impasses can be openly acknowledged and discussed, without defensiveness on the caregiver's part. There is evidence that outcome is improved for patients with positive alliances with their therapist.

Recovery from Mental or Substance Use Disorders

■ THE CONCEPT OF RECOVERY

The concept of "recovery" originated in the field of substance abuse treatment, but has been expanded to the field of mental health treatment in recent years. Recovery refers to the process of the patient learning to accept and manage his or her disorders and to make changes in self and lifestyle to reduce the risk of relapse. Table 1-6 summarizes some of the key themes related to physical, psychological, family, social, and spiritual recovery.

The patient assumes a major role in his or her recovery, identifying problems and goals, and takes responsibility for making

TABLE 1-6. PSYCHOSOCIAL ISSUES IN RECOVERY FROM MENTAL HEALTH OR SUBSTANCE USE DISORDERS

Physical/lifestyle	*Behavioral/cognitive*
Exercise	Accept the disorder(s) or problem(s)
Follow a healthy diet	Control urges to drink alcohol or use drugs
Rest and relaxation	Change unhealthy beliefs and thoughts
Take medications (if needed)	Reduce depressed thoughts
Take care of medical problem	Increase pleasant thoughts
Learn to structure time	Reduce violent thoughts
Engage in pleasant activities	Control violent impulses
Achieve balance in life	Develop motivation to change
	Change self-defeating patterns of behavior
Psychological	*Family/interpersonal/social*
Monitor moods	Identify effects on family and significant
Manage negative moods	relationships
Reduce anxiety	Involve family in treatment/recovery
Reduce boredom and emptiness	Resolve family/marital conflicts
Reduce guilt and shame	Make amends to family or other significant people
Control anger/rage	harmed
Address "losses" (grief)	Manage high-risk people, places, and events
	Engage in non-drinking activities or healthy leisure
Personal growth/maintenance	interests
Address spirituality issues	Address relationship problems or deficits
Engage in meditation	Resist social pressures to drink alcohol or use
Develop relapse prevention plan for all	other drugs
disorders or problems	Resolve work, school, financial, legal problems
Develop relapse interruption plan for all	Learn to face vs. avoid interpersonal conflicts
disorders or problems	Learn to ask for help and support
Use "recovery tools" on ongoing basis	Seek and use an A.A. or N.A. sponsor

changes in any of the domains of recovery. Such active involvement empowers the patient and builds on his or her strengths. Recovery is viewed as an active process involving:

- *Learning information:* becoming educated about the mental and/or substance use disorder(s), the role and limitations of professional treatment (therapy and medications), the process of recovery, and the process of relapse.
- *Self-awareness:* understanding the impact of the disorder(s) on self and others, motivation to change, personal coping mechanisms, and personal barriers to change.
- *Coping skills:* developing or strengthening behavioral, cognitive, and interpersonal skills to effectively manage symptoms of the disorder(s), and making changes pertinent to treatment goals.
- *Family or significant other involvement:* including others in treatment and the recovery process in order to reduce their burden, elicit their support, and provide them an opportunity to work through personal feelings and problems.
- *Self-help programs:* participating in a self-help program for a mental disorder, substance use disorder, or a dual disorder.
- *Relapse:* anticipating the possibility of relapse and reducing risk through early identification and management of relapse warning signs and personal high-risk factors.

■ FACTORS MEDIATING RECOVERY

There are many similar elements to recovery despite the specific type(s) or combinations of mental and substance use disorders. The recovery process, however, will vary among patients and will be mediated by a variety of illness, patient, family, and social system factors including (Daley et al., 1993; Daley et al., in press):

1. *Type and severity of the mental disorders:* patients with more chronic and severe mental disorders such as schizophrenia,

recurrent depression, or obsessive–compulsive disorder often require more extensive professional treatment or higher levels of care, particularly during periods in which symptoms worsen and cause more severe adverse effects on the patient or others. These patients, especially those with multiple disorders, are more likely to experience struggles or complications in the recovery process such as poor judgment, low motivation, suicidality, lethality, or poor adherence to treatment.

2. *Type and severity of the substance use disorder(s)*: patients with mental disorders who have comorbid substance use disorders often have more psychopathology, greater impairment, poorer treatment adherence rates, and higher rates of relapse and rehospitalization compared to those without substance abuse problems. Active substance use causes its own set of problems and difficulties. Substance use also adversely affects psychiatric symptoms and recovery, interferes with the efficacy of psychiatric medications and/or psychotherapy.

3. *Level of social anxiety*: many patients with mental and/or substance use disorders have significant symptoms of social anxiety or social phobias as well as avoidance behaviors. These symptoms can interfere with the patient's ability to participate in group treatment and self-help programs.

4. *Effects of disorders on current functioning*: patients with multiple psychosocial problems often struggle in their recovery due to the effects of these problems on their motivation, mood, and ability to function.

5. *Effects of disorders on family and significant relationships*: mental and substance use disorders can have major adverse effects on relationships with family and significant others and can cause guilt and shame in the patient. A patient who lacks supportive relationships, or is subject to criticism, hostility, or sabotage from a family member or significant other, is at increased risk of relapse.

6. *Demographic characteristics* (*age, gender, employment status, ethnicity*): unemployed patients and those from lower socioeconomic backgrounds often experience problems with housing, money, child care, and transportation that affect their ability to

attend professional treatment and self-help programs. They may not gain optimum benefits and experience more difficulties in recovery as a result. For example, in one of our recent studies of psychiatric inpatients, we found that patients who were unemployed, single, or African-American were less likely to follow-up with aftercare treatment after hospital discharge compared to others.

7. *Level of acceptance of disorder and professional help:* denial of illness and low motivation to change are common with psychiatric and substance use disorders. Individuals who do not believe they have a mental and/or substance use disorder will have little or no motivation to change, engage in professional treatment, or the process of recovery. Also, individuals who accept their disorder(s) but do not believe they need professional help are less likely to engage in treatment. External motivation or pressure from the family, the legal system, or an employer often are needed before some patients engage in treatment or get involved in a recovery program.

8. *Personality factors:* many patients with mood, anxiety, psychotic and/or substance use disorders have personality disorders or specific traits that interfere with their judgment, perception, motivation, interpersonal relationships, moods, coping abilities, and, hence, their ability to engage in recovery. For example, a stubborn patient may resist professional advice on the need to change, how to change, or the need for involvement in a recovery program. Or, an antisocial patient may resist all efforts of a professional to help.

9. *Cognitive factors:* cognitive impairment can interfere with an individual's ability to learn information and acquire recovery skills needed to cope with a mental and/or substance use disorder. Persistent and severe psychotic symptoms may adversely impact on the patient's ability to manage the disorder(s) and engage in a recovery program.

10. *Current family and social supports:* patients with positive family and social support systems tend to function better than those lacking support or those involved in negative social networks.

11. Therapeutic alliance with professional caregiver(s): patients who develop a strong working alliance with their therapist or treatment team have better collaboration, adherence, and completion rates, and hence better clinical outcomes than those who do not like or trust their caregiver. A positive alliance is one in which the patient feels accepted, understood, and not judged for his behaviors or mistakes. This is characterized by a sense of working as a team to address the problems and concerns of the patient.

12. Appropriateness of treatment: recovery is moderated by the clinical services and specific treatment provided. For example, if a high level of care is needed but not offered or not available, the patient may not get sufficient help in stabilizing from the acute symptoms of the disorder(s).

■ SUICIDE

Suicide is a serious problem for some patients with mental health or substance use disorders (Bongar, Berman, Maris, Silverman, Harris & Packman, 1998; Shea, 1999; Jamison, 1999). Rates of suicide are highest among patients with affective disorders, schizophrenia, and alcoholism. Depression and alcoholism are the leading causes of completed suicide with lifetime rates that are significantly higher than the general population. Having a comorbid substance use disorder increases suicidal risk even further. The risk of completion of suicide increases when more violent means are used such as a gun. Following are some of the more common risk factors associated with suicide:

- Depression with feelings of hopelessness
- Recent heavy drinking
- Suicidal threats or gestures
- Prior attempts or multiple attempts
- Suicide within the family
- Lack of social support
- Unemployment
- Living alone

- Presence of a serious medical problem or chronic illness
- Poor coping skills.

Suicidal behavior is one of the leading causes of psychiatric hospitalization. Patients with a plan or intent who are unable to guarantee their safety should be hospitalized in order to provide safety until there is no longer intent or a specific plan. Eliciting family support, helping the patient through the crisis precipitating suicidal feelings through extra telephone contact or treatment sessions, encouraging abstinence from alcohol or other drugs, the use of medications to treat depressive and other psychiatric syndromes contributing to suicidality, and the use of an anti-suicide contract are interventions that can reduce the likelihood that the patient will act on suicidal thoughts or feelings.

■ VIOLENCE

Violence is also a significant problem for some individuals with a mental health, substance use, or dual disorder (Salloum, Daley & Thase, 2000; Stoff, Breiling & Maser, 1997). Violence shows in many ways including child abuse, spousal abuse, elder abuse, sexual abuse, assault, and homicide. Often, the patient who is violent in one area evidences violence in another area. Diagnoses that increase the risk of violence include:

- Schizophrenia, paranoid type
- Bipolar disorder
- Major depression
- Intermittent explosive disorder
- Post-traumatic stress disorder
- Cluster B personality disorders: especially antisocial, borderline, and narcissistic personality disorders
- Substance use especially alcohol abuse, stimulant intoxication, hallucinogens; phencyclidine, inhalants, and other depressants
- Conduct disorders and attention deficit disorders

- Delirium, dementia, mental retardation, and seizure disorders.

Treatment can help the patient change beliefs, control violent impulses, and learn to manage feelings and problems without acting out in violent ways toward others. For example, men who abused their spouse and believed they were justified, wronged, or the spouse deserved the abuse have to alter these beliefs in order to help them gain control over violent behaviors. These men often need help in identifying triggers to acting out, containing negative affect, and learning cognitive and behavioral skills to manage their feelings and negotiate interpersonal conflicts. Medications such as SSRI antidepressants, mood stabilizers, antipsychotics, and axiolytics may also be used as part of the treatment approach when violence is a significant problem (Karper & Krystal, 1997).

■ FAMILY ISSUES

There is considerable evidence that families are affected by a mental, substance use, or combination of disorders (Mueser & Glynn, 1999; Miklowitz & Goldstein, 1997; Daley et al., 1993; Daley & Miller, 1993; Daley & Raskin, 1991; Hatfield, 1990; Hatfield & Lefley, 1987; Anderson & Stewart, 1983; Anderson, Reiss & Hogarty, 1986). The entire family system as well as individual members may experience any number of adverse effects from exposure to patients, particularly those who display low motivation to change; poor judgment; violent, suicidal, homicidal, intoxicated, bizarre, or unpredictable behavior; or whose functioning is severely impaired. Any area of functioning of the family member—physical, emotional, social, interpersonal, occupational, spiritual or financial—can be affected. The burden on the family can be great, and some members may even experience their own mental disorders, such as depression or anxiety, or abuse substances.

Family involvement in assessment and treatment is helpful to both the patient and the family. The family can provide important assessment information, influence the patient to adhere to the treatment plan, and provide support during the patient's recovery.

The family can also become educated about the illness, learning what they can and cannot do to help their affected member, and what they can do to deal with their own emotional or personal reactions (e.g., anxiety and worry, fear, anger, etc.). There is considerable evidence that family psychoeducational programs and various forms of marital and family therapy are beneficial to families and patients.

■ RELAPSE ISSUES

All patients with mental or substance use disorders face the possibility of a relapse or recurrence of illness after a period of recovery or significantly improved functioning (Marlatt & Gordon, 1984; Wilson, 1992; Daley & Marlatt, 1997a–c). A major focus of psychiatric and substance abuse treatment is helping patients anticipate and prepare for the possibility of relapse by learning how to identify and manage obvious and subtle signs of relapse and to identify and manage high-risk factors that increase relapse risk. Patients are also taught how to intervene early in the relapse process should it occur in order to minimize adverse effects of a relapse and to stabilize symptoms. The more chronic and persistent forms of disorders often involve multiple episodes over time.

■ SELF-HELP PROGRAMS

Self-help programs are supportive recovery resources for many patients with mental and substance use disorders. These include: (1) programs for substance abuse such as Alcoholics Anonymous, Narcotics Anonymous, Cocaine Anonymous, Rational Recovery, SMART Recovery, and Women for Sobriety; (2) programs for mental health problems such as Recovery, Inc., Emotional Health Anonymous, Emotions Anonymous or programs for specific types of mental disorders; and (3) programs for patients with comorbid psychiatric and substance use disorders such as Dual Recovery Anonymous, Double Trouble, or special groups within A.A. or N.A. Self-help programs help the patient learn valuable information, adopt positive recovery attitudes, learn skills to manage the illness, provide ongoing social support from others with similar problems, and provide "mentors" who can help the patient utilize the specific "tools" of the self-help program. As managed care limits the number of treatment sessions, self-help programs are all the more important in helping patients recover from mental and substance use disorders.

Caregivers can facilitate the use of self-help programs by:

- Educating the patient on the purpose and structure of the specific self-help program to which he or she is being encouraged to participate. Providing brochures, written information, and meeting lists can aid in this process.
- Discussing and acknowledging the patient's resistances, questions, or concerns regarding self-help programs.
- Helping to correct misconceptions that the patient may have about self-help programs (e.g., you have to stand up and tell your life story to a bunch of strangers, these programs are run by religious fanatics, etc.).
- Helping the patient overcome reluctance or social anxiety to attend self-help group programs. Our research shows that about one-third of patients have very high levels of social anxiety and often avoid group situations as a result.
- Discussing potential ways in which a self-help program can aid the patient's recovery.
- Providing specific recommendations regarding a type of self-help program or particular meetings.
- Negotiating an agreement in which the patient will attend a certain number of meetings before making a judgment about the potential usefulness of a self-help program.
- Linking the patient with members of self-help programs who volunteer to help newcomers get acclimated into the programs. Some patients are more likely to attend a self-help program if they do not go alone.
- Monitoring participation and discussing both positive and negative experiences of the patient who attends meetings.

■ MEASURING OUTCOME

Measuring outcome of mental health and substance abuse treatment is important in order to demonstrate the effectiveness of care. Outcomes can relate to the patient's symptoms or problems or participation in treatment (referred to as process measures). Desired clinical outcomes for treatment for a given patient may include:

- Remission or reduction of psychiatric symptoms
- Remission or reduction of substance use
- Reduction of specific problems
- Reduction of high-risk behaviors
- Improvement in overall functioning
- Improvement in quality of life
- Reduced hospitalization rates
- Reduced relapse rates
- Satisfaction with treatment.

Outcomes can be measured by using specific clinical questionnaires such as psychiatric symptom inventories (e.g., Beck depression or anxiety), substance abuse inventories (e.g., Addiction Severity Index) or global measures such as the Global Assessment of Functioning score (Axis V of DSM-IV) or Clinical Global Impressions scale at baseline, at various points in treatment and at termination. In addition, biological measures can be used with patients on certain types of psychiatric medication to determine if they are adhering to treatment, or with substance abusing patients to assess recent alcohol or drug use. Patient satisfaction questionnaires and adherence with treatment sessions are other ways to gather important information from a patient. Poor session attendance, for example, is correlated with symptom exacerbation.

REFERENCES

American Psychiatric Association (APA) (1994). *Diagnostic and statistical manual of mental disorders* (4th ed.). Washington, DC: APA.

American Society of Addiction Medicine, Inc. (ASAM) (1998). *Principles of addiction medicine* (2nd ed.). Chevy Chase, MD: ASAM.

Anderson, C. M., Reiss, D. J., & Hogarty, G. E. (1986). *Schizophrenia and the family.* New York, NY: Guilford Press.

Anderson, C. M., & Stewart, S. (1983). *Mastering resistance.* New York, NY: Guilford Press.

Anthenelli, R. M., & Schuckit, M. A. (1997). Genetics. In: J. H. Lowinson, P. Ruiz, R. B. Millman & J. G. Langrod (Eds.), *Substance abuse: A comprehensive textbook* (3rd ed., pp. 41–50). Baltimore, MD: Williams & Wilkins.

Basco, M. R., & Rush, A. J. (1996). *Cognitive-behavioral therapy for bipolar disorder.* New York, NY: Guilford Press.

Beck, A. T. (1976). *Cognitive therapy of the emotional disorders.* New York, NY: International Universities Press.

Beck, A. T., & Freeman, A. (1990). *Cognitive therapy of personality disorders.* New York, NY: Guilford Press.

Beck, A. T., Wright, F. D., Newman, C. F., & Liese, B. S. (1993). *Cognitive therapy of substance abuse.* New York, NY: Guilford Press.

Bellack, A. S., Mueser, K.T., Gingerich, S., & Agresta, J. (1997). *Social skills training for schizophrenia.* New York, NY: Guilford Press.

Blackwell, B. (1997). *Treatment compliance and the therapeutic alliance.* The Netherlands: Harwood Academic Publishers.

Bongar, B., Berman, A. L., Maris, R. W., Silverman, M. M., Harris, E. A., & Packman, W. L. (Eds.) (1998). *Risk management with suicidal patients.* New York, NY: Guilford Press.

Carroll, K. (1997). *Improving compliance with alcoholism treatment.* Rockville, MD: U.S. Department of Health and Human Services.

Daley, D. C. (1999). *A comparison of aftercare compliance and rehospitalization rates between psychiatric patients with and without comorbid substance use disorders.* Santa Ana, CA: California Coast University.

Daley, D. C., & Marlatt, G. A. (1997a). *Managing your drug or alcohol problem—Client workbook.* San Antonio, TX: Psychological Corporation.

Daley, D. C., & Marlatt, G. A. (1997b). *Managing your drug or alcohol problem—Therapist's guide.* San Antonio, TX: Psychological Corporation.

Daley, D. C., & Marlatt, G. A. (1997c). Relapse prevention. In: J. H. Lowinson, P. Ruiz, R. B. Millman & J. G. Langrod (Eds.), *Substance abuse: A comprehensive textbook* (3rd ed., pp. 458–466). Baltimore, MD: Williams & Wilkins.

Daley, D. C., Mercer, D., & Carpenter, G. (1998). *Group drug counseling manual.* Holmes Beach, FL: Learning Publications, Inc.

Daley, D. C., & Miller, J. (1993). *Taking control: A practical family guide to dealing with chemical dependency.* Holmes Beach, FL: Learning Publications.

Daley, D. C., Moss, H. B., & Campbell, F. (1993). *Dual disorders: Counseling clients with chemical dependency and mental illness* (2nd ed.). Center City, MN: Hazelden.

Daley, D. C., & Raskin, M. (Eds.) (1991). *Treating the chemically dependent and their families.* Newbury Park, CA: Sage Publications.

Daley, D. C., Salloum, I. M., & Thase, M. E. (in press). Improving treatment adherence among patients with comorbid psychiatric and substance use disorders. In: D. F. O'Connell (Ed.), *Managing the dually diagnosed patient: Current issues and clinical approaches.* New York, NY: Haworth Press.

Daley, D. C., Salloum, I. M., Zuckoff, A., Kirisci, L., & Thase, M. (1998). Increasing treatment compliance among outpatients with depression and cocaine dependence. Results of a pilot study. American Journal of Psychiatry, *155*, 1611–1613.

Daley, D. C., & Thase, M. E. (2000). *Dual disorders recovery counseling: Integrated treatment for substance use and mental health disorders* (2nd ed.). Independence, MO: Independence Press.

Daley, D. C., & Zuckoff, A. (1999). *Improving treatment compliance: Counseling and system strategies for substance use and dual disorders.* Center City, MN: Hazelden.

Ellis, A., McInerney, J. F., DiGiuseppe, R., & Yeager, R. J. (1988). *Rational-emotive therapy with alcoholics and substance abusers.* New York, NY: Pergamon Press.

Foy, D. W. (1992). *Treating PTSD: Cognitive-behavioral strategies.* New York, NY: Guilford Press.

Frank, E., Kupfer, D. J., & Siegel, L. R. (1995). Alliance not compliance: a philosophy of outpatient care. *Journal of Clinical Psychiatry,* *56* (Suppl. 1), 11–16.

Frank, E., Swartz, H. A., & Kupfer, D. J. (2000). Interpersonal and social rhythm therapy: managing the chaos of bipolar disorder. *Biological Psychiatry, 48*, 593–604.

Galanter, M., & Kleber, H. D. (Eds.) (1999). *Textbook of substance abuse treatment* (2nd ed.). Washington, DC: American Psychiatric Press Inc.

Hatfield, A. B. (1990). *Family education in mental illness.* New York, NY: Guilford Press.

Hatfield, A. B., & Lefley, H. P. (Eds.) (1987). *Families of the mentally ill: Coping and adaptation.* New York, NY: Guilford Press.

Hester, R. K., & Miller, W. R. (Eds.) (1995). *Handbook of alcoholism treatment approaches: Effective alternatives* (2nd ed.). Boston, MA: Allyn and Bacon.

Jamison, K. R. (1999). *Night falls fast: Understanding suicide.* New York, NY: Alfred A. Knopf.

Karper, L. P., & Krystal, J. H. (1997). Pharmacotherapy of violent behavior. In: D. M. Stoff, J. Breiling, & J. D. Maser (Eds.), *Handbook of antisocial behavior* (pp. 436–444). New York, NY: John Wiley & Sons.

Kendall, P. C., Foster, S. C., Lambert, M. J., Haaga, D. A., & Smith, T. W. (Eds.) (1998). Empirically supported psychological therapies. *Journal of Consulting and Clinical Psychology, 66*(1), 1–209.

Klerman, G. L., Weissman, M. M., Roussaville, B. J., & Chevron, E. S. (1984). *Interpersonal psychotherapy of depression.* New York, NY: Basic Books.

Kozak, M. J., & Foa, E. B. (1997). *Mastery of obsessive-compulsive disorder: A cognitive-behavioral approach. Therapist guide.* San Antonio, TX: Psychological Corporation.

Layden, M. A., Newman, C. F., Freeman, A., & Morse, S. B. (1993). *Cognitive therapy of borderline personality disorders.* Boston, MA: Allyn and Bacon.

Liberman, R. B., DeRisi, W. J., & Mueser, K. T. (1989). *Social skills training for psychiatric patients.* New York, NY: Pergamon Press.

Linehan, M. M. (1993). *Cognitive-behavioral treatment of borderline personality disorder.* New York, NY: Guilford Press..

Lowinson, J. H., Ruiz, P., Millman, R. B., & Langrod, J. G. (Eds.) (1997). *Substance abuse: A comprehensive textbook* (3rd ed.). Baltimore, MD: Williams & Wilkins.

Luborsky, L. (1984). *Principles of supportive-expressive psychotherapy*. New York, NY: Basic Books.

McCrady, B. S., & Epstein, E. E. (Eds.) (1999). *Addictions: A comprehensive guidebook*. London: Oxford University Press.

Marlatt, G. A., & Gordon, J. R. (Eds.) (1984). *Relapse prevention: Maintenance strategies in the treatment of addictive behaviors*. New York, NY: Guilford Press.

Meichenbaum, D., & Turk, K. (1987). *Facilitating treatment adherence: A practitioner's guidebook*. New York, NY: Plenum Press.

Meyers, R. J., & Smith, J. E. (1995). *Clinical guide to alcohol treatment: The community reinforcement approach*. New York, NY: Guilford Press.

Miklowitz, D. J., & Goldstein, M. J. (1997). *Bipolar disorder: A family-focused treatment approach*. New York, NY: Guilford Press.

Miller, W. R., & Rollnick, S. (1991). *Motivational interviewing: Preparing people to change addictive behavior*. New York, NY: Guilford Press

Minkoff, K., & Drake, R. E. (1991). *Dual diagnosis of major mental illness and substance disorder*. San Francisco, CA: Jossey-Bass, Inc.

Monti, P. M., Abrams, D. B., Kadden, R. M., & Cooney, N. L. (1989). *Treatment of alcohol dependence*. New York, NY: Guilford Press.

Montrose, K., & Daley, D. C. (1995). *Celebrating small victories: A primer of approaches and attitudes for helping clients with dual disorders*. Center City, MN: Hazelden.

Mueser, K. T., & Glynn, S. M. (1999). *Behavioral family therapy for psychiatric disorders* (2nd ed.). Oakland, CA: New Harbinger.

Nathan, P. E., & Gorman, J. M. (Eds.) (1998). *A guide to treatments that work*. New York, NY: Oxford University Press.

National Institute on Alcohol Abuse and Alcoholism (NIAAA) (1995a). Project Match Series, Volume 1: *Twelve step facilitation therapy manual*. Rockville, MD: U.S. Department of Health and Human Services.

National Institute on Alcohol Abuse and Alcoholism (NIAAA) (1995b). Project Match Series, Volume 2: *Motivational enhancement therapy manual*. Rockville, MD: U.S. Department of Health and Human Services.

National Institute on Alcohol Abuse and Alcoholism (NIAAA) (1995c). Project Match Series, Volume 3: *Cognitive-behavioral coping skills therapy manual*. Rockville, MD: U.S. Department of Health and Human Services.

National Institute on Alcohol Abuse and Alcoholism (NIAAA) (1997). *Alcohol and health: Ninth special report to the U.S. Congress*. Rockville, MD: U.S. Department of Health and Human Services.

National Institute on Drug Abuse (NIDA) (1993). *Cue extinction*. Rockville, MD: U.S. Department of Health and Human Services.

National Institute on Drug Abuse (NIDA) (1998a). Therapy Manuals for Drug Addiction, Manual 1: *A cognitive behavioral approach: Treating cocaine addiction*. Rockville, MD: U.S. Department of Health and Human Services.

National Institute on Drug Abuse (NIDA) (1998b). Therapy Manuals for Drug Addiction, Manual 2: *A community reinforcement plus vouchers approach: Treating cocaine addiction*. Rockville, MD: U.S. Department of Health and Human Services.

National Institute on Drug Abuse (NIDA) (1999). Therapy Manuals for Drug Addiction, Manual 3: *An individual drug counseling approach to treat cocaine addiction: The collaborative cocaine treatment study model*. Rockville, MD: U.S. Department of Health and Human Services.

National Institute on Drug Abuse (NIDA) (2001). Therapy Manuals for Drug Addiction, Manual 4: *A group drug counseling approach to treat cocaine addiction: The collaborative cocaine treatment study model*. Rockville, MD: U.S. Department of Health and Human Services.

O'Connell, D. F. (in press). *Managing the dually diagnosed patient: Current issues and clinical approaches* (2nd ed.). New York, NY: Haworth Press.

O'Farrell, T. J., & Fals-Stewart, W. (1999). Treatment models and methods: Family models. In B. S. McCrady & E. E. Epstein (Eds.), *Addictions: A comprehensive guidebook* (pp. 287–305). London: Oxford University Press.

Onken, L. S., Blaine, J. D., & Boren, J. (1997). *Beyond the therapeutic alliance: Keeping the drug-dependent individual in treatment*. NIDA Research Monograph 165. Rockville, MD: U.S. Department of Health and Human Services.

Onken, L. S., Blaine, J. D., Genser, S., & Horton, Jr, A. M. (1997). *Treatment of drug-dependent individuals with comorbid mental disorders:* NIDA Research Monograph 172. Rockville, MD: U.S. Department of Health and Human Services.

Ott, P. J., Tarter, R. E., & Ammerman, R. T. (Eds.) (1999). *Sourcebook on substance abuse: Etiology, epidemiology, assessment, and treatment.* Needham Heights, MA: Allyn & Bacon.

Ries, R. (1995). *Assessment and treatment of patients with coexisting mental illness and alcohol and other drug abuse.* Treatment improvement protocol (TIP) Series. Rockville, MD: U.S. Department of Health and Human Services.

Robins, L. N., & Regier, D. A. (Eds.) (1991). *Psychiatric disorders in America: The epidemiologic catchment area study.* New York, NY: The Free Press.

Roberts, L. J., Shaner, A., & Eckman, T. A. (1999). *Overcoming addictions: Skills training for people with schizophrenia.* New York, NY: W.W. Norton & Company.

Ryglewicz, H., & Pepper, B. (1996). *Lives at risk: Understanding and treating young people with dual disorders.* New York, NY: The Free Press.

Sadock, B. J., & Sadock, V. A. (Eds.) (2000). *Comprehensive textbook of psychiatry* (7th ed.). New York, NY: Lippincott, Williams and Wilkins.

Salloum, I. M., Daley, D. C., & Thase, M. E. (2000). *Male alcoholism, violence, and depression.* Malden, MA: Blackwell Science, Inc.

Shea, S. C. (1999). *The practical art of suicide assessment: A guide for mental health professionals and substance abuse counselors.* New York, NY: John Wiley & Sons.

Steketee, G. S. (1993). *Treatment of obsessive compulsive disorder.* New York, NY: Guilford Press.

Stoff, D. M., Breiling, J., & Maser, J. D. (Eds.) (1997). *Handbook of antisocial behavior.* New York , NY: John Wiley & Sons.

Washton, A. M. (Ed.) (1995). *Psychotherapy and substance abuse: A practitioner's handbook.* New York, NY: Guilford Press.

Weissman, M. M., Markowitz, J. C., & Klerman, G. L. (2000). *Comprehensive guide to interpersonal psychotherapy.* New York, NY: Basic Books.

Wilson, P. (Ed.) (1992). *Principles and practice of relapse prevention.* New York, NY: Guilford Press.

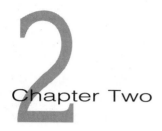

Chapter Two

Substance Use Disorders

Dennis C. Daley • Ihsan M. Salloum • Tad Gorske

Introduction and Overview

■ SUBSTANCES OF ABUSE AND ROUTES OF ADMINISTRATION

Millions of citizens in the United States will experience a substance use disorder of some kind during their lifetime. Substance use disorders refer to clinical syndromes such as intoxication, withdrawal, abuse or dependence. Each syndrome is defined by specific symptoms by the American Psychiatric Association *Diagnostic and Statistical Manual of Mental Disorders* (1994).

Virtually any compound or drug may be used by individuals with substance use disorders. Substances of abuse include legal drugs, such as prescription and over-the-counter medications as well as illicit drugs. Types of legal substances or prescribed drugs include alcohol, nicotine, caffeine, amphetamines, certain opioids, sedatives, hypnotics, and anxioltyics. Types of illegal or street drugs include cannabis, cocaine, heroin, hallucinogens, inhalants and phencyclidine. While many patients abuse or are dependent on a single substance, substantial numbers of patients use and abuse multiple substances from these various classifications. For example, the majority of patients with cocaine dependence have problems with alcohol abuse or dependence. Some patients mix drugs to boost the effects, others use anything or everything available without regard to what specific compound they are using or to what street drugs are "cut" with.

The actual effects of a given substance use episode depend on the type and amount of drug(s) used, level of tolerance, expectations, social setting, and route of administration. Substances may be taken orally (e.g., alcohol or pills), snorted (e.g., cocaine or heroin), smoked (e.g., marijuana or cocaine) or injected with a needle (e.g., opiates, cocaine, or stimulants). Substances that are rapidly absorbed into the bloodstream through smoking, snorting or injecting have a more immediate effect than those taken orally and are more likely to lead to more intense intoxication as well as increased risk of developing a dependency on the substance. The patient who ingests drugs through smoking, snorting or IV use often consumes large quantities and increases the risk of toxic effects or overdose. Rapidly acting substances such as diazepam and alprazolam that produce immediate intoxication are more likely than slower-acting ones to lead to abuse or dependence (APA, 1994, p. 186).

■ PREVALENCE OF ALCOHOL AND DRUG USE DISORDERS

Numerous studies of community and clinical populations show that lifetime and current rates of substance use disorders are high and represent a significant public health problem in our country. The Epidemiologic Catchment Area study found a 13.7 percent lifetime prevalence of alcohol abuse or dependence and 6.1 percent of drug abuse or dependence among adults in the United States (Robins & Regier, 1991). The National Comorbidity survey found that 20 million people, or 11.3 percent of 15–54 year olds in the US had a substance abuse or dependence problem within the past year (Kessler, McGonagle & Zhao, 1994). Clinical studies of psychiatric patients indicate that significant numbers of patients also suffer from substance use disorders in addition to mental health disorders (Daley, Moss & Campbell, 1993; O'Connell, in press).

■ CLASSIFICATION OF SUBSTANCE USE DISORDERS

Following are categories of substance-related diagnoses according to *Diagnostic and Statistical Manual of Mental Disorders* (APA, 1994) (see Table 2-1):

1. Intoxication. This is a reversible syndrome caused by recent ingestion of a substance or exposure to certain substances. Physiological signs vary depending on the substances used and may include slurred speech, incoordination, unsteady gait, nystagmus, flushed face, and impairment of memory or attention. Behavioral or psychological signs also vary according to substances used and may include mood lability, elation, grandiosity, euphoria, dysphoria, apathy, belligerence, agitation or irritability, increased talkativeness, hypervigilance, impaired judgment, or impaired functioning at school, work, or in the family. The effects of intoxication may last hours or even longer and put the patient at risk for accidents, medical problems or complications, or difficulty in any area of functioning.

2. Withdrawal. This is a substance-specific syndrome caused by reducing or stopping substance use that leads to significant distress or impairment. Withdrawal occurs when the patient with physiological dependence stops or reduces heavy or prolonged substance use. Withdrawal symptoms vary greatly

---

TABLE 2-1. DSM-IV SUBSTANCE ABUSE AND DEPENDENCE DISORDERS

Substance dependence	*Substance abuse*
1. Tolerance	1. Recurrent alcohol use resulting in a failure to fulfill major role obligations at work, school, or home
2. Withdrawal	
3. Alcohol taken in larger amount or over a longer period than was intended	2. Recurrent use of alcohol in situations in which it is physically hazardous
4. Persistent desire or unsuccessful efforts to cut down or control use	3. Recurrent alcohol-related legal problems
5. A great deal of time is spent on activities necessary to obtain alcohol	4. Continued alcohol use despite having persistent or recurrent social or interpersonal problems caused or exacerbated by the effects of alcohol
6. Important social, occupational, or recreational activities are given up or reduced because of alcohol use	
7. Alcohol use is continued despite knowledge of having a persistent or recurrent physical or psychological problem caused or exacerbated by alcohol	

across the different classification of substances and are more easily observed or measured with certain drugs such as alcohol, opiates, and sedatives, hypnotics, or anxiolytics. Cocaine and other stimulants have withdrawal symptoms but they are often less apparent than with other substances. Symptoms of *alcohol withdrawal* include coarse tremor of hands, tongue, and eyelids and one of the following symptoms: nausea and vomiting, malaise or weakness, tachycardia, sweating or elevated blood pressure, anxiety, depressed mood or irritability, or orthostatic hypotension. Symptoms of *barbiturate or similarly acting sedative or hypnotic withdrawal* include three of the following: nausea and vomiting, malaise or weakness, tachycardia, sweating or elevated blood pressure, anxiety, depressed mood or irritability, orthostatic hypotension, or coarse tremor of hands, tongue, and eyelids. Symptoms of *opioid withdrawal* include four of the following: lacrimation, rhinorrhea, pupillary dilation, piloerection, sweating, diarrhea, yawning, mild hypertension, tachycardia, fever and insomnia. Symptoms of *amphetamine or similarly acting sympathomimetic drug withdrawal* include depressed mood and two of the following: fatigue, disturbed sleep, or increased dreaming.

3. *Substance abuse.* This involves a maladaptive pattern of substance use leading to distress or impairment with at least one of four symptoms occurring within a 12-month period: failure to fulfill obligations at home, work or school, recurrent substance use in hazardous situations, recurrent legal problems, or continued substance use despite the persistence of problems caused by such use. Abuse does not include withdrawal, tolerance, or compulsive use and instead refers to repeated use that includes only harmful consequences.

4. *Substance dependence.* This involves a maladaptive pattern of substance use leading to distress or impairment with at least three or more of these symptoms occurring within a 12-month period: increased or decreased tolerance; withdrawal symptoms or using substances to avoid or relieve withdrawal; loss of control or inability to cut down or control use; spending a great deal of time to obtain or recover from the substance; giving

up or reducing important activities because of substance use; and continued use despite knowledge of a persistent or recurrent physical or psychological problem caused or exacerbated by the substance use.

5. *Mood, anxiety, psychotic induced disorders*. These refer to prominent psychiatric symptoms that are due to the physiological effects of substances. The acute or protracted effects of substances can cause symptoms that may remit when the patient's system is free of substances. In some instances, symptoms may remit fairly rapidly where in other instances it may take several weeks or more of continuous abstinence before substance-induced psychiatric symptoms remit.

■ EFFECTS OF SUBSTANCE USE DISORDERS

Substance use disorders are associated with significant morbidity and mortality as affected individuals are at increased risk for medical or psychiatric disorders. Such individuals are more likely to engage in high-risk behaviors such as driving under the influence, swimming alone, damaging property, provoking violent altercations, unprotected sex or multiple sexual partners, and using or sharing needles, cotton, or rinsing water (for IV drug users) (Daley & Marlatt, 1997a; NIAAA, 1997). Some of the specific adverse effects on the patient, family, and society include:

1. *Medical*: deleterious effects on tissues and organs of the body leading to medical and dental diseases; early death due to conditions caused or worsened by substance use, drug overdoses, vehicular accidents, industrial accidents, falls, drownings and fires, or homicide; acquisition and transmission of HIV; damage to the fetus and increased risk of infant mortality; and sexual problems.

2. *Psychiatric:* increased risk of psychiatric disorders, suicidality, interpersonal violence, or visit to a psychiatric emergency room; or, poor adherence to treatment, which increases the risk of poor response to medications and/or therapy as well as psychiatric hospitalization.

3. Social and family: accidents on the job, lost productivity, unemployment, school dropout or poor performance, criminal behaviors and arrests, family and domestic violence, child abuse and neglect, family break-ups, homelessness, physical and developmental disabilities of children, and psychiatric or substance abuse among offspring or other family members.

4. Economic: increased financial costs to employers, the government and insurance companies due to lost or reduced productivity, health care costs associated with medical or psychiatric disorders, social service costs (e.g., welfare), and costs associated with crime and the criminal justice system.

Substance abuse can cause tremendous personal suffering and distress for the abuser as well as the family member. While the personal, subjective experience may vary from one person to the next, it is clear that substance use disorders are associated with serious emotional and spiritual effects that cannot be adequately conveyed in data or an objective listing of problems. Books written about recovery, such as the "Big Book" of Alcoholics Anonymous (1976) and the "Basic Text" of Narcotics Anonymous (1988), contain a wealth of personal stories that convey the personal experiences and suffering of the substance abuser and family.

Assessment Strategies

1. Patient interview. Eliciting a history of alcohol or drug use may generate defensiveness, particularly among patients who deny or minimize their problem. A non-judgmental and matter-of-fact approach can help reduce defensiveness and facilitate compliance with treatment recommendations. A comprehensive assessment of substance use includes a review of the following:

- Quantity and frequency of substances currently and previously used, methods of use (oral, smoking, intramuscular, intravenous), and preferred substance(s) of choice.
- The presence of tolerance and withdrawal symptoms.

- Medical and psychiatric history to determine if significant comorbidity exists or if there are viruses or diseases present (e.g., HIV, tuberculosis, hepatitis).
- Negative consequences of substance use.
- Presence of obsessions and compulsions to use, attempts to cut down or stop, and experiences with relapse.
- How the substance problem is perceived and motivation to change.
- Family history of substance abuse or dependence.
- History of previous treatment attempts and outcome of treatment.
- Participation in high-risk behaviors (e.g., IV drug use, sharing needles or paraphernalia, unprotected sex, promiscuous sex, prostitution, selling drugs, committing crimes to get money for drugs).

2. Informant or collateral interviews with family members, significant others, or health care professionals. These often provide additional information about the patient. Family and significant others can also play a role in the recovery process by influencing the patient to seek and comply with treatment and by providing support.

3. A physical examination and a comprehensive medical history. These are used to assess signs of substance intoxication or withdrawal, medical consequences of substance use, and to rule out medical problems that can complicate withdrawal. Alcohol withdrawal complications such as seizures or delirium tremens, for example, are more likely to occur in patients with compromised physical health problems.

4. Laboratory tests. These help rule out the likelihood of alcohol or drug overdose. Breath alcohol levels or blood alcohol concentration (BAC) provide objective measurements of the intoxication state and the levels of tolerance. A BAC of 200–300 mg/ml in a patient who shows only minor signs of intoxication indicates a high level of tolerance, and the patient may be vulnerable to severe withdrawal when substances are reduced or stopped. An initial test battery may include urinalysis, complete blood count with differential, blood chemistry, serology, and liver enzymes. Hepatitis screen and HIV testing should also be performed in high-risk groups such as those with other drug use, especially intravenous drug users. These tests, conducted regularly and/or randomly, are also useful during treatment to monitor alcohol and other substance use.

5. *Pen and paper screening instruments.* Simple, time-efficient, reliable, and widely used pen and paper screening instruments can be used to assess substance use problems. These include the CAGE questionnaire (Mayfield, McLeod & Hall, 1974), the Brief Michigan alcoholism screening test (MAST) (Selzer, 1971), the AUDIT (Saunders, Aasland, Babor et al., 1993), and the drug abuse screening test (DAST) (Skinner & Allen, 1982). The CAGE is a very brief, four-item, widely used screening instrument; the MAST is a brief questionnaire about alcohol use behaviors, the DAST is a brief questionnaire about drug use behaviors, and the AUDIT is a 10-item questionnaire that provides information on the amount and frequency, the alcohol dependence syndrome, and on problems caused by alcohol.

6. *Rating scales and structured diagnostic interviews.* The alcohol dependence scale (ADS) and the severity of alcohol dependence questionnaire (SADQ) (Stockwell, Murphy & Hodgson, 1983) provide a measure of the severity of the dependence syndrome. The Structured Clinical Interview for DSM-IV (SCID) (First, Spitzer, Gibbon & Williams, 1994) and the Psychiatric Research Interview for Substance and Mental Disorders (PRISM) (Hasin, Trautman, Miele, Samet, Smith & Endicott, 1996) provide reliable DSM-IV psychiatric diagnoses, including substance use disorders. These instruments, however, are very time intensive, although primary care versions of the SCID is now available.

Other instruments, such as the alcohol timeline followback (TLFB) (Sobell, Sobell, Leo & Cancilla, 1988), the addiction severity index (ASI) (McLellan, Luborsky, Woody & O'Brien, 1980), and drinker inventory of consequences (DrinC) (Miller, Tonigan & Longabaugh, 1995) assess drinking or other drug use behavior, treatment planning, treatment process, and treatment outcome. For example, the ASI provides indices of severity in seven health-related domains including alcohol, other drugs, psychiatric, medical, family, social, and legal areas. The ASI also provides a measure of change over time in terms of severity and frequency of alcohol and drug use.

■ ASSESSMENT OF WITHDRAWAL

The Clinical Institute Withdrawal Assessment Scale for Alcohol-Revised version (CIWA-r) (Sullivan, Sykora, Schneiderman, Naranjo & Sellers, 1989) provides a comprehensive assessment of the withdrawal syndrome and it requires approximately 5–7 minutes to administer. Versions of this instrument have been found to be useful in dual diagnosis patients as well (Handelsman, Cochrane, Aronson, Ness, Rubinsten & Kanof, 1987). Opiate withdrawal may be monitored using a short 10-item validated scale called the Short Opiate Withdrawal Scale (Gossop, 1990). The patient self-rates the intensity of symptoms on a scale from scale 0 (not at all) to 4 (extremely). The Objective Opiate Withdrawal Scale (Handelsman et al., 1987) is an observer-rated scale that assesses 13 physical signs of opiate withdrawal.

■ COMORBIDITY WITH PSYCHIATRIC DISORDERS

The ECA study found that 53 percent of individuals meeting criteria for a drug abuse or dependence disorder, and 37 percent meeting criteria for an alcohol abuse or dependence disorder also met lifetime criteria for a psychiatric disorder (Robins & Regier, 1991). Specific rates of substance abuse or dependence was as follows for these psychiatric diagnoses:

- Antisocial personality disorder   84 percent
- Bipolar disorder   61 percent
- Schizophrenia   47 percent
- Depressive disorders   28 percent
- Anxiety disorders   24 percent

Numerous studies of patients in substance abuse or psychiatric treatment programs also found high rates of comorbidity (Daley et al., 1993; O'Connell, in press). These dual disordered patients are at risk for a number of problems including poor treatment adherence, suicidality, relapse, and hospitalization. Due to the very high rates of substance abuse and psychiatric comorbidity, a number of integrated treatment approaches have been developed to address both psychiatric and substance abuse issues in the same treatment program. Integrated treatment is generally seen as the preferable model of care for more severe cases of comorbidity.

■ MOTIVATING SUBSTANCE ABUSING PATIENTS TO ACCEPT TREATMENT

Patients with substance use disorders often deny or minimize their problems or the adverse effects of these problems on their lives or the lives of family members. As a result, they may believe they do not need any type of treatment. Or, they may believe that they can change on their own without the help of others. By using motivational enhancement strategies, the clinician can increase the likelihood that the patient will follow through with the recommendations to seek specialized help. These strategies have been used successfully with a variety of problems including alcohol use disorders (Bien, Miller & Toniga, 1993), opiate addiction (Saunders, Wilkinson & Phillips, 1995), patients with the dual disorders of substance abuse and depressive illness (Daley et al., 1998), and patients with psychotic disorders (Miner et al., 1997). These motivational strategies, developed by Miller and Rollnick (1991), aim to increase patients' readiness for treatment and motivation to change. Motivation is viewed as a "state" that can be affected by the clinician. Low motivation is a clinical problem to be addressed and resolved rather than a reason not to engage the patient in treatment.

While more extensive information is available elsewhere describing motivational interventions, the key components are summarized in the acronym FRAMES:

1. _Feedback_: the physician or other caregiver provides the patient with specific objective feedback about diagnosis or problems assessed through clinical interviews, medical records, laboratory reports and/or collateral data (e.g., from a family member). This feedback gives the patient valuable information about the diagnoses, effects of the problem(s), possible interactions among several problems that may lead the patient to agree to accept a referral for specialized treatment. With substance use problems, feedback can incorporate any significant laboratory findings. Examples include high blood alcohol levels, elevated liver enzymes, related medical disorders that are caused or exacerbated by substance abuse, urinalysis results and others. Other feedback items may include the assessment of withdrawal symptoms, changes in tolerance, and behaviors or problems associated with the substance use (e.g., family, legal, work, etc.). For example, the caregiver may say to a patient "Ms. Blake, our laboratory results show high levels of cocaine in your urine. Also, you and your husband both told us that you've been using large amounts of cocaine every day, you can't seem to stop for more than a few days at a time even though you want to, you feel depressed and suicidal when you run out of drugs, you're getting into arguments with your husband, you've missed a lot of work, and spent a lot of money on drugs. All of these symptoms and behaviors, taken together, mean you meet criteria for cocaine dependence. You even said yourself that you were addicted, so you know there's a serious problem with your drug use. The amount of cocaine that you are using and the frequency at which you use indicate a very serious level of addiction."

2. _Responsibility_: the decision to seek help or change is the sole responsibility of the patient. While recommendations can be provided about treatment programs or change strategies, the patient must bear the responsibility for the disorder(s) and for making the decision to engage in treatment. Specific and concrete

feedback regarding diagnoses and problems caused by the patient's substance may instill guilt and motivate the patient to take responsibility for seeking further help.

3. _Advice:_ the patient is given specific advice on how to deal with his problem. For example, to the patient who has a problem with alcohol, the physician might say, "We've seen other people like yourself who've had trouble controlling their drinking really benefit from professional treatment. I'd strongly advise you to get help and would like to recommend you see . . . or attend the program at . . ." Or, "You told me you're worried about your drinking and how it's affecting your health and family. I would recommend you stop drinking altogether since there's a good chance your liver would return to normal, and you could also begin to work out your problems with your wife. I think you would gain a lot by getting involved in treatment at . . ."

4. _Menu_: different treatment or change options are provided to the patient, who chooses from among them. The physician might say to a patient with moderate problem with marijuana or alcohol abuse: "I can refer you to a private therapist or to the local drug and alcohol treatment clinic for counseling. This can help you address your concerns about marijuana (or alcohol) abuse." Or, for a more severe type of substance dependence the caregiver may say, "You describe a severe problem with heroin in which you've been injecting large amounts of the drug every day for almost two years. I would like to refer you for detoxification and a rehabilitation program. Let me tell you about treatment programs and you can decide which one to attend."

5. _Empathy:_ a positive therapeutic alliance or relationship with a patient is built on empathy. This refers to the caregiver's ability to accept, understand, and have a sincere desire to help the patient and to convey this to the patient. Judgmentalism and negative attitudes or reactions will impede the ability to help these patients, so the physician or caregiver must be aware of personal attitudes, perceptions, and beliefs regarding these types of problems. If, for example, alcohol or other drug dependence is viewed as bad behavior and a flaw in the individual rather than a serious biopsychosocial disorder, the professional will be less

able to help the affected patient. Health and mental health care professionals sometimes struggle with this issue because they view the addicted patient as manipulative, unmotivated, antisocial, or a hassle to deal with. They judge the patient based on the behavior shown. Rather than see the behavior as part of the addiction, which is amenable to change, some clinicians react negatively and push the patient away. Accepting the patient and conveying empathy are needed in order to influence the patient to participate in treatment or change.

6. *Self-efficacy:* the caregiver supports the patient's belief in the ability to make positive changes whenever possible. Realistic optimism that things can get better is conveyed. For example, the patient may be told, "It sounds like you've succeeded in the past coping with your addiction when you had the support of your wife, saw a therapist regularly, and went to NA meetings. You're in a good position to do this again, which I think will help you get back on the recovery track." Or, "You've been very honest about how close you came to drinking again. The fact that you didn't drink, even though you wanted very badly to do so, is a good sign that you have both the desire and ability to stay sober. Let's talk more about other things that can help you stay sober and prevent a relapse."

Principles of Effective Treatment

A recent research-based guide published by the National Institute on Drug Abuse (NIDA, 1999a) delineated the following principles for effective treatment of substance use disorders.

- *No single treatment is appropriate for all individuals.* A variety of different treatments have been used successfully for both alcohol and drug abuse problems.
- *Treatment needs to be readily available.* The caregiver must "strike when the iron is hot" so to speak. Helping the patient access treatment in a timely manner will improve outcome. The patient who has to wait for an opening before

a treatment program will accept him or her can be strongly encouraged to attend a self-help program such as Alcoholics Anonymous, Narcotics Anonymous, or Cocaine Anonymous.

- *Effective treatment addresses other needs and problems in addition to substance use.* Substance abuse is seldom the only problem that the patient will have. While other problems usually should not be the main focus of treatment, addressing these may be critical to the success of substance abuse treatment.

- *The treatment plan must be assessed and changed continually to meet the patient's changing needs.* Treatment is a "dynamic" process and the focus may shift from time to time as the patient's problems and needs change. However, the clinician must always insure that the substance abuse problem receives proper attention since too much focus on "other" problems can contribute to the patient's lack of focus on the importance of abstaining from the substance use disorder.

- *Remaining in treatment for an adequate period of time is critical for treatment effectiveness.* For many people, substance dependence is a long-term, chronic condition. While professional treatment may be limited in terms of time, the patient always has the option of continuing to receive support in self-help programs. While brief treatments have been show to be effective with alcohol use disorders, there are no demonstrated effective brief treatments for drug abuse. Evidence shows that at least 90 days in outpatient care is needed at a minimum for the drug abusing patient to benefit (Simpson et al., 1995). Therefore, one of the early important treatment goals is retaining the patient in treatment.

- *Counseling and therapy are critical components of effective treatment for addiction.* While medications are sometimes helpful for certain types of addiction, individual, group or family treatments are often needed to help the patient accept the substance use disorder, address problems contributing to and resulting from the substance abuse, and learn coping skills to stay sober and make positive lifestyle changes.

- *Medications may be an important element of treatment for many patients, especially when combined with counseling or therapy.* Some providers may choose medications such as Naltrexone hydrochloride or Antabuse reduce cravings and relapse risk for some alcoholics. Opiate replacement therapy such as methadone or L-a-Alethymethadol (LAAM) help some narcotic addicts avoid using heroin or other opiates, thus reducing the need to engage in illegal activities to secure money to pay for expensive drugs, and reducing involvement in high-risk behaviors such as IV drug use, sharing needles, cotton, or rinsing water.

- *Drug abusing or dependent patients with comorbid psychiatric disorders need to have both disorders treated in an integrated way.* Treatment that focuses only on substance abuse or psychiatric illness is often inadequate since comorbid disorders are often linked in many ways (Minkoff, 1999; Daley & Thase, 2000).

- *Medical detoxification* (see also Pharmacological Treatment of Substance Abuse Disorders, pp. 78–79) *is only the first stage of treatment and by itself does little to change long-term substance use.* Detoxification simply allows the patient to withdraw safely from alcohol or other drugs. It paves the way for ongoing treatment and involvement in recovery. Patients referred for detoxification should be told that this is only one aspect of treatment, and that follow-up care in a residential, partial hospital, or outpatient program is needed in order to reduce relapse risk.

- *Treatment does not need to be voluntary to be effective.* Many patients enter substance abuse treatment as a result of external pressure from employers, the legal system, or family members. Once the patient participates in treatment, motivation may shift from external to internal. Since treatment effectiveness is correlated with the amount of time spent in treatment, involuntary patients who have to stay in treatment over a long period of time actually are in a good position to internalize the desire to change.

- *Possible substance use during treatment should be monitored continuously.* While the majority of patients will be honest about substance use, some will lie, minimize, or deny any use, especially if they believe there will be an adverse outcome for using substances. Regular and random use of breathlyzers or urine drug screens can be used as an objective way to monitor substance use. Caregivers should also routinely ask substance abusing patients about episodes of use, strong cravings and close calls. Persistent strong cravings and frequent close calls often signal that a particular patient is at high-risk for relapse.

- *Treatment programs should assess for HIV/AIDS, Hepatitis B and C, Tuberculosis and other infectious diseases, and provide counseling to help patients change behaviors placing themselves or others at risk of infection.* These diseases are common among substance abusers, particularly those who use drugs intravenously, share needles or paraphernalia, or engage in high-risk behaviors such as unprotected sex or sex with strangers, prostitutes, or multiple partners. Both acquiring and transmitting diseases are important issues to address with patients. It is not unusual for some substance abusing patients to react fatalistically when they discover they are HIV+ and use this as an excuse not to say sober or change. Anger, depression, and despair are common reactions and can be addressed in therapy.

- *Recovery is a long-term process that frequently requires multiple episodes of treatment.* For many patients, substance use disorders are chronic and life-long disorders. While some patients establish and maintain long periods of continuous sobriety, many experience periods of remission followed by episodes of relapse to substance use. Therefore, many patients need to return to treatment to stabilize from periods of relapse.

Psychosocial Treatments for Substance Use Disorders....

This section will present some of the more common treatments for substance use disorders. Many of these treatments have demonstrated empirical success through the Project Match Therapy Manual series from NIAAA (1995a–c) or the "Therapy Manuals for Drug Addiction Series" through NIDA (1998a,b, 1999, 2000). The treatments will be divided into three categories. The first, Disease Model Treatments, will include Individual Drug Counseling and Twelve-Step Facilitation Therapy. The second category of treatment will be Behavioral and Cognitive Interventions. This will include Cognitive Behavioral Coping Skills Treatment, Cue Exposure, and Contingency Management. The third category will be systems approaches. This will include family systems approaches, therapeutic communities, and group treatments. Finally a special section will present Motivational Enhancement Therapy and Dual Diagnoses Recovery Counseling. This chapter is meant to present brief explanations in order to encourage readers to explore these treatments further.

■ DISEASE MODEL TREATMENT

A treatment philosophy based on the disease model conceptualizes alcohol and drug addiction as a biopsychosocial illness that affects social, psychological, spiritual, and physical dimensions. Rush introduced this concept in the 18th century but Jellinek elaborated the disease theory in 1946. Alcoholism is seen as an illness that progresses in phases. The first is the pre-alcoholic phase where substance use produces initial rewards such as relaxation and sedation. The prodromal phase is where the drinker begins to experience negative consequences from drinking and yet drinks excessively. The crucial phase is when loss of control becomes overt and the person's lifestyle centers around drinking. The chronic phase is characterized by extreme deterioration in functioning with prolonged periods of intoxication. The person is now drinking to feel normal. There is no cure for the disease but it can be arrested through treatment and life-long abstinence. The best known and widely used disease approach is based on Twelve-Step philosophy, which calls for broad life changes that reflect a new, more spiritual way of living. Such changes are key to maintaining abstinence from chemicals.

■ INDIVIDUAL DRUG COUNSELING (IDC) (NIDA, 1999b)

IDC is a model developed for the treatment of cocaine addiction but applicable to other types of substance use disorders. The approach is based on the disease model of addiction and reflects the Twelve-Step philosophy. Addiction is viewed as a biopsycho-social disease that affects many areas of functioning. These areas must all be addressed for successful treatment. The Twelve-Step component represents the spiritual focus of the approach. IDC is different from typical psychotherapy because it focuses on developing short-term behavioral goals that specifically target substance use. IDC focuses primarily on present issues and behavior and does not delve much into issues of the past.

The focus of treatment is on the symptoms of substance abuse and the areas of impaired functioning. The treatment emphasizes specific behavioral change with the primary goal of achieving and maintaining abstinence from all substances. Patients are successful in treatment when they recognize the existence of a problem and the addictive thinking that supports the problem. Through therapy, patients learn coping strategies and "tools" for ongoing sobriety. Patients are also encouraged to engage in support groups and follow a Twelve-Step program.

There are four stages of treatment. In the *initiation* stage, therapists deal with patient denial and ambivalence about entering a recovery program. The goal is to help them realize they suffer from an incurable disease and need to break the addictive cycle. In the *early recovery* stage, patients learn about potential triggers and gain skills to successfully deal with those triggers. In the *main-*

tenance stage, the patient continues to learn about the relapse process, which includes identifying and coping with triggers, cravings, and urges. The patient continually practices learned skills and makes ongoing changes to support sobriety. Finally, *advanced recovery* is a lifelong commitment to change and growth. Formal treatment may end at this stage but the patient continues to engage in activities to support sobriety and enhance life fulfillment.

Each session adheres to the following format:

- Inquiring as to the last time patient used substances
- Current substance use
- Any urgent problems the patient has
- Feedback about drug screens
- Relevant recovery related topics.

Sessions are scheduled twice a week for 3 months, weekly for 3 months, and monthly for 3 months (NIDA, 1999b).

■ TWELVE-STEP FACILITATION THERAPY (TSF) (NIAAA, 1995a)

TSF is a treatment based on the Twelve-Step philosophy of Alcoholics Anonymous (A.A). The primary objective is to facilitate patient participation in Twelve-Step programs. This is accomplished by helping the patient accept addiction as a progressive illness. By accepting that they have an illness, patients break through their denial and open themselves to the Twelve-Step program. Patients must admit that that they have lost all control over their substance use and their life in general. They must accept that there is no cure for the illness and only lifelong abstinence and recovery will arrest the disease process.

Each session has an agenda based on topics related to Twelve-Step philosophy. The patient is required to attend Twelve-Step meetings, maintain a journal of their reactions to meetings, and read Twelve-step materials. A maximum of 12 sessions is allowed with two extra "emergency" sessions, if needed. An introductory session includes an alcohol use history, previous treatment experiences, and a determination of a diagnosis. Topics that are covered in session include negative consequences, tolerance levels, and examples where the patient lost control of their usage. Sessions 2–11 cover various topics of Twelve-Step recovery. Each session adheres to the following format:

- Review of the patient's journal
- Review of any substance use episodes the patient may have had
- Review of urges or cravings to use chemicals
- Assessment of the number of sober days the patient has (Categories 1–4 take about 10–15 minutes)
- Introduction of new topic material (30 minutes)
- Assignment of recovery tasks (10 minutes)
- Summary of session (5 minutes).

The sessions are active and focused. Following the patient's lead is generally discouraged. However, the therapist will consider personal issues the patient is dealing with in recovery. These issues will not be dwelled upon for the majority of the session. A therapist who follows this program should have a good working knowledge of the Twelve Steps, readings, meeting places, and networking with other Twelve-Step members.

Behavioral and Cognitive Treatments

Behavioral and cognitive approaches include a broad range of interventions that share a common origin in learning theory. In learning theory, human behavior is learned versus being genetically determined and is affected by environmental factors. Learning principles are applied in treatment to enact cognitive and behavioral changes. Therapy tends to be highly focused on treatment approaches that target specific behaviors, beliefs, or cognitions. Examples of such approaches include cognitive-behavioral coping skills treatments, contingency management, and cue exposure interventions.

■ COGNITIVE-BEHAVIORAL COPING SKILLS TREATMENT

This is a structured and time-limited treatment where the goal is to teach coping skills that will help patients maintain abstinence from drugs and alcohol (NIAAA, 1995c; Monti, Abrams, Kadden & Cooney, 1989). Substance abuse is viewed from a social learning perspective. Patients learn harmful behaviors, such as substance use, in order to change the way they feel. Over time, patients begin to expect positive feelings from substance use and this motivates their substance-seeking behavior. As the addiction progresses, patients have less confidence in their ability to cope without the use of chemicals, known as low self-efficacy.

The goal of treatment is to identify high-risk environmental cues that increase the likelihood the patient will use chemicals. Through treatment, the patient learns problem-solving and behavioral skills to effectively cope with situations and feelings. A second goal is to examine the patient's thoughts, feelings, and beliefs about these situations. The therapist can then teach the patient to counteract self-defeating cognitions.

The treatment is conducted in 12 sessions. First there is an introductory session where the therapist establishes rapport and explains the rationale for treatment. The next 8 sessions are the "core" sessions where various topics are covered. Topics include: (1) coping with cravings and urges, (2) managing thoughts about chemical use, (3) problem solving high-risk situations, (4) drinking refusal skills, (5) planning for emergencies, and (6) seemingly irrelevant decisions. There are numerous other "elective" topics discussed along with a final termination session.

Strategies that are used in sessions include role plays and homework assignments. Role plays are viewed as critical because they facilitate the use of coping skills in real-life situations. Homework is used to encourage the practice of skills in real-life situations outside the therapy office. Skills are also taught through therapist modeling, verbal presentation, treatment contracts, and self-monitoring forms. The therapist is active and directive in carrying out the treatment protocol and encouraging active collaboration with the patient.

CBT has also been used as a treatment for cocaine addiction (NIDA, 1998a). Learning procedures are used to reduce cocaine use. First a functional analysis is conducted for the reasons patients use cocaine. This includes an analysis of obstacles to maintaining abstinence, strengths the patient possesses that foster abstinence, and determinants of cocaine use. Patients then learn skills and strategies that focus on stopping behaviors that support cocaine use. This approach differs from traditional cognitive therapy (CT) in that CT focuses on increasing personal control over urges and cravings by modifying dysfunctional attitudes and beliefs about substance use (Beck, Wright, Newman & Liese, 1993). CBT will work on modifying these cognitions but the initial focus is on developing healthy coping behaviors.

■ CUE EXPOSURE TREATMENT (NIDA, 1993)

Substance abusers are faced with a variety of internal and external stimuli, known as cues, which increase arousal and trigger craving to use chemicals. Stimuli that trigger cravings are varied and often depend on the individual. Typical approaches encourage people in recovery to avoid "slippery people, places, and things," but this is not always possible.

Cue exposure is a relapse prevention approach that combines learning theory and behavior modification techniques. The technique involves presenting cues to patients, when they are in a protected setting, while working to reduce craving for the drug. The theory states that when a patient is repeatedly exposed to a cue (drug or alcohol trigger) without the presence of a reinforcer (the substance), the response (arousal, drug craving) will gradually diminish and the patient will become desensitized to the cue or trigger. Cue exposure treatment also teaches the patient to reduce the drug craving by learning alternative responses to the cue.

The two main goals for treatment are to identify triggers and to master or control the patient's responses to those triggers. The first stage of treatment is to help the patient identify potential triggers. Triggers may be internal (thoughts, feelings, moods, physical sensations) or external (people, places, and things). Second, the patient is taught to rate the intensity of the trigger. Next, a cue extinction tool is introduced. Cue extinction tools are responses that are incompatible with drug cravings and arousal. Examples are as follows:

- Deep relaxation techniques
- Delay of responding to craving
- Thinking of positive consequences to not using and negative consequences to using
- Imagery techniques
- Master imagery: patient pictures a powerful person to help battle craving
- Cognitive interventions to counteract negative thinking.

Once a cue extinction tool is utilized, the intensity of the craving is reassessed. If the intervention is unsuccessful, the appropriateness of a tool, or the patient's ability to use the tool, is assessed. After the introduction and completion of the technique, any lingering feelings or arousal states are processed and dealt with prior to termination of the session. A plan for practicing the tools is developed between sessions.

Cue exposure is best used in individual therapy. Group treatments are appropriate for teaching coping tools but it is not recommended that cravings be induced. This is because some patients will experience cravings and triggers more intensely than others. Cue exposure can be conducted at all levels of care but is best used during inpatient treatment because of the safe environment. Patients best suited for cue exposure are not actively using substances for at least a week following their last usage or medical detoxification.

■ CONTINGENCY MANAGEMENT APPROACHES (HIGGINS & SILVERMAN, 1999)

Individuals with substance abuse problems often find few rewards in their initial attempts to achieve abstinence from chemicals. Contingency management is a behavioral approach that uses positive incentives to help patients maintain abstinence from substances of abuse. Also known as a community reinforcement approach (CRA) (Meyers & Smith, 1995), the program utilizes individual counseling and disulfiram to assist patients in making lifestyle changes. In the CRA, abstinence is positively reinforced while drug use leads to loss of reinforcement. The goal is to develop reinforcers that effectively compete with the reinforcing properties of drug abuse. An example of such a program is the Community Reinforcement plus Vouchers approach with cocaine addiction (NIDA, 1998b).

In the CRA plus vouchers approach, patients earn points toward exchangeable retail items by remaining abstinent from drugs. Along with abstinence, patients are encouraged to make major lifestyle changes to support sobriety. Progress is measured through urine drug screens. A negative drug screen is a basis for positive reinforcement while a positive drug screen leads to an absence of reinforcement and a need to problem solve regarding relapse prevention.

In the skills training component, patients are taught to identify their substance use patterns and develop drug refusal skills. They also learn strategies to cope with high-risk situations and learn other skills as needed (communication, assertiveness, interpersonal, etc.). Treatment is provided through individual counseling. The counseling style is flexible, active, and collaborative. Counselors should have an adequate knowledge of behavioral principles and be able to use them effectively in treatment. Primarily, counselors need to socially reinforce any apparent efforts by the patient to change. Other techniques include behavioral contracting, goal setting, modeling, and shaping.

The counseling is active and focused. If patients have particular issues or crises, they will be addressed but the particular focus of the session remains primary. A session protocol will first review urinalysis results. A negative result is reinforced in contrast to a positive result that removes reinforcement. If a drug screen is positive, then the counselor and patient will analyze the relapse process to determine problem areas. The rest of the session reviews progress with treatment goals, problem solving around the goals, skill training, and establishing new goals if necessary. The skills training aspect of the program develops behaviors conducive to the maintenance of sobriety. These include practical avoidance or refusal skills, recreational planning, vocational counseling, and social skills training.

Systems Approaches

■ FAMILY TREATMENT APPROACHES

The family systems model and behavioral model of marital treatment assume that there is a reciprocal relationship between substance use and the quality of family/marital interactions. The substance abuser's behavior affects the way family members interact with each other. Likewise, the family interactions punish or reinforce the behavior of the substance abuser. Therefore, treatment must focus on changing the behavior of the substance abuser and the family members in order to enhance recovery efforts.

Family interventions began in the late 1800s, when psychoanalytic theory determined that family interactions had a significant influence in the shaping of personality. Between the 1930s and 1950s, clinicians became aware of the effect alcoholic men had on the emotional health of their spouses. The Family Disease Model arose from A.A. outreach to family members and gave rise to the concepts of co-dependents, and to children and adult children of alcoholics. Alcoholism was viewed as a family disease and this led to groups such as Al-Anon, Al-Ateen, and Adult Children of Alcoholics groups (McCrady & Epstein, 1999). These groups emphasized the need for family members to change attitudes and behaviors developed in the alcoholic family system. Members following the Twelve-Step philosophy and realizing they cannot control the behavior of the alcoholic accomplish this change.

The Family Systems Model views families in terms of developmental issues. Families are constantly changing to meet the needs of their members and the goal is to maintain stability or homeostasis. In order to maintain this, families develop unwritten rules, family roles, and develop family boundaries in order to maintain stability. In alcoholic families, alcohol is the focal point through which these concepts are organized. The family system is organized in order to maintain drinking behavior. The family rules and roles serve to distract families from the main problem, alcohol. Families are thought to have slowed or stopped their developmental movement in order to maintain pathological drinking behavior (Ott, Tarter & Ammerman, 1999).

The goals of family therapy are to eliminate the drinking behavior of the identified alcoholic and then to change the family system, which has been organized to accommodate the alcoholic. This occurs in two primary ways. First, the alcoholism must be removed from the family through intervention and treatment. This disrupts the family system and often leaves the family unstable. The second goal is to stabilize and reorganize the family. This is accomplished through a restructuring of family roles and rules while developing developmentally appropriate family boundaries.

Therapy is often very difficult because families are entrenched in their unhealthy interaction patterns and any change is threatening to the family homeostasis. The therapist must tolerate the families expressed emotion, ambivalence, and what often seems like tremendous effort to keep the family in the previous unhealthy patterns. It is important to recognize the fears that change represents because family member's identities are often determined by the alcoholic interaction patterns. Therapists may use a variety of strategies to change these patterns but must progress at a pace tolerable to the family.

■ BEHAVIORAL MARITAL TREATMENT

Behavioral models stem from learning theory which states behavior is maintained through reinforcement or punishment. In regard to substance abuse, drinking behavior is reinforced through familial interaction. Drinking can be reinforced through positive attention or caretaking, which protects the alcoholic from the negative consequences of drinking behavior. Therapy focuses on changing the drinking behavior and the familial interaction that reinforces drinking and may trigger relapse. Behavioral marital therapy (BMT) is one empirically supported treatment for family interventions (O'Farrell & Fals-Stewart, 1999).

BMT utilizes both couples therapy and group therapy to address the alcoholic's drinking and change the interaction styles within a marriage to support sobriety. Alcohol use is viewed from a social learning perspective where interaction styles support drinking behavior. The goals are to support sobriety by decreasing negative interactions that may trigger relapse and increasing positive interactions that support an improved marital relationship. This will be accomplished through various behavioral and problem-solving strategies. First a functional analysis of the behaviors, within the relationship, that may trigger chemical usage is conducted. Then the therapist would help the couple develop new interaction styles that are less likely to trigger usage. This may be accomplished by planning behavioral alternatives to current interaction styles. The couple will learn which communication styles are most likely to create stress in the relationship and therefore be a trigger for relapse. The therapist will then teach ways to alter these communication styles through behavioral experiments. For example, a spouse will purposely search for positive behaviors in the other spouse and provide positive reinforcement. The couple will be encouraged to plan rewarding activities versus constantly arguing about substance use. The therapist may explore spouse's thoughts regarding new behaviors and utilize cognitive restructuring techniques to alter faulty assumptions about the new behaviors.

■ THERAPEUTIC COMMUNITIES (DeLEON, 1999)

A therapeutic community (TC) is a group of people who share a common problem, such as substance abuse, living together in a house or facility run by a staff of professionals and recovering substance abusers. Individuals in TCs usually have histories of multiple drug use, poor coping skills, antisocial character traits, and few support systems. TCs typically have an "open door" policy but would consider risk factors and individual motivation as criteria for admission. Risk factors refer to the degree an individual would be a behavioral management problem within the community. This may include serious violent behavior, suicide attempts, or severe psychiatric problems, such as psychotic disorders. Motivation issues would include acceptance of the addiction problem and willingness to conform to the TC.

Although each program has its own individual philosophy, all communities follow social-psychological and self-help theories. In the TC approach, substance abuse is viewed as a deviant behavior reflecting abnormal personality development and/or deficits in various life skills. The primary goal is a global lifestyle change in all areas of functioning. This includes abstinence from substances, development of functional life skills, and a change in antisocial attitudes and values. The TC approach has beginnings in the A.A program of recovery. More specifically its roots stem from Synanon in 1958.

The TC approach sees substance abuse as a disorder of the whole person, involving multiple physical, psychological, and spiritual areas of functioning. The problem of addiction is within the person, therefore treatment focuses on changing various psychological dysfunctions and social deficits. Recovery is viewed as a developmental process where the person makes changes in lifestyle and personal identity. This is accomplished by following TC values and beliefs that are viewed as essential to personal growth and healthy living. The TC approach calls this the "View of Right Living."

The main concepts of TC reflect a focus on group membership and participation. Individuals define themselves and their particular roles in reference to the community. Particular members who reflect positive progress serve as role models within the community. Members are expected to adhere to the community norms and values while using these guidelines as a basis for evaluating individual growth and change. The community facilitates individual growth through open communication in the context of group relationships. Members are given feedback from other members about their progress. This exemplifies the philosophy of the "community as context and method." This means that the community is the agent through which change takes place.

The ways which TC creates change through community, is by using a variety of activities aimed at facilitating movement through the stages of change. The stages of change vary depending on individual programming but generally reflect an initial orientation, a primary treatment component, and a re-entry phase into society. One way change is accomplished is through individual engagement in the group milieu. Patients attend meetings and activities aimed at enhancing group cohesion and reinforcing the group structure and goals. Another method is through group behavior management. This occurs through the use of privileges and disciplinary procedures. Members are rewarded for prosocial behavior and lose privileges for negative or antisocial behavior. Change occurs when members are successfully socialized to the TC philosophy of living. This can be evaluated through overt behavioral change or change in attitudes and perceptions. The goal is for the individual to internalize the concepts taught while involved in the TC. Internalization is important because the person has then incorporated the values as their own and is more likely to use them after treatment termination.

■ GROUP DRUG COUNSELING (DALEY, MERCER & CARPENTER, 1998; NIDA, 2001).

Group treatment is a modality frequently used in substance abuse treatment. Groups are often preferred because they provide a forum for peer feedback and support with individuals recovering from substance abuse. Through groups, individuals can hear other people's experiences and learn ways to change behaviors. Peer feedback about someone's behavior is often more powerful than feedback from professionals whom patients sometimes view as different from them. This section describes a particular group approach, Group Drug Counseling (GDC).

GDC is a manualized group counseling approach for patients recovering from an addiction. The approach views addiction as a biopsychosocial disease that affects all areas of functioning. Treatment must therefore address issues within various domains of functioning. Abstinence along with personal and lifestyle changes are the main goals of treatment.

The GDC approach is divided into two phases. During phase one, group members meet for 12 weeks and receive information about addiction and recovery. This phase of the treatment is psychoeducational in nature and patients receive information about various topics on recovery. Group members are encouraged to interact with each other and share experiences regarding the topics. In this way they can develop relationships when provided encouragement and support. Each topic has a format for lecture discussion along with handouts and written assignments to facilitate learning. Therapist should have experience in dealing with group content and process. Group content refers to what is being said in the group regarding the topic. Process refers to the way information is presented and the member's reactions to the topic. Both provide useful information for group dialogue.

The second phase of treatment is the problem-solving group. This phase of group lasts from weeks 13 to 24 and is a semistructured group where members problem solve various life issues without resorting to chemical use. Group members are encouraged to discuss current problems or concerns for group. The group leader can then facilitate feedback, encouragement, confrontation, or any other form of interaction among group members to help with these problems. In this phase, members are more likely to interact with each other, giving the therapist a chance to teach skills and problem solve immediate issues within the group.

Specialized Treatment Interventions

This section will focus on two specific treatments, motivational enhancement therapy (MET) (NIAAA, 1995b) and dual diagnosis recovery counseling (DDRC) (Daley & Thase, 2000). These treatments are considered specialized because they were developed for specific purposes. MET was developed specifically to increase motivation in difficult patient populations so that they follow through with treatment. DDRC was developed to treat patients with psychiatric and comorbid substance abuse disorders. Such patients are very difficult to treat and often fall through the cracks of the behavioral health delivery systems.

■ MOTIVATIONAL ENHANCEMENT THERAPY (NIAAA, 1995b)

Motivational Enhancement Therapy (MET) is an intervention designed specifically to increase motivation for change in problem drinkers. The therapy follows the change model of Prochaska, Norcross & DiClemente (1994), who discovered through empirical research that change in humans occurs in stages. In the precontemplation stage, the patient is not considering change of problem behaviors. The contemplation stage is where the patient begins to consider that they might have a problem. The patient makes a decision to take action toward change in the determination stage. In the action stage they begin to actually take steps to modify their behavior. The final phase, maintenance, is where the patient works to maintain the changes that have occurred.

MET attempts to facilitate the change process through a series of interventions, usually within 3–4 sessions, designed to create ambivalence about patient's current behavior, mobilize motivation for change, and encourage steps to change. In doing so, the therapist creates conditions conducive to exploration and change. MET is both patient centered and directive. It utilizes non-directive interventions consistent with patient centered therapy which makes it different from typical substance abuse interventions that tend to be confrontive. At the same time therapists ask questions that challenge the patient to look at the discrepancies in their current behavior in comparison to their personal goals. Therapists will enhance discrepancy by providing non-judgmental and objective feedback about the patient's behavior. The two main issues that patients are asked to consider are: (1) How much is their drinking behavior affecting them and causing problems? and (2) what are the costs and benefits of changing problematic behavior? If the patient becomes motivated to change, the therapist can offer advice and possible alternatives in order to create change. The therapist always emphasizes that change is the patient's personal decision.

There are three primary phases of MET treatment. In the first phase, the therapist attempts to build motivation within the patient to change. This is accomplished by understanding the patient's perceptions and feelings about the situation. The therapist then attempts to elicit self-motivating statements by creating ambivalence through feedback, questioning, and reframing situations. The therapist is always looking for discrepancies between the patient's behavior and their goals. Resistance is dealt non-defensively and is considered a natural part of the change process. In the second phase the therapist attempts to strengthen the patient's commitment to change. This is accomplished by weighing consequences of change versus no change, offering information and advice, dealing with resistance, and communicating the patient's free choice in the change process. In the final phase, the patient and therapist review progress and renew the commitment to change. Further interventions to increase motivation are utilized as necessary. The basic motivational principles underlying the approach are to (1) express empathy, (2) develop discrepancy, (3) avoid argumentation, (4) roll with the resistance, and (5) support self-efficacy (NIAAA, 1995; Miller & Rollnick, 1991).

■ DUAL DISORDERS RECOVERY COUNSELING (DALEY & THASE, 2000; MONTROSE & DALEY, 1995)

Individuals diagnosed with comorbid psychiatric and a substance use disorder have typically received inadequate treatment from mental health and substance abuse delivery systems. Historically, such individuals received treatment in mental health settings, usually with psychotherapy. This method, proved ineffective because therapists were not trained in addiction and often missed critical issues. Likewise, individuals receiving standard addiction counseling did not receive adequate treatment for their psychiatric issues. DDRC grew out of the need to combine mental health and substance abuse delivery systems (Daley & Thase, 2000).

DDRC is a developmental treatment approach that is comprehensive, flexible, and integrates addiction, psychiatric, and dual disorder literature. Dual disorders are seen as bio-psychosocial illnesses that require integrated approaches focusing on psychiatric and substance abuse issues. Recovery occurs in six stages: (1) transition and engagement (several weeks or more), (2) stabilization (few weeks to several months), (3) early recovery (3–6 months), (4) middle recovery (6–12 months), (5) late recovery (1–2 years), and (6) maintenance (ongoing). In each stage there are tasks to be accomplished that depend on the patient's presenting problems, symptoms, and the protocol of the treatment setting where the intervention is conducted (Daley & Thase, 2000). DDRC is flexible and makes use of a variety of theoretical interventions. Possible interventions depend on the patient's stage of recovery and the individual issues brought into treatment.

The main goals of DDRC are to stabilize psychiatric symptoms, achieve abstinence, and improve functioning in various life domains. This includes the development of cognitive, behavioral, and interpersonal skills. Another objective of DDRC is to intervene in the relapse process of substance abuse or psychiatric disorders. Patients are encouraged to make positive lifestyle changes that support recovery. Such changes result from a positive and collaborative relationship between the counselor and patient. The counselor empathizes with the patient's personal struggles in recovery and encourages movement through the developmental stages. Other community and professional support systems can be used to support recovery.

DDRC can be adapted to all levels of care and is compatible with other treatment modalities such as pharmacotherapy, family treatment, and group treatment. Patients best suited for DDRC have mood disorders, anxiety disorders, schizophrenia, and personality adjustment issues. Patients least appropriate for DDRC are diagnosed with mental retardation, have organic impairment, or severe thought disorders.

■ PHARMACOLOGICAL TREATMENT OF SUBSTANCE USE DISORDERS

Detoxification

The major goals of detoxification are to prevent or reduce withdrawal symptoms, prevent withdrawal complications, and persuade the patient to get involved in treatment and an ongoing program of recovery. Benzodiazepines are the medications of choice to treat alcohol withdrawal. The most frequently used include long-acting compounds such as diazepam and chlordiazepoxide, and intermediate-acting compounds such as lorazepam, oxazepam, and temazepam. The pharmacokinetic profile of the long-acting diazepam and chlordiazepoxide, and their active metabolites, provide improved control over the withdrawal symptoms (Litten, Allen & Fertig, 1997). Intermediate-acting benzodiazepines are particularly useful in patients with compromised liver function.

An effective method for managing alcohol withdrawal is the use of objective assessment scales such as the diazepam loading-dose method, which can guide medication administration. This method allows for frequent and more reliable assessment of withdrawal syndrome progression, thus preventing the development of either withdrawal complications or side effects caused by excessive medication dose. We have used this procedure successfully in a large group of comorbid psychiatric and alcohol-dependent patients, most of whom had major depression. See Table 2-2 for stategies in prescribing medication for substance abusers.

TABLE 2-2. PRESCRIBING MEDICATIONS IN THE CONTEXT OF ALCOHOL OR DRUG ABUSE

Ascertain the diagnosis
Prescribe medications with low abuse potential (e.g. avoid narcotics or benzodiazepines)
Prescribe medications that have low lethality on overdose (e.g. SSRIs)
Dispense limited amount
Maintain frequent contact and monitor closely medication side effects and treatment compliance
Encourage initial involvement with a structured, intensive treatment program (e.g. several meetings per week)
Educate patient on medication effects, side effects, and expected response
Discuss patient's attitude, thoughts, and feelings regarding medication
Prepare the patient for the possibility of getting pressure from self-help group members to stop taking medications
Perform random urine or plasma toxicology screens

Pharmacotherapy of Alcoholism

Some providers may choose pharmacological agents to treat alcoholism: (1) the aversive agent disulfiram (Table 2-3), (2) the opioid antagonist naltrexone hydrochloride (Table 2-4), and (3) the GABA analogue acamprosate (available in many European countries) (Karper & Krystal, 1997; Hasin et al., 1996). Disulfiram is useful in a subgroup of select patients, but side effects and potential extensive interaction with other medications limit its usefulness in alcoholism treatment, especially those with other psychiatric or medical comorbidity and those with poor impulse control (Ciraulo, Barnhill & Jaffe, 1988). Naltrexone appears to be safe in combination with antidepressant medications, especially of the SSRI class. Acamprosate has a favorable side-effect profile, and has no interactions with alcohol as it is eliminated, unchanged, through the kidney, and it may prove very useful in dual diagnosis patients.

■ PSYCHOSOCIAL ISSUES IN RECOVERY

The goals of a treatment are to help dependent patients abstain from substances and address problems contributing to or resulting from their substance abuse problems, and make specific intrapersonal or interpersonal changes. Patients with less severe types of substance use problems may adopt the goal of reducing the amount and frequency of use. Involvement in professional treatment provides the patient with the opportunity to begin the process

TABLE 2-3. DISULFIRAM FOR ALCOHOLICS

Aversive agent
Irreversible inhibition of the enzyme aldehyde dehydrogenase
Accumulation of acetaldehyde causes the acetaldehyde syndrome or disulfiram–ethanol reaction
Dose range 125–250 mg/day
Problematic side-effects profile with liver toxicity and neuropathy
Generalized enzyme inhibitors
Liver toxicity monitoring is essential
May precipitate psychopathology including psychosis or depression
Contraindicated in severely ill patients
May be used in mild non-psychotic depressive or anxiety disorders
Generalized enzyme inhibitors
Multiple medication/medication interactions

of recovery and make changes. The major issues in recovery that the patient may address relate to physical, behavioral, cognitive, family, interpersonal, and social functioning, personal growth and lifestyle (see Table 2-5). Specific areas of focus in therapy will depend on the motivation, and unique problems and needs of the patient.

■ SELF-HELP PROGRAMS

Self-help programs such as A.A, N.A., Rational Recovery, SMART Recovery, Women for Sobriety and Men for Sobriety are commonly used with substance use problems. Self-help programs such as Dual Recovery Anonymous or Double Trouble are also available for individuals with substance use and psychiatric disorders. The caregiver can help the patient by providing education

TABLE 2-4. NALTREXONE HYDROCHLORIDE FOR ALCOHOLICS

Pure opiate antagonist
Decreases alcohol use and alcohol relapse probably by influencing the positive reinforcing effects of alcohol
Dose is 50 mg/day
Appears safe mixed with alcohol
Limited side effects profile mostly nausea and anxiety
Reported liver damage at higher dosage
Precipitates severe opiate withdrawal
Blocks the effects of opiate analgesia
Does not worsen depression
Well tolerated in combination with antidepressants

TABLE 2-5. PSYCHOSOCIAL ISSUES IN RECOVERY

Physical/lifestyle	*Behavioral/cognitive*
Exercise	Accept the disorder(s) or problem(s)
Follow a healthy diet	Control urges to drink alcohol or use drugs
Rest and relaxation	Change unhealthy beliefs and thoughts
Take medications (if needed)	Reduce depressed thoughts
Take care of medical problem	Increase pleasant thoughts
Learn to structure time	Reduce violent thoughts
Engage in pleasant activities	Control violent impulses
Achieve balance in life	Develop motivation to change
Engage in meditation	Change self-defeating patterns of behavior
Psychological	*Family/interpersonal/social*
Monitor moods	Identify effects on family and significant
Manage negative	relationships
Reduce anxiety	Involve family in treatment/recovery
Reduce boredom and emptiness	Resolve family/marital conflicts
Reduce guilt and shame	Make amends to family or other significant people
Control anger/rage	harmed
Address "losses" (grief)	Manage high-risk people, places and events
	Engage in non-drinking activities or healthy leisure
Personal growth/maintenance	interests
Address spirituality issues	Address relationship problems or deficits
Develop relapse prevention plan for all disorders	Resist social pressures to drink alcohol
or problems	Resolve work, school, financial, legal problems
Develop relapse interruption plan for all disorders	Learn to face vs. avoid interpersonal conflicts
or problems	Learn to ask for help and support
Use "recovery tools" on ongoing basis	Seek and use an A.A. sponsor

about self-help programs, identifying and discussing resistances, questions or concerns regarding these programs, examining how these programs can help the patient with his or her specific disorders or problems, and facilitating entry into specific types of self-help groups. In some cases, it helps to have contacts in self-help programs so that the patient can be called by other members of self-help groups or the patient can be given names of specific individuals to call.

■ SUBSTANCE USE LAPSE AND RELAPSE

Many individuals with alcohol problems who quit for a period of time drink again at some point in their lives (Daley & Marlatt,

1997a–c). Some *lapse,* or have a single episode of use that does not lead to continued use and an eventual relapse in which drinking escalates. Others *relapse,* or experience ongoing use of substances once they resume drinking again. Lapses and relapses can vary from mild to severe in terms of quantity of alcohol used, duration of the drinking episode and adverse effects on the person's life. The greatest risk period during treatment or recovery for relapse is the first three months. Most lapses and relapses occur early because during this time, patients are most likely to feel ambivalent about abstinence, have not developed a strong commitment to change, or do not have the coping skills needed to meet the many demands and challenges of recovery (e.g., managing strong cravings, dealing with negative affect without drinking, using a support system, etc.). Although there are many commonalties across relapse situations, each patient needs an individualized plan that helps him or her anticipate and prepare for the possibility of relapse.

■ CAUSES OF LAPSE OR RELAPSE

It is usually a combination of factors rather than one that contributes to alcohol relapse. For example, an alcoholic at a party may respond to pressures to drink alcohol from others only during times in which he or she feels anxious or bored. Drinking may be an attempt to reduce anxiety or boredom and feel part of a group that is perceived to be having fun. Or, an alcoholic may drink mainly when upset and angry at a spouse following an argument because coping skills are lacking in managing interpersonal conflict. Therefore, it is not only the "high-risk" situation that is a mediator of relapse, but the alcoholic's ability to use coping skills to manage the situation. The most common factors contributing to relapse are negative emotional states, social pressures to engage in substance use, interpersonal conflict, positive emotions, and urges, temptations or cravings.

■ RELAPSE PREVENTION STRATEGIES

Relapse prevention (RP) strategies focus on key issues associated with relapse and long-term recovery (Marlatt & Gordon, 1984; Daley & Marlatt, 1997). These RP strategies help the patient prepare for the possibility of relapse and hence reduce relapse risk by (1) identifying and managing individual high-risk relapse factors, (2) identifying and managing early warning signs of relapse, (3) intervening early should a lapse or relapse actually occur, and (4) making broader changes in order to achieve a more balanced lifestyle so that alcohol is not desired.

- *Identifying and managing high-risk situations:* negative emotional states such as anxiety, anger, boredom, emptiness, depression, guilt, shame and loneliness are the most common factors contributing to relapse. Interpersonal situations such as direct or indirect social pressures to drink alcohol or conflicts with another person are the second and third most common precipitants of relapse. The caregiver can help the patient reduce relapse risk by first examining which emotions or interpersonal situations are perceived to be high-risk for relapse. Then, specific strategies can be taught related to these high-risk situations. Strategies should be adapted based on the unique features of the high-risk situation for the patient. For example, anger problems with one alcoholic patient may require helping this individual learn to accept and express anger appropriately. Anger problems with another patient may require helping this individual to control anger and rage, and not express it in interpersonal encounters. Boredom for one individual may be a function of lacking interesting hobbies or activities whereas with another, boredom may represent a serious problem in a job in which this person feels underused, underemployed, and not challenged.

- *Identifying and managing relapse warning signs:* obvious and subtle warning signs often show prior to an alcohol relapse. These signs show in changes in attitudes, thoughts, feelings, and behaviors. For example, a patient's lower motivation may show in an increase in negative attitudes toward recovery or A.A, which may eventually lead to relapse. Or, a patient may reduce or stop attending alcoholism treatment and/or A.A meetings without first discussing this with someone knowledgeable about his or her situation such as a therapist or A.A sponsor. Another common warning sign is putting oneself in high-risk situations such as socializing with old drinking partners. A patient may not be consciously aware of "a relapse set-up" in this example. Patients can be taught common relapse warning signs and ways to manage these. Patients who have had previous relapse experiences can complete a microanalysis of these experiences in order to become aware of the warning signs that were ignored. Hence, they can learn from past mistakes. Family members can play a helpful role by pointing out warning signs they have observed in the past preceding relapse, and by agreeing to let the addict know if they see any current potential relapse warning signs. The following shows a visual representation of the "road to relapse."

- *Managing lapses and relapses:* patients need to prepare to intervene early in the process in order to prevent a lapse from becoming a relapse, or stopping a relapse before it gets out of hand. At the fork in the road in the previous figure, the patient's initial emotional and cognitive response to a lapse largely determines whether there is a return to recovery or movement further down the road to a full-blown relapse. Patients may feel angry, depressed, guilty or shameful following a lapse or relapse. They may think *I'm a failure, I'm incapable of changing, I just can't do it, or why even bother trying* that can fuel the relapse further. Teaching patients to challenge such negative thoughts and rehearsing a plan to interrupt a lapse or relapse ahead of time can prepare patients to take action rather than passively accept that there is nothing they can do.
- *Lifestyle balance:* in addition to specific RP strategies to manage high-risk situations, patients can benefit from

broader strategies that reduce stress, improve coping ability, or improve health. These include exercise, meditation, focusing on spirituality, or focusing on achieving a better balance between "obligations" in life (shoulds) and "desires" (wants).

■ FAMILY ISSUES

Substance use disorders often have an adverse effect on the family system as well as individual members (Daley & Miller, 1993). Families can be helped in a number of ways:

- Involving them in assessment and ongoing treatment
- Addressing their questions and concerns
- Addressing family burden (e.g., anger, anxiety, worry, etc.)
- Providing education on substance use disorders, recovery, and various treatments available for patients and family members
- Eliciting the family's support for the patient to improve adherence to treatment and involvement in recovery
- Reducing family enabling behaviors
- Preparing the family for potential setbacks (lapses or relapses)
- Linking the family with needed resources
- Involving the family in ongoing sessions to address specific problems
- Encouraging participation in self-help programs (Al-anon, Nar-anon, etc.).

■ AFTERCARE AND MEASURING OUTCOME

Patients with substance use disorders typically are referred to aftercare following completion of a professional treatment program. Aftercare for patients completing a residential or day rehabilitation program may include outpatient counselor as well as ongoing self-help meetings. Aftercare for patients completing outpatient treatment usually involves self-help program participation.

Outcome of substance abuse can be measured by

- Reduction of substance use
- Reduction of negative consequences associated with substance abuse
- Improvement or resolution of specific problems
- Improvement in functioning
- Increased adherence to professional treatment or self-help program attendance.

REFERENCES

Alcoholics Anonymous (1976). *Big book*. New York, NY: A.A. World Services, Inc.

American Psychiatric Association (APA) (1994). *Diagnostic and statistical manual of mental disorders* (4th ed.). Washington, DC: APA.

Beck, A. T., Wright, F. D., Newman, C. F., & Liese, B. S. (1993). *Cognitive therapy of substance abuse*. New York, NY: Guilford Press.

Bien, T. H., Miller, W. R., & Toniga, J. S. (1993). Brief interventions for alcohol problems: A review. *Addiction, 88*, 315–336.

Ciraulo, D. A., Barnhill, J. G., & Jaffe, J. H. (1988). Clinical pharmacokinetics of imipramine and desipramine in alcoholics and normal volunteers. *Clinical Pharmacology and Therapeutics, 43*, 509–518.

Daley, D. C., & Marlatt, G. A. (1997a). *Managing your drug or alcohol problem—Client workbook*. San Antonio, TX: Psychological Corporation.

Daley, D. C., & Marlatt, G. A. (1997b). *Managing your drug or alcohol problem—Therapist's guide*. San Antonio, TX: Psychological Corporation.

Daley, D. C., & Marlatt, G. A. (1997c). Relapse prevention. In: J. H. Lowinson, P. Ruiz, R. B. Millman, & J. G. Langrod (Eds.), *Substance abuse: A comprehensive textbook* (3rd ed., pp. 458–466). Baltimore, MD: Williams & Wilkins.

Daley, D. C., Mercer, D., & Carpenter, G. (1998). *Group drug counseling manual*. Holmes Beach, FL: Learning Publications, Inc.

Daley, D. C., & Miller, J. (1993). *Taking control: A practical family guide to dealing with chemical dependency.* Holmes Beach, FL: Learning Publications.

Daley, D. C., Moss, H. B., & Campbell, F. (1993). *Dual disorders: Counseling clients with chemical dependency and mental illness* (2nd ed.). Center City, MN: Hazelden.

Daley, D. C., Salloum, I. M., Zuckoff, A., Kirisci, L., & Thase, M. (1998). Increasing treatment compliance among outpatients with depression and cocaine dependence: Results of a pilot study. *American Journal of Psychiatry, 155*(11), 1611–1613.

Daley, D. C., & Thase, M. E. (2000). *Dual disorders recovery counseling: Integrated treatment for substance use and mental health disorders* (2nd ed.). Independence, MO: Independence Press.

DeLeon, G. (1999). The therapeutic community treatment model. In: B. S. McCrady & E. E. Epstein (Eds.), *Addictions: A comprehensive guidebook* (pp. 306–307). London: Oxford University Press.

First, M. B., Spitzer, R. L., Gibbon, M., & Williams, J. B. (1994). *Structured clinical interview for DSM-IV, Axis I disorders.* New York, NY: New York State Psychiatric Institute.

Gossop, M. (1990). The development of a Short Opiate Withdrawal Scale (SOWS). *Addictive Behaviors, 15,* 487–490.

Handelsman, L., Cochrane, K. J., Aronson, M. J., Ness, R., Rubinstein, K. J., & Kanof, P. D. (1987). Two new rating scales for opiate withdrawal. *American Journal of Drug and Alcohol Abuse, 13*(3), 293–308.

Hasin, D. S., Trautman, K. D., Miele, G. M., Samet, S., Smith, M., & Endicott, J. (1996). *Psychiatric Research Interview for Substance and Mental Disorders (PRISM).*

Higgins, S. T., & Silverman, K. (Eds.) (1999). *Motivating behavior change among illicit drug abusers: Research on contingency management.* Washington, DC: American Psychological Association.

Karper, L. P., & Krystal, J. H. (1997). Pharmacotherapy of violent behavior. In: D. M. Stoff, J. Breiling, & J. D. Maser (Eds.), *Handbook of antisocial behavior* (pp. 436–444). New York, NY: John Wiley & Sons.

Litten, R. Z., Allen, J., & Fertig, J. (1996). Pharmacotherapies for alcohol problems: a review of research with focus on developments since 1991. *Alcoholism: Clinical and Experimental Research, 20,* 859–876.

Marlatt, G. A., & Gordon, J. R. (Eds.) (1984). *Relapse prevention: Maintenance strategies in the treatment of addictive behaviors.* New York, NY: Guilford Press.

Mayfield, D., McLeod, G., & Hall, P. (1974). The CAGE questionnaire: validation of a new alcoholism screening instrument. *American Journal of Psychiatry, 131*, 1121–1123.

McCrady, B. S., & Epstein, E. E. (Eds.) (1999). *Addictions: A comprehensive guidebook*. London: Oxford University Press.

McLellan, A. T., Luborsky, L., Woody, G. E., & O'Brien, C. P. (1980). An improved diagnostic evaluation instrument for substance abuse patients. The addiction severity index. *Journal of Nervous and Mental Disease, 168*, 26–33.

Meyers, R. J., & Smith, J. E. (1995). *Clinical guide to alcohol treatment: The community reinforcement approach*. New York, NY: Guilford Press.

Miller, W. R., & Rollnick, S. (1991). *Motivational interviewing: Preparing people to change addictive behavior*. New York, NY: Guilford Press.

Miller, W. R., Tonigan, J. S., & Longabaugh, R. (1995). *The Drinker Inventory of Consequences (DrinC): An instrument for assessing adverse consequences of alcohol abuse. Test Manual*. NIAAA Project MATCH Monograph Series, Vol. 4. NIH Pub. No. 95–3911. Washington, DC: U.S. Government Printing Office.

Monti, P. M., Abrams, D. B., Kadden, R. M., & Cooney, N. L. (1989). *Treatment of alcohol dependence*. New York: NY: Guilford Press.

Montrose, K., & Daley, D. C. (1995). *Celebrating small victories: A primer of approaches and attitudes for helping clients with dual disorders*. Center City, MN: Hazelden.

Narcotics Anonymous (1988). *Basic text*. Van Nuys, CA: World Service Office, Inc.

National Institute on Alcohol Abuse and Alcoholism (NIAAA) (1995a). Project Match Series, Volume 1: *Twelve step facilitation therapy manual*. Rockville, MD: U.S. Department of Health and Human Services.

National Institute on Alcohol Abuse and Alcoholism (NIAAA) (1995b). Project Match Series, Volume 2: *Motivational enhancement therapy manual*. Rockville, MD: U.S. Department of Health and Human Services.

National Institute on Alcohol Abuse and Alcoholism (NIAAA) (1995c). Project Match Series, Volume 3: *Cognitive-behavioral coping skills therapy manual*. Rockville, MD: U.S. Department of Health and Human Services.

National Institute on Alcohol Abuse and Alcoholism (NIAA) (1997). *Alcohol and health: Ninth special report to the U.S. Congress.* Rockville, MD: U.S. Department of Health and Human Services.

National Institute on Drug Abuse (NIDA) (1993). *Cue extinction.* Rockville, MD: U.S. Department of Health and Human Services.

National Institute on Drug Abuse (NIDA) (1998a). Therapy manuals for drug addiction, Manual 1: *A cognitive behavioral approach: Treating cocaine addiction.* Rockville, MD: U.S. Department of Health and Human Services.

National Institute on Drug Abuse (NIDA) (1998b) Therapy manuals for drug addiction, Manual 2: *A community reinforcement plus vouchers approach: Treating cocaine addiction.* Rockville, MD: U.S. Department of Health and Human Services.

National Institute on Drug Abuse (1999a). *Principles of drug addiction treatment: A research-based guide.* Rockville, MD: U.S. Department of Health and Human Services.

National Institute on Drug Abuse (NIDA) (1999b) Therapy manuals for drug addiction, Manual 3: *An individual drug counseling approach to treat cocaine addiction: The collaborative cocaine treatment study model.* Rockville, MD: U.S. Department of Health and Human Services.

National Institute on Drug Abuse (NIDA) (2001). Therapy manuals for drug addiction, Manual 4: *A group drug counseling approach to treat cocaine addiction: The collaborative cocaine treatment study model.* Rockville, MD: U.S. Department of Health and Human Services.

O'Connell, D. F. (in press). *Managing the dually diagnosed patient: Current issues and clinical approaches* (2nd ed.). New York, NY: Haworth Press.

O'Farrell, T. J., & Fals-Stewart, W. (1999). Treatment models and methods: Family models. In: B. S. McCrady & E. E. Epstein (Eds.) *Addictions: A comprehensive guidebook* (pp. 287–305). London: Oxford University Press.

Ott, P. J., Tarter, R. E., & Ammerman, R. T. (Eds.) (1999). *Sourcebook on substance abuse: Etiology, epidemiology, assessment, and treatment.* Needham Heights, MA: Allyn & Bacon.

Prochaska, J. O., Norcross, J. C., & DiClemente, C. C. (1994). *Changing for good.* New York, NY: William Morrow.

Robins, L. N., & Regier, D. A. (Eds.) (1991). *Psychiatric disorders in America: The epidemiologic catchment area study.* New York, NY: The Free Press.

Saunders, J. B., Aasland, O. G., Babor, T. F., et al. (1993). Development of the alcohol use disorders identification test (AUDIT): WHO collaborative project on early detection of persons with harmful alcohol consumption. *Addiction, 88,* 791–804.

Selzer, M. L. (1971). The Michigan Alcoholism Screening Test: The quest for a new diagnostic instrument. *American Journal of Psychiatry, 127,* 1653–1658.

Skinner, H. A., & Allen, B. A. (1982). Alcohol dependence syndrome: measurement and validation. *Journal of Abnormal Psychology, 91,* 199–209.

Sobell, L. C., Sobell, M. B., Leo, G. I., & Cancilla, A. (1988). Reliability of a timeline method: Assessing normal drinkers' reports of recent drinking and a comparative evaluation across several populations. *British Journal of Addiction, 83,* 393–402.

Stockwell, T., Murphy, D., & Hodgson, R. (1983). The severity of alcohol dependence questionnaire: its use, reliability and validity. *British Journal of Addiction, 78,* 145–155.

Sullivan, J. T., Sykora, K., Schneiderman, J., Naranjo, C. A., & Sellers, E. M. (1989). Assessment of alcohol withdrawal: The revised clinical institute withdrawal assessment for alcohol scale (CIWA-Ar). *British Journal of Addiction, 84,* 1353–1357.

3

Chapter Three

Mood Disorders

Ihsan M. Salloum • Dennis C. Daley • Roger Haskett •
Tad Gorske

Introduction and Overview

Mood refers to a prolonged emotion that affects a person's thoughts,
judgement, behaviors, interpersonal relationships, and overall
functioning. Mood disorders refer to psychiatric illnesses characterized by a prominent disturbance of mood. These are divided into
two main categories: (1) depressive disorders in which depression
or sadness is the essential feature of the disorder; and (2) bipolar
disorders in which elation, depression or both are the essential features of the disorder. Each category includes a cluster of symptoms
in addition to the disturbance of mood. Bipolar disorders are distin-
guished from depressive disorders by the presence or history of a
manic, hypomanic or mixed episode, usually in addition to depressive episodes. In this chapter, we present an overview of clinical,
epidemiological, etiologic, diagnostic, prognostic, and treatment
issues of these categories of mood disorders.

Depressive disorders are among the most frequent psychiatric illnesses affecting all age groups. Depressed patients present
with a wide variety, range, and severity of clinical symptoms.
Depressive disorders are among the most successfully treated
psychiatric conditions with increasing availability of effective
treatment options. Bipolar disorders are less common, are recurrent conditions, and will generally require lifelong maintenance
pharmacological treatment. In addition to clear depressive,

manic or hypomanic episodes, patients with bipolar disorders often experience transitional and rapidly fluctuating changes in their mental state which, if inadequately treated, are very disruptive and sometimes life threatening.

While clinical depression has been recognized since antiquity, the current concept of manic-depressive illness was established by Emil Kraepelin at the beginning of the 20th century. The subsequent distinction between unipolar and bipolar disorders proved to be useful for both clinicians and researchers, but did not adequately address the wide range of depressive disorders included in the unipolar category. Many attempts at classifying the different types of depression have been advanced recently. For an extensive discussion of the evolution of the nomenclature and classification of depressive disorder the reader is referred to several authoritative reviews on the topic (Akiskal & Cassano, 1997; Kocsis & Klein, 1995; Paykel, 1998). Table 3-1 lists the *Diagnostic and Statistical Manual of Mental Disorders* edition classification of mood disorders (APA, 1994).

■ DEPRESSIVE DISORDERS

The core features of depressive disorders are sustained feelings of despondency, sadness, anhedonia, changes in sleep and appetite,

---

TABLE 3-1. DSM-IV MOOD DISORDERS

A. *Primary depressive disorders*
  1. Major depressive disorder
     Single episode
     Recurrent
  2. Dysthymic disorder
  3. Depressive disorder not otherwise specified

B. *Bipolar disorders*
  1. Bipolar I disorder
  2. Bipolar II disorder
  3. Cyclothymic disorder
  4. Bipolar disorder not otherwise specified

C. *Induced mood disorders*
  1. Due to a general medical condition
  2. Psychoactive substance-induced

---

and feelings of hopelessness that result in significant distress or changes in the individual's ability to function. Tables 3-2 and 3-3 list the essential features of the two primary depressive disorders, major depression and dysthymia. Depressive disorders tend to reoccur in almost two-thirds of the cases, and in a substantial minority, is a chronic and lifelong condition.

■ BIPOLAR DISORDERS

The defining feature of a bipolar disorder is a manic episode, which is a distinct period with abnormally and persistently elevated, expansive, or irritable mood. This may be accompanied by grandiosity and disinhibited behavior, increased activity and decreased need for sleep, pressured speech, flight of ideas, and distractibility. Table 3-4 lists the essential features for a manic episode that result in marked impairment in occupational functioning, social activities

TABLE 3-2. DSM-IV SYMPTOMS OF MAJOR DEPRESSION (FIVE OR MORE SYMPTOMS FOR 2+ WEEKS)

1. Depressed mood for 2 weeks
2. Markedly diminished interest or pleasure in all, or almost all, activities
3. Significant weight loss when not dieting or weight gain (e.g., a change of more than 5 percent of body weight in a month), or decrease or increase in appetite
4. Insomnia or hypersomnia
5. Psychomotor agitation or retardation
6. Fatigue or loss of energy
7. Feelings of worthlessness or excessive or inappropriate guilt (which may be delusional)
8. Diminished ability to think or concentrate, or indecisiveness
9. Recurrent thoughts of death, recurrent suicidal ideation without a specific plan, or a suicide attempt or a specific plan for committing suicide

TABLE 3-3. DSM-IV SYMPTOMS FOR DYSTHYMIC DISORDER

Depressed mood for at least 2 years.
Presence, while depressed, of two (or more) of the following
    Poor appetite or overeating
    Insomnia or hypersomnia
    Low energy or fatigue
    Low self-esteem
    Poor concentration or difficulty making decisions
    Feelings of hopelessness

TABLE 3-4. DSM-IV SYMPTOMS OF A MANIC EPISODE (THREE OR MORE SYMPTOMS FOR 1+ WEEKS)

1. Elevated, expansive or irritable mood for 1 week
2. Inflated self-esteem or grandiosity
3. Decreased need for sleep
4. More talkative or pressure to keep talking
5. Flight of ideas or racing thoughts
6. Distractibility
7. Increase in goal-directed activity or psychomotor agitation
8. Excessive involvement in pleasurable activities with high potential for painful consequences

or relationships, necessitate hospitalization to prevent harm to self or others, or are accompanied by psychotic features. Although hypomanic episodes have the same list of characteristic symptoms, they may be of shorter duration, minimum of 4 days, and while there needs to be an unequivocal change in functioning that is uncharacteristic and observable by others, they are not severe enough to cause marked impairment in functioning or require hospitalization. Hypomanic episodes are often difficult to distinguish from the normal range of behaviors when viewed at a single point in time and are most commonly diagnosed using a longitudinal perspective of the individual's illness. Mixed episodes are characterized by at least one week in which the individual meets criteria for both a manic episode and a depressive episode every day.

Prevalence and Public Health Significance of Mood Disorders

Large community surveys show high rates of lifetime major depression for both men and women. The frequency of depression for women is almost double than that of men. Women have a lifetime risk that ranges from 10 to 25 percent, and men from 5 to 10 percent. It is estimated that at any one time, 5–9 percent of women and 2–3 percent of men have a current major depressive disorder. These rates appear to be unrelated to marital status, ethnic background, income, or educational attainment. The lifetime rate of dysthymic disorder is about 8 percent for women and 5 percent for men. The current rate of dysthymic disorder in the general population is 3 percent. Current epidemiological trends indicate that the rate of new cases of depression has been increasing throughout this century.

The lifetime prevalence of bipolar disorder is at least 1.2 percent and appears to be equally common in men and women. There are no clear differences in the frequency of the disorder across culture, marital status, or racial or socioeconomic group. While many individuals with bipolar disorder achieve a full remission between episodes of mania or depression, with return to optimal functioning, up to one-third of patients will have chronic symptoms and social impairment. This is particularly likely in patients with comorbid illness, rapid cycling of episodes, and those patients who are either noncompliant or not receiving adequate prophylactic treatment.

Mood disorders represent a major public health concern due to their high prevalence, the personal suffering experienced by affected individuals, the adverse impact on the family, and the adverse effects on society. Despite the high frequency of mood disorders, they are still unrecognized and most cases go untreated.

Both depressive and bipolar disorders often carry a high level of disability and severe complications such as suicide. The lifetime risk for suicide among major depressive disorder patients is 15 percent, which is among the highest of any other psychiatric illness. Moreover, in a considerable number of patients, high levels of residual symptoms may persist despite adequate treatment, and in many cases depression may become chronic (Angst, 1997). Suicide attempts and suicide are of comparable frequency among individuals with bipolar disorders.

Etiology

Mood disorders are believed to be a heterogeneous group of disorders that have multiple etiologies. Theories of the etiology of mood disorders have evolved throughout this century, with shifting emphasis from psychological to genetic and biomedical factors. Current theories of etiology focus on the relative contribution of these factors to the manifestation and expression of mood disorders. Table 3-5 lists the most frequently discussed etiologically important genetic, biochemical, psychological and environmental factors of mood disorders.

■ GENETIC FACTORS

The role of genetic factors in the etiology of depressive disorders has been highlighted using several study designs. These include familial pedigree studies, twin studies (comparing monozygotic or identical to dizygotic or fraternal twins), adoption studies, linkage studies, and general population studies. These studies have all underscored the importance of genetic factors in the etiology of depression. For example, first-degree relatives of patients with recurrent depression have 2–3 times the risk of developing depression than the general population. Monozygotic twins, whether reared together or apart, have similar concordance rates of developing depressive disorders, which is higher than dizygotic twins (41 percent versus 13 per-

---

TABLE 3-5. ETIOLOGY OF MOOD DISORDERS

A. *Genetic factors*
1. Familial pedigree studies
2. Twin studies
3. Adoption studies

B. *Biochemical factors*
1. Biogenic amines hypothesis
2. Neuroendocrine regulation abnormalities
3. Neurophysiological abnormalities

C. *Psychological and environmental factors*
1. Psychoanalytic constructs
2. Cognitive model and learned helplessness
3. Reinforcement and depression
4. Temperament
5. Life events-loss

---

cent). Biological parents of adopted-out children have a greater prevalence of depressive disorder than adopting parents. Also, adopted-away children of parents with mood disorders are more likely than adopted-away children of normal controls to develop a mood disorder.

■ BIOCHEMICAL FACTORS

The biogenic amines hypothesis points to dysfunction in the mono-amine neurotransmitter system. Neurotransmitters are chemical messengers that regulate the transmissions of impulses between nerve cells. Four major neurotransmitters have been implicated in the pathophysiology of depression. These include norepine-phrine, serotonin (5-hydroxytryptamine), acetylcholine–adrener-gic balance, and dopamine. Both deficiencies in norepinephrine and serotonin, as well as changes in receptor sensitivity and num-ber appear to be involved in the mechanisms underlying major depressive disorders.

Other pathophysiological changes including a host of patho-physiological abnormalities are present in major depression. These include neuroendocrine abnormalities such as increased secretion of cortisol, alterations in the pituitary-adrenal axis, ele-vation in serum thyroid hormones (triiodothyronine and thyrox-ine), and blunting of the response of thyroid-stimulating hormone to thyrotropin-releasing hormone. Neurophysiological abnormal-ities such as sleep dysregulation have been consistently demon-strated in major depression. These include decreased total sleep, shortening the period from sleep onset to the first rapid eye move-ment (REM) sleep, and increased the ratio of REM activity to REM time (REM density), and decreased stage-4 delta sleep. These abnormalities have been found to predict response to antidepres-sant medications.

■ PSYCHOLOGICAL AND ENVIRONMENTAL FACTORS

Early psychoanalytic constructs including Freud's concept of aggression turned-inward, later object loss, such as traumatic separation from a significant object of attachment, and depression as collapse of self-esteem have been advanced as causes of depression. The role of temperamental traits, negative cognitive schemata, "learned helplessness," life events and environmental stress, especially loss, have all been implicated as causative or contributing factors in precipitating depressive disorders.

Clinical Presentation of Mood Disorders

Patients with depressive disorders present with a variety of signs and symptoms in a broad range of clinical situations which may be challenging for the clinician to recognize. The most frequent reported symptoms include persistent sad mood, characterized by feeling sad, blue, and hopeless. Other symptoms include changes in the patients' demeanor such as stooped posture, sad or blunted facial expression, neglect of grooming and self-care, and general slowness in motor behavior, speech, and in thought processes manifested as delayed reaction time, delayed response to questions, and poverty of speech content. Furthermore, anhedonia, or lack of ability to enjoy previously pleasurable activities, fatigue, lethargy, feelings of exhaustion, and reductions in overall activities are also prominent, which may result in withdrawal from social activities and significant isolation. Other very frequent signs and symptoms include decreased or increased appetite with weight loss or gain, difficulty initiating and maintaining sleep, early morning awakening or hypersomnia, and loss of interest in most activities, including sexual interest. Depressed patients may have excessive guilt, with constant rumination and self-reproach. They frequently have difficulty concentrating, in addition to generalized bodily complaints. About 60–70 percent of patients with major depression also have anxiety symptoms, and some experience severe agitation. Low self-esteem, feeling of helplessness, pessimism and hopelessness, suicidal thoughts and intent are also characteristics of acute major depressive episode. A severe depressive episode may manifest with "depressive stupor," characterized by severe psychomotor retardation, mutism, and inactivity, a state which may be confused with catatonic syndrome. Furthermore, guilt and self-reproach may assume delusional proportions, as also disturbances in reality testing with frank nihilistic delusions and mood congruent hallucinations.

Patients with hypomania are usually euphoric, self-confident, and expansive, the latter appearing as increased enthusiasm for a range of interactions and plans. Interspersed with this positive state however, patients may demonstrate increased emotional lability and irritability. Speech is often rapid and loud, with clear evidence of humor in the patient's use of words and phrases. Perhaps the most characteristic and specific feature is the decreased need for sleep, associated with increased energy and absence of fatigue, which often leads to increased productivity. Patients in a manic episode demonstrate similar moods to hypomania, although anger and lability are likely to be more apparent, especially when the individual is opposed or set limits. More noticeable, however, are the changes in cognition and psychomotor function. The individual's self-confidence increases to the point of grandiosity, which may be delusional, thoughts are rapid, often disjointed and the ability to focus on a single thought or theme is lost. Speech is pressured, difficult to interrupt, and may become disorganized or incoherent. Behavioral change is characterized by increased goal-directed activity in social, interpersonal, or financial situations with a high potential for damaging consequences. Anger may result in explicit threats or physical violence. Abuse of alcohol and other drugs is common and consistent with the individual's apparent inability to anticipate the painful consequences of their behavior. Severe or repeated manic episodes may result in financial ruin, legal difficulties, social disgrace, and loss of employment, professional certification, and major interpersonal relationships. These outcomes are catastrophic not only for the individual, but also result in serious hardship for their family members.

Diagnosis

The DSM-IV diagnostic system requires that 5 or more out of 9 criteria be present for a period of 2 weeks, and in the absence of any other cause that may account for the major depressive episode (Table 3-2). This is further specified for severity, predominant clinical features, and longitudinal course.

The diagnosis of major depressive disorder is made in the presence of one or more episodes of major depression that is not due to other causes such as substance use disorders, medications, or medical disorders, and in the absence of a history of mania or hypomania. Major depressive episode is single, or recurrent if there has been a period of two consecutive months with either complete or partial remission of symptoms. The severity of the depressive disorder is further documented as mild, moderate, and severe, with or without psychotic features, and in partial or full remission. In addition to the severity ratings of the depressive episode, the DSM-IV also allows for further specification of the depressive episode according to the predominance of the presenting features. These include chronic, with catatonic features, with melancholic features, with atypical features, and with postpartum onset. The longitudinal course of the disorder is also specified as with or without full interepisode recovery and with seasonal pattern (Tables 3-6 and 3-7 display specifiers used in DSM-IV).

Assessment

A primary task in the assessment of major depressive disorder is to formulate the diagnosis and develop an individualized treatment plan, including the type and intensity of services needed. Several factors may interfere with the recognition of major depression. First, most common major depressive symptoms are also within the range of normal emotional experiences; therefore, recognition of the pathological nature of the mood states may be difficult.

TABLE 3-6. DSM-IV SPECIFIERS FOR CURRENT OR MOST RECENT EPISODE OF MAJOR DEPRESSIVE DISORDER

Coded specifiers	
Severity	
Mild	Meet diagnosis; minor impairment
Moderate	
Severe without psychotic features	Symptoms exceeds diagnosis; markedly impaired
Severe with psychotic features	Presence of mood congruent or mood incongruent delusions or hallucinations
In partial remission	Symptomatic but does not criteria
In full remission	No symptoms during past 2 months
Non-coded specifiers	
Chronic	Two years of full criteria present
With catatonic features	See Table 3-7
With melancholic features	See Table 3-7
With atypical features	See Table 3-7
With postpartum onset	Within 4 weeks postpartum
Longitudinal course specifiers	
With interepisode recovery	Full remission between the two most recent episodes
Without interepisode recovery	Persistent symptoms between the two most recent episodes
With seasonal pattern	See Table 3-7

Pathological mood states are characterized by an increase in duration, intensity, pervasiveness, and persistence of depressed mood, resulting in distress and disability. Second, depressive symptoms may vary according to the cultural background of the patient. Cultural context influences symptom presentation, expression of distress, and subjective experiences and explanation of the pathological mood state. In some cultures somatic complaints may be the predominant symptoms as opposed to feeling of sadness. Thus, attention to the cultural background of the patient is a key factor in accurately recognizing major depression among these patients. Furthermore, major depressive disorder, as one the most common psychiatric disorders, may co-exist with multiple other disorders. Many of the comorbid conditions change the manifestations of the depressive disorder with symptoms that overlap, mimic, mask, or exacerbate the depressive symptoms.

Dysthymic disorder may be even more problematic than a major depressive disorder in terms of its differentiation from nor-

TABLE 3-7. DSM-IV CURRENT OR MOST RECENT EPISODE OF MAJOR DEPRESSIVE DISORDER FEATURE SUBTYPES

Catatonic features are characterized by specific motor behavior including the following symptoms:
1. Extreme hypoactivity manifested as catalepsy or stupor
2. Extreme, purposeless, hyperactivity, not influenced by external stimuli.
3. Extreme negativism or mutism
4. Posturing (inappropriate or bizarre postures), stereotyped movements, prominent mannerisms, or prominent grimacing
5. Echolalia or echopraxia

Melancholic features are characterized by the following symptoms:
1. Loss of pleasure
2. Lack of reactivity to pleasurable stimuli
3. Distinct quality of depressed mood
4. Depression regularly worse in the morning
5. Early morning awakening
6. Marked psychomotor retardation or agitation
7. Significant anorexia or weight loss
8. Excessive or inappropriate guilt

Atypical features include the following symptoms:
1. Reactive mood
2. Significant weight gain or increase in appetite
3. Hypersomnia
4. Leaden paralysis
5. Pattern of interpersonal rejection sensitivity resulting in significant social or occupational impairment

Seasonal pattern is characterized by the following symptoms:
1. Regular temporal relationship between the onset of major depressive episodes and a particular time of the year
2. Full remissions also occur at a characteristic time of the year (e.g., depression disappears in the spring)
3. In the last 2 years, two major depressive episodes have occurred that demonstrate the temporal seasonal relationships described above, and no non-seasonal major depressive episodes have occurred during that same period

Lifetime seasonal major depressive episodes substantially outnumber the nonseasonal major depressive episodes

mal mood state, as symptoms are usually milder, yet have been present for a long period of time (over 2 years). Symptom onset, intensity and the resulting functional impairment become more ingrained in the patient's personality, blurring the boundaries between psychopathology and usual functioning.

Assessment of manic episodes is usually characterized by the patient's lack of cooperation. Loss of insight is common, even in individuals with only a moderate level of impairment and disturbance. Recognition of the inappropriateness of their behavior may be absent and efforts to provide treatment are often rejected. Access to another source of historical information, like a spouse or family member, is often crucial in obtaining relevant past history, as well as a clear description of recent changes. Characterization of the progress of symptoms from depression or hypomania to mania, as well as the change in severity of the disturbance over time, are often crucial to establishing the diagnosis. In patients who are grossly or psychotically disorganized, an account of the preceding symptoms or description of earlier episodes and remissions is often of great value in differentiating a manic episode with psychotic features from schizophrenia. Finally, considering the high comorbidity of alcohol and drug abuse with bipolar illness, and the adverse effect on response to treatment and outcome if not addressed, it is essential to obtain reliable information about the individual's drug and alcohol use, both during the current episode and during periods of remission.

Following are key elements of a comprehensive initial diagnostic assessment for patients with major mood disorder (Table 3-8).

Patient interview. While patients usually feel comfortable discussing their distress, they may be unaware of the significance of their symptoms or may minimize or deny their mood disorder. Therefore, the clinician's task is to elicit the pertinent depressive or manic symptoms, both current and past, including the predominant feature and its severity, as well as the degree of distress and impairment.

TABLE 3-8. DIAGNOSTIC ASSESSMENT OF MOOD DISORDER

Patient interview
Informant interview (significant others, referring agencies, other health provider)
Sign and symptoms of depression or bipolar disorder
Alcohol and drug use history (to rule out substance-induced disorder)
Mental status examination
Medical information review
Physical examination
Laboratory tests
History of current and past stress
Medical, occupational, social, legal problems, and family history
The use of screening instruments, rating scales, and structured clinical interviews

Informant or collateral interviews with family members, significant others, or health care professionals often provide additional pertinent information about the patient. Family and significant others can also play a positive role in the treatment process by influencing the patient to seek and adhere to treatment, and by providing support. Family and significant others, on the other hand, may sometimes minimize the significance of the depressive or hypomanic symptoms, believing that these symptoms are experienced as normal part of mood states.

A comprehensive medical history and physical examination are important to assess the presence of any general medical or neurological condition that may induce a major mood disorder (see Table 3-9). An individual presenting with a first manic episode after age 50 should be carefully evaluated for the presence of an identifiable etiology, such as a general medical condition, medication, or substance-induced disorder.

Laboratory tests may include drug and alcohol screening, urinalysis, complete blood count with differential, blood chemistry, serology, and liver and thyroid screens.

Assessment instruments provide a validated approach to the identification, diagnosis, and measure the severity of major depression and mania. These can also be used in treatment planning and in assessing outcome. Among the most widely used assessment instruments include the self-rated Beck Depression Inventory and the interviewer administered Hamilton Rating Scale for Depression. Both scales assess the presence and severity of depressive symptoms and help to monitor the

---

TABLE 3-9. GENERAL MEDICAL CONDITIONS INDUCING MOOD DISORDERS

Endocrine disorders (e.g., hypothyroidism, diabetes, Cushings disease)
Metabolic disorders (e.g., severe anemia, vitamin deficiencies)
Neurologic disorders (e.g., multiple sclerosis, dementia)
Infectious diseases (e.g., hepatitis, mononucleosis)
Connective tissue diseases (e.g., systemic lupus erythematosus)
Neoplastic disorders (e.g., pancreatic or CNS tumors)
Digestive disorders (e.g., hepatic and pancreatic diseases)
Substance use disorders (e.g., alcohol intoxication/withdrawal, stimulant withdrawal)
Certain medications and toxins (e.g., corticosteroids, propranolol, steroids, lead poisoning)

progress of depression during treatment. For assessment of mania, self-ratings are rarely useful and the common interviewer administered instruments are the Mania Rating Scale and the Bech–Rafaelsen Mania Scale. The Structured Clinical Interview for DSM-IV (SCID) provides reliable DSM- IV psychiatric diagnoses (First, Spitzer, Gibbon & Williams, 1994). This later instrument, however, is very time intensive, although primary care version of the SCID is now available.

Assessment of Suicidal Behavior

Major depressive and bipolar disorders are among the highest risks for suicide compared to other psychiatric diagnoses. An evaluation of suicidal behavior is an essential element of the evaluation of a mood disorder. Evaluation of suicidality should include the assessment of current suicidal ideation, plan, and intent, the circumstance, severity, and lethality of any suicidal gesture or attempt, the availability of suicide method, and the presence of risk factors for suicide. While suicide during a manic episode is rare, the risk during the depressive episode which commonly follows requires careful evaluation.

Differential Diagnosis

Depressive symptoms may occur in the context of a wide variety of general medical, neurological, and psychiatric conditions (see Table 3-10). In some instances of co-occurrence, the associated disorder appears to have an etiological role, e.g., endocrine disorders (hypothyroidism and Cushing's syndrome), and in substance-induced depressive syndromes. The course, severity, onset, and associated features and prior history are used to distinguish major depression from other conditions. For example, the severity and duration of the symptoms distinguish major

TABLE 3-10. GENERAL PROFILE OF MAJOR CLASSES OF ANTIDEPRESSANT MEDICATIONS

	Tricyclics[1]	MAO-I[2]	SSRI[3]	Other recent antidepressants[4]
Efficacy	High	High	High	High
Dosing convenience	Low to moderate	Low	High	Moderate to high
Side effects	High	High	Low	Low to moderate
Potential interaction	High	High/may be lethal	Low	Low to moderate
Lethality on overdose	Very high	Very high	Low	Low to moderate

[1] Tricyclics antidepressants: amytriptyline, Imipramine, desipramine, nortriptyline, doxepin, protriptyline, trimipramine, chlomipramine, maprotiline.
[2] Monoamine-oxidase inhibitors (MAO-I): phenelzine, tranylcypramine.
[3] Selective serotonin reuptake inhibitors: fluoxetine, sertraline, paroxatine, fluvoxamine, citalopram.
[4] Other recent antidepressants: venlafaxine, mirtazapine, buprpion, nefazodone.

depressive disorder from dysthymia, while the failure to spontaneously remit after 3–6 months differentiates a major depressive episode from grief reaction.

Comorbidity with Psychiatric and Substance Use Disorders

Mood disorders have a high frequency of comorbid psychiatric and substance use disorders (Kessler, McGonagle, Zhao et al., 1994; Salloum, Mezzich, Cornelius, Day, Daley & Kirisci, 1995; Daley, Salloum & Thase, in press). Usually, comorbid conditions have a negative impact on the course and prognosis of mood disorders and complicate their clinical presentation as well as response to treatment. For example, major depression is highly associated with anxiety disorders. Studies have shown that anxiety disorders significantly increase the risk for completed suicide among depressed patients. The likelihood of alcohol and substance use disorders among individuals with mood disorders is higher than that expected to occur by chance alone. The rate of substance abuse and dependence in patients with bipolar disorder is estimated to be as high as 60 percent (Robins & Regier, 1991; Goodwin & Jamison, 1990) although widely varying frequencies have been reported. In patients with bipolar disorder, alcohol and drug abuse are more common during manic than depressive episodes.

Patients with both mood and substance use disorders do poorly in treatment if both disorders are not addressed, preferably, within the framework of an integrated treatment approach (Daley & Thase, 2000). Comorbid substance use disorders are associated with treatment noncompliance and increase the likelihood of adverse legal situations during manic episodes (Daley & Zuckoff, 1999). The presence of a substance use disorder is a strong predictor of suicide in patients with mood disorders, particularly in males. Furthermore, a substantial minority of patients with mood disorders have comorbid personality disorders, high levels of social stressors, and impaired functioning.

Course and Outcome

The average age of onset of major depression is around 40 years old, although it may occur at any age. The onset and progression of the depressive episode may vary from a slow and gradual worsening of symptoms over a period of weeks to months, to an abrupt and rapid progression over a short period of time. The duration of the depressive episode varies from a few weeks to 8 months. An early age of onset, as well as an onset after the age of 60 years, is associated with higher frequency of recurrent depression. Depression is a chronic and relapsing illness for many patients (Frank, Kupfer, Perel et al., 1990; Maj, Veltro, Pirozzi, Lobrace & Magliano, 1992; Thase, 1999). It is estimated that around one-third have only a single episode, while two-thirds develop recurrent episodes, with an expected 5–6 episodes throughout the lifetime (Akiskal, 2000).

The median age of onset of bipolar disorder is in the early to mid-20s, although onset in adolescence is not uncommon. This disorder is almost universally recurrent but patients vary in the severity and duration of manic and depressive episodes. Variation over a patient's course of illness appears to be significantly less than variation between patients. In some individuals only the manic or the depressive episodes will be severe enough to produce marked impairment and require hospitalization. Males are more likely to have predominantly manic forms of bipolar disorder, while prominent depressive episodes are more common in females. Depressive episodes are usually of longer duration than manic episodes.

Maintenance treatment after remission of the acute episode is indicated for a significant percentage of patients with major depressive disorder as it considerably reduces the risk of future episodes (Frank et al., 1990; Kupfer, Frank, Perel et al., 1992). The relapse rate within one year after discontinuation of antidepressant medication is above 50 percent, and nearly three-quarters of the patients relapse by the second year. The relapse rate reaches 85 percent by the third year of medication discontinuation. Maintenance antidepressant treatment is recommended for patients who have had two recent episodes (within the past 5 years) or more than two lifetime episodes of depression (Kupfer, 1993). Maintenance treatment is indicated for the majority of patients with bipolar disorder.

Factors associated with increased risk of recurrent major depression include an early age of onset of the first depressive episode or a first depressive episode occurring after the age of 60, familial and genetic factors, comorbid anxiety disorders, substance abuse, and psychosis (Maj et al., 1992). The risk of recurrence is also associated with the presence of chronic and long-standing conditions such as dysthymic disorder, personality disorders, and depressive characterological traits, as well as early exposure to environmental stressors. Furthermore, the number of prior episodes correlates with shorter periods of remission with a potential acceleration of the course of illness.

Other strong predictors of recurrences include the persistence of subsyndromal depressive symptoms, and a history of two or more depressive episodes, or chronic mood symptoms. For example, in one study the presence of subsyndromal symptoms in recovered individuals shortened the "well time" threefold (68 versus 231 weeks). In another study, subjects with both two or more prior episodes and chronic mood symptoms were 3 times as likely to relapse. The recurrences of suicidal symptoms and severe psychosis in successive episodes also indicate poor prognosis.

Long-term antidepressant pharmacotherapy helps the patient to maintain a state of well-being and to prevent relapse. Chronic depression, recurrent depression, severe and protracted episodes of depression, double depression (major depression and dysthymia), and residual dysthymia are all indications for maintenance antidepressant therapy.

Over one-fifth of depressed patients develop a manic or hypomanic episode over time, that is, their diagnosis changes from a major depressive disorder to a bipolar disorder. Development of these episodes is associated with young age of onset of the major depressive episode (below 25 years), particularly with psychotic features, the use of antidepressant medications, and with postpartum depression.

Treatment of Mood Disorders

There are a number of psychological, pharmacotherapy and combined treatment approaches for mood disorders that have empirical support for their effectiveness (Basco & Rush, 1996; Nathan & Gorman, 1998; Kendall, Foster, Haaga, Lambert & Smith, 1998; Bergin & Garfield, 1994; Weissman, Markowitz & Klerman, 2000; Beck, 1995). Treatment of mood disorders can be viewed as occurring in phases according to the natural course of the illness. These phases include (Thase, 1999):

1. *Acute treatment* aimed at stabilizing the patient and ameliorating the acute symptoms of the episode of the mood disorder.
2. *Continuation treatment*, which follows symptom remission and continues until the untreated patient would be expected to recover spontaneously. This treatment is aimed at preventing relapse into either a depressive or manic episode.

3. *Maintenance treatment*, which follows a period of sustained recovery and is aimed at preventing recurrences of future episodes of mania and/or depression.

The goals of treatment for a depressive disorder are to attain remission of symptoms and associated disabilities, and to prevent relapse and recurrences of the depressive episodes. The acuity of the depressive symptoms, the presence of suicidal behavior, the degree of resulting disability, along with the availability of psychosocial support and resources, dictate the intensity of services required. For example, inpatient hospitalization may be used for an acutely suicidal patient as opposed to outpatient treatment for a moderately depressed patient who does not present any suicidal risk. The goals and principles of treatment for bipolar disorder are very similar to those described above, particularly for depressive episodes occurring during bipolar disorder. Bipolar disorder does however require additional emphasis on the importance of maintenance treatment and the long-term alliance between the clinician and the patient.

There are increasing options of effective treatments available for major depression. These include a number of antidepressants of equivalent efficacy, as well as several specific psychotherapeutic modalities with proven effectiveness for major depression. Although mild to moderately severe major depressive disorders respond to psychotherapy alone, pharmacotherapy is indicated for the treatment of moderate to severe forms. Combined antidepressant medication and psychotherapy may be required in more complicated subtypes of major depression. Other forms of treatment may be necessary in certain subtypes of depressive disorder. For example, electroconvulsive therapy (ECT) is the treatment of choice for persistent and severe mood disorders that resistant to medications. ECT involves the passage of a brief electrical current through the patient's brain in order to induce a seizure (Isenberg & Zorumski, 2000). Light therapy is indicated for seasonal affective disorder. Furthermore, pharmacotherapy is indicated as maintenance treatment to prevent recurrences of major depressive episodes.

Interpersonal and social rhythm therapy (IPSRT; Frank, Swartz & Kupfer, 2000) is an adjunct to pharmacotherapy that integrates behavioral, interpersonal, and psychoeducational approaches for the treatment of bipolar disorder. IPSRT involves educating the patient about bipolar disorder and the relationships between mood, life events, circadian, and sleep–wake rhythms. The patient is taught to record daily activities, and monitor and rate moods with a Social Rhythm Metric. IPSRT also involves helping the patient develop strategies to manage moods, stabilize daily rhythms, and resolve interpersonal problem areas that are potential triggers for social rhythm dysregulation. These include behavioral and self-management strategies to maintain circadian and sleep–wake cycle integrity, and resolving interpersonal problems. Grief issues (e.g., loss of healthy self or relationships), interpersonal role disputes or deficits, and role transitions may be addressed. The final, preventative phase involves continued work on maintaining regular social rhythms and dealing with interpersonal problems. Preliminary reports indicate that patients treated with IPSRT show greater stability in routine, decreased time to remission of symptoms, lower rates of recurrence, and decreased levels of symptomology.

Treatment adherence has a major impact on treatment response for both depression and bipolar disorders. Patients may deny, minimize, or have misconceptions regarding the severity of their disorders as well as the need for treatment, including medications. They may experience severe side effects or discontinue treatment following early signs of improvement. Patient education about the clinical features of major depression and mania, medication response, and side effects is essential in enhancing treatment adherence. Response to treatment should be monitored with a comprehensive assessment of the symptoms. In the treatment of depressive episodes, the use of rating scales such as the Beck Depression Inventory may also improve the clinical evaluation of residual depressive symptoms and the degree of remission.

Pharmacotherapy

All available antidepressant agents have comparable efficacy; however, they differ in their side effects profile, tolerability, dosing convenience, and potential interactions with other medications and safety profile (Table 3-10). A consideration in selecting an antidepressant medication is to attempt to match the pharmacological effects of the medication to prominent symptom clusters of the current depressive episode. For example, anxiety and sleep disturbances may be addressed by selecting a more sedating antidepressant agent, while anergia and lack of energy may benefit from activating agents. The SSRI and the other more recent classes of antidepressant agents have a more favorable safety and medication interaction profile than either the tricyclics or the MAO-I antidepressants. Some of the new agents, however, have problematic pharmacodynamic interactions due to their effects on the liver metabolism of other medication through the CYP450 enzyme system. Furthermore, with the frequent use of the SSRI class of medication, there is an increased likelihood of occurrence of a serotonergic syndrome. This syndrome is caused by a state of increased serotonin function—a sort of serotonin intoxication—and is manifested by symptoms of restlessness, anxiety, tremulousness, briks reflexes, changes and unstable vital signs among other symtpoms. This syndrome may require emergency medical treatment. Low lethality on overdose and ease of use has been an important factor in the popularity of the SSRI and other newer antidepressant medications.

The effective pharmacological treatment of patients with bipolar disorder involves the use of mood stabilizers. Other medications such as antipsychotics, hypnotics, and antianxiety agents are also useful in many patients during the treatment of bipolar disorder. Mood stabilizers are used for the acute treatment of manic, hypomanic, or mixed episodes, as well as for prophylaxis during the continuation and maintenance phases. Lithium remains the first choice for the acute treatment of mania and for prophylaxis in many patients. In recent years, anticonvulsants have been increasingly used in patients who either do not have an optimal response to lithium or who have unacceptable side effects. These include valproate, carbamazepine, gabapentin, lamotrigine and topiramate. Some anticonvulsants may be more effective than lithium in patients with mixed episodes or who are rapid cycling.

Patients with mania will usually respond more rapidly if a neuroleptic and benzodiazepine, such as lorazepam or clonazepam, are added to the mood stabilizer during the initial weeks of treatment. Use of the older "typical" neuroleptics is being replaced in many patients with the newer "atypical" neuroleptics, such as risperidone and olanzapine, due to the lower frequency of extrapyramidal side effects and tardive dyskinesia with the latter medications. Patients with bipolar disorder who become depressed raise some important clinical questions. While these patients are commonly treated with the same antidepressants given to patients with major depressive disorder, the risk that antidepressants will precipitate mania in bipolar I disorder, requires several important steps prior to starting antidepressant medication. It is essential to first evaluate the patient for poor compliance with mood stabilizer treatment, possible drug or alcohol abuse, and increase in psychosocial stressors. Antidepressants should only be started after the administration of adequate doses of mood stabilizer, since this will decrease the risk of precipitating mania. In addition, some patients with bipolar I disorder will have an antidepressant response to lithium or anticonvulsant treatment alone, which will remove the need for addition of antidepressants.

ECT has both antimanic and antidepressant properties. Unfortunately, the loss of insight in manic patients commonly is associated with refusal to consent to ECT and probably results in the less frequent use of this modality than the actual risk–benefit relationship would predict. In addition, while transient hypomania is common during a course of ECT, precipitation of mania does not appear to be a significant problem.

Optimizing pharmacological treatment and maintaining a therapeutic dose of a mood stabilizer or antidepressant, in addition to effective treatment of residual symptoms, are crucial to maintain remission and recovery from depressive and manic episodes and avoiding recurrences. The key to the successful treatment is a collaborative relationship between the clinician and patient. In many instances this relationship will be long standing and mutual respect and sharing of information become central. Patients should be encouraged to become experts about the course and features of their illness and to readily express concerns about their illness or its treatment. A major issue is medication compliance, as patients may question the role of the medication after a period of stability, sometimes leading to medication discontinuation. Apart from the increased risk of relapse or recurrence that this raises, there are more concerning reports that, following a period of discontinuation, some patients with bipolar disorder will not respond to agents that were previously effective. Management of side effects is a key aspect of maintaining optimal compliance in the long-term treatment of mood disorder. Patients must be fully informed of potential side effects prior to starting a medication and the clinician must be ready to address constructively, any unwelcome changes that appear during treatment.

Psychotherapy

Specific psychotherapies alone have been shown to be effective for mild to moderate forms of depression. However, psychotherapy is commonly indicated in conjunction with pharmacotherapy for a substantial number of patients with depressive and bipolar disorders. Combined psychotherapy with medication is indicated for those with underlying personality or characterological difficulties, for those who need to enhance their interpersonal effectiveness or for those with concomitant family or marital problems.

A number of effective specific psychotherapeutic approaches have been used in patients with depressive or bipolar disorder. Cognitive therapy, interpersonal psychotherapy, and behavior therapy are the most widely used and extensively studied therapies. The following sections will present these therapies in more detail. The last two sections will discuss family interventions and the outpatient treatment of suicidality.

■ COGNITIVE THERAPY (BECK, 1967)

Cognitive therapy was developed from a reformulation of depressive psychopathology. Previously, patients treated with psychoanalytic therapy were thought to have a masochistic need to suffer. Beck focused on a patient's tendency to view daily experiences in a globally negative way. By focusing on patients negative cognitive distortions of reality, he developed methods to help patients restructure their interpretations and therefore change their feelings about situations. As a result, patients significantly improved in alleviating depressive symptoms. Beck's work led to the development and refinement of cognitive therapy.

Cognitive therapy is an active, directive, and time-limited therapy that focuses on how patient's mentally structure their world. A basic assumption is that human perception is an active process that includes the influence of internal messages and the perception of external events. The way a person interprets reality can be understood by exploring and understanding their cognitions (thoughts and mental images). There are three concepts that represent a person's mental structure: the cognitive triad, cognitive schemas, and cognitive errors.

Cognitive triad: Three major cognitive patterns influence how humans perceive reality. The first is a *view of self*. In depression, a person has a negative view of self as flawed, defective, or inadequate. The second is a *view of daily experience*. A depressed person interprets daily situations as negative despite evidence of alternative explanations. The third is a *view of the future*. The depressed person anticipates that current suffering will continue indefinitely and expects failure in daily tasks. Signs and symptoms of depression can be explained through the cognitive triad.

Cognitive schemas: Schemas are stable cognitive patterns, developed from life experiences that function as a filter through which patients interpret daily events. Individuals categorize events through schemas in order to make sense of them. Depressed patient schemas have a negative bias, which is why they focus on negative details of a particular event.

Cognitive errors: Cognitive errors are specific ways of thinking that reflect the negative bias through which depressed patients process information. Cognitive errors reflect broad, global thought processes that are absolute, rigid, and negative. These are reflected in automatic negative thoughts (ANTs). ANTs are specific thoughts that are mood-dependent errors in information processing. Examples include "all or nothing thinking, over-generalization, and personalization."

A detailed description of the process of cognitive therapy is beyond the scope of this book. The following will present a summary of the therapy process based on Beck (1995). The primary goals of cognitive therapy are to alleviate depressive symptoms, increase mastery in management of daily problems, and increase self-confidence. This is accomplished by changing thinking errors based on the therapist's conceptualization of the cognitive triad and developing effective problem-solving skills. The therapist helps the patient identify negative cognitions and then test the reality of these cognitions through probing questions that try to determine how a patient came to believe their current interpretations of reality. This is accomplished by identifying negative mood states and the accompanying ANTs. The therapist and patient collaboratively evaluate the validity of ANTs and work to develop more realistic ways of perceiving reality. This can be accomplished through in-session dialogue and the use of homework where the patient systematically tests the validity of their cognitions in daily life.

A cognitive therapy session always begins with the setting of an agenda. The agenda includes a mood check, along with an objective assessment of depressive symptoms with the Beck Depression Inventory (BDI). There will be a review of the patient's presenting problem and progress toward goals previously developed for that problem. The therapist and patient collaboratively set goals for the session based on the patient's needs and description of the presenting problem. After a discussion of issues on the agenda there is a review of homework and the setting of new homework assignments. The session ends with a summary and feedback from both therapist and patient.

■ INTERPERSONAL PSYCHOTHERAPY (KLERMAN & WEISSMAN, 1993; WEISSMAN, MARKOWITZ & KLERMAN, 2000)

Interpersonal psychotherapy (IPT) emphasizes interpersonal and social factors in understanding and treating depression. IPT theory is derived from the works of Adolf Meyer, Harry Stack Sullivan, and Frieda Fromm-Reichmann, all of whom focused on the patient's relationships in their environment and social groups as related to psychopathology. IPT is a time-limited therapy that focuses on the patient's current life circumstances where the main goals are to alleviate depressive symptoms and improve interpersonal functioning. IPT is conducted by explicitly diagnosing and educating the patient about depression. Patient's must accept a "sick role," which means the patient admits to having a condition that requires professional help. Therapy continues by identifying the interpersonal context of depression and developing strategies to deal with these issues.

IPT does not make explicit assumptions regarding depressive etiology and acknowledges the multifaceted nature of depression, including biological, genetic, and psychological aspects. IPT conceptualizes depression as having three processes: (1) symptom formation; (2) social functioning; and (3) personality. Symptom formation includes the signs and symptoms of depression including depressive affect. Social functioning involves interpersonal interactions with significant others in the patient's social milieu. The way a patient interacts with others is learned from childhood and relies on the quality of attachment bonds and social learning experiences. Personality refers to an individual's unique traits and characteristics that determine how they interact with their environment. IPT focuses on symptom formation and social functioning. IPT works to alleviate symptoms by educating the patient on the disorder and ensuring that there is a good prognosis. Interpersonal difficulties are dealt with during the middle phase of treatment and generally cover four problem areas: (1) grief; (2) role disputes; (3) role transitions; and (4) interpersonal deficits. Specific techniques employed include an exploration of interpersonal areas, encouraging the patient to express affect, analysis of communication difficulties, and specific behavioral techniques. The therapeutic relationship is used as a model for other interpersonal relations.

■ BEHAVIORAL THERAPY (REHM, 1981)

Behavioral treatments are based on the application of classical conditioning theory from Pavlov, operant conditioning theory from Skinner, and social learning theory of Bandura. Behavioral treatments for depression began in the late 1960s, whereas previously, behavioral interventions focused on anxiety, the social behavior of institutionalized persons, and the behavior of children. Behavioral therapy has shown some positive effects in depression treatment, yet, in general, the results are inconclusive.

The etiology of depression is complex, from a behavioral standpoint. Predisposing factors for depression include deficits in adaptive learning. Patients have not learned adaptive behavioral skills to meet their needs and instead have learned that they are helpless actors within their environment (learned helplessness). Other factors include a lack of environmental reinforcers for adaptive behavior, modeling of depressive behavior by family or significant others, and biological/genetic variables. The lack of positive reinforcement for adaptive behaviors leads to depressive syndromes and the attribution of negative labels. Symptoms of the depressive syndrome are maintained through social reinforcement by significant others, the medical/psychiatric community, or through avoidance of situations that are unpleasant or difficult.

Treatment of depression with behavior therapy involves a functional analysis of contingencies that maintain the maladaptive behavior and then working toward overt behavior change. Behavioral therapy relies on many techniques to change behavior, including social problem solving, skills training, and contingency management.

Problem solving: A functional analysis of a current life problem is conducted, including the patient symptoms involved in the problem, coinciding impairments, and the antecedents and consequences of the behavior. Once this occurs, goals are set reflecting possible alternative behaviors to the situation at hand. Once alternatives are generated the possible advantages and disadvantages of the new behavior is discussed.

Skills training: Skills training involves teaching the patient personal and interpersonal skills in order to adaptively function in their environment. Examples include assertion training to counteract learned helplessness, interpersonal skills such as giving compliments or other adaptive verbal behavior, and learning effective communication skills to request help or ask for behavior change in others.

Contingency management: This technique can be used in therapy sessions and as a self-control technique. Contingencies are reinforcers for adaptive behavioral responses. Therapists can use reinforcing verbal behaviors (praise, attention) for adaptive behavior in session. Patients can be trained to use their own reinforcers in daily life to increase adaptive responses. An example would be a patient who is allowed to revert to an old behavior provided he performs a new undesirable behavior that is more adaptive.

The above techniques are only a sample of behavioral interventions. The main ingredients include a functional analysis of maladaptive behavior that maintains the depressive symptoms and that treatment focuses on overt behavior change in order to reduce symptoms and lead to more adaptive environmental responses.

■ ROLE OF THE FAMILY IN THE TREATMENT OF MOOD DISORDER

Family members are often markedly affected by a mood disorder in their relative and its consequences (Keitner, 1990; Rosen & Amador, 1996; Miklowitz & Goldstein, 1997; Jamison, 1999). Understanding the needs, strengths, and weaknesses of family members is crucial to the care of patients with major mood disorders. These stresses on relationships and individuals may result in additional suffering and treating clinicians should be sensitive to this and respond appropriately. Joint interventions with the patient and the family members or individual treatment for the relative may be indicated. Clinicians should also recognize the important contribution that family members can make to the treatment of patients with mood disorders. Their observations of changes in a patient's emotions and behaviors are important in the early recognition of relapse and in monitoring compliance.

Family members will be able to contribute most effectively to their relative's care if they are educated about the disorder and its treatments. A better understanding of the disorder will often increase acceptance of the patient's dysfunctional behaviors and decrease conflict. Recognition that mood disorders are treatable and that recovery is common increases hope. Support and education for patients and their families can be accessed through national and local support organizations such as the National Depressive and Manic-Depressive Association (NDMDA) and the National Alliance for the Mentally Ill (NAMI). These organizations provide excellent support groups, educational programs, newsletters, and referral information. Many patients and family members find it particularly helpful to share experiences and coping strategies with others dealing with similar situations. The contributions of these organizations supplement the efforts of the treatment teams and are becoming increasingly important in the quality of care provided to patients with severe mood disorders.

Issues of confidentiality of clinical information within families should be addressed explicitly early in treatment. The timing of this discussion may need to be coordinated with the course of the patient's illness. During manic episodes, patients may express more anger and lack of trust with family members than when their illness is in remission. Clinicians should discuss with patients the nature of information that they want to be shared with family and which specific individuals they would like to be involved. It is also important to help patients and relatives understand that clinicians need information to provide optimal care and that receiving reports from family members about a patient's behavior does not violate confidentiality.

In some families, the interaction between the patient and family may not only result in significant distress for the family members, but also interfere with the patient's response to treatment. Depression colors patient perceptions such that they frequently have negative views of their world and their relationships with significant others. As a result, their interpersonal behavior is often viewed negatively by others and elicits negative reactions. This creates a self-fulfilling prophecy that reinforces depressed patients' views. In families of depressed patients, this reciprocal process may lead to decompensation and relapse, further reinforcing the hopelessness that patients and family members often share. The interpersonal, behavioral, and financial consequences of a depressive episode may also lead to marital or family conflict or aggravate long-standing conflicts. Family members, who cope with the resulting crises using communication styles that increase interpersonal conflict within the family, may increase the likelihood of further decompensation by the patient. In these families, treatment that directly addresses family interactions and relationships may be indicated.

Family treatment seeks to support recovery by assisting family members to distinguish the features of a mood disorder from other negative behaviors by the patient, to understand the link between functional deficits produced by depression or mania and behavioral changes, and to emphasize responses that decrease symptoms and optimize patient functioning. This family approach to the management of a mood disorder assumes that multiple biologic, genetic, and psychologic factors play a role in the etiology of depression. Family influence is not seen as the cause of a depressive or manic episode and this is often an important message to family members who experience inappropriate guilt and feelings of responsibility for their relative's condition. In some circumstances, however, the interactive styles of family members can add to stressors acting on the patient and intensify symptoms of the mood disorder. Examples of such communication styles are high expressed emotion, judgmentalism, advice giving, and criticism. The primary goals of family treatment are to help increase understanding between the family and the patient regarding the mood disorder and to support and increase adaptive family interaction and communication styles that will support recovery. This can be accomplished in several ways: (1) providing education to the family on mood disorders, treatment, and the course of recovery; (2) instilling hope so that the family accepts the reality that mood disorders are treatable conditions, regardless of the severity of their loved one's illness; (3) decreasing stressful interactions between patient and family members (e.g., reducing critical comments or negative interactives); and (4) learning new skills to facilitate improved communication between family members and the patient.

■ TREATMENT OF SUICIDAL BEHAVIOR

This section will focus on the treatment of the suicidal patient in an outpatient setting and will provide only a brief overview of some of the principles of suicide assessment and treatment. Additional information on assessment and treatment of suicidality can be found in several publications (Chiles & Strosahl, 1995; Bongar et al., 1998; Jamison, 1999; Shea, 1999).

A patient who expresses suicidal ideation creates a great deal of anxiety for health professionals. Each year about 30,000 people die to suicides, so a complete assessment along with swift and appropriate intervention must be conducted to ensure safety.

Although a fail-proof prediction of suicide is not possible, high-risk factors include being a male over age 45, a history of alcohol dependence, a history of suicidal and/or violent behavior, and prior psychiatric hospitalizations. Warning signs that may indicate an increased risk of suicide include previous attempts, depression, availability of a method, verbalized suicide ideation, a recent life crisis, pervasive hopelessness, and a family history of suicide. Another high-risk indicator is when a patient exhibits behavior indicating plans for their death, such as making out a will or giving away possessions.

When treating a suicidal patient in crises, a clinician must check their own attitudes about the situation at hand. It is important not to judge, moralize, criticize, or make light of the situations or feelings leading to suicidal ideation. It is also important not to over-react with excessive anxiety. Most patients are looking for some-one who can be stable and confident that help is available. Suicidal thoughts should be elicited through straightforward ques-tioning. It is often best to view thoughts of suicide as a patient's method to confront a problem that they feel is inescapable, intoler-able, and will never end. The clinician's goal is to change the patient's perception that the problem is overwhelming and unsol-vable. This can be accomplished by instilling hope that problems can be resolved and painful feelings can be tolerated with help. The primary interventions can be categorized as follows:

1. Reduce psychological pain through modification of percep-tions or environment.
2. Enlist the aid of significant other that the patient trusts.
3. Build up a support system.
4. Offer alternatives to suicide.

Some specific principles of intervention include *validating* the pain that the patient is in while acknowledging that suicide is a *per-manent* solution to a temporary problem. Such a solution brings about more problems in the long run. Avoid *power struggles* about the patient's attitude toward problems and suicide as a solution. Instead take a *collaborative* approach by helping the patient to understand the problems and generate *alternative solutions*. Such solutions might include *skill training, stress management*, or *problem-solving* interventions. Finally, if the patient commits to a plan of action and is able to control suicidal impulses, a *crisis plan* can be developed should the patient decompensate. In such cases, the therapist may need to have 24-hour availability to facilitate safety management. If the patient cannot commit to a safety plan, is actively suicidal, and has other strong indicators of lethality as previously specified, inpatient hospitalization should be sought.

REFERENCES

Akiskal, H. S. (2000). Mood disorders. In: B. J. Sadock & V. A. Sadock (Eds.), *Comprehensive textbook of psychiatry* (7th ed., pp. 1284–1297). New York, NY: Lippincott Williams & Wilkins.

Akiskal, H. S., & Cassano, G. B. (Eds.) (1997). *Dysthymia and the spectrum of chronic depressions.* New York, NY: Guilford Press.

American Psychiatric Association (APA) (1994). *DSM-IV: Diagnostic and statistical manual of mental disorders* (4th ed.). Washington, DC: APA.

Angst, J. (1997). Fortnightly review. A regular review of the long-term follow up of depression. *BMJ, 315,* 1143–1146.

Basco, M. R., & Rush, A. J. (1996). *Cognitive-behavioral therapy for bipolar disorder.* New York, NY: Guilford Press.

Beck, A.T. (1967). *Cognitive therapy and the emotional disorders.* New York, NY: International Universities Press.

Beck, J. S. (1995). *Cognitive therapy: Basics and beyond.* New York, NY: Guilford Press.

Bergin, A. E., & Garfield S. L. (1994). *Handbook of psychotherapy and behavior change* (4th ed.). New York, NY: John Wiley & Sons.

Bongar, B. B., Berman, A. L., Maris, R. W., Silverman, M. M., Harris, E. A., & Packman, W. L. (1998). *Risk management with suicidal patients.* New York, NY: Guilford Press.

Chiles, J. A., & Strosahl, K. (1995). *The suicidal patient: Principles of assessment, treatment, and case management.* Washington, DC; American Psychiatric Press Inc.

Daley, D. C., Salloum, I. M., & Thase, M. E. (in press). Improving treatment adherence among patients with comorbid psychiatric and substance use disorders. In: D. F. O'Connell (Ed.), *Managing the dually diagnosed patient: Current issues and clinical approaches.* New York, NY: Haworth.

Daley, D. C., & Thase, M. E. (2000). *Dual disorders recovery counseling: Integrated treatment for substance use and mental health disorders* (2nd ed.). Independence, MO: Independence Press.

Daley, D. C., & Zuckoff, A. (1999). *Improving treatment compliance: Counseling and system strategies for substance use and dual disorders.* Center City, MN: Hazelden.

First, M. B., Spitzer, R. L., Gibbon, M., & Williams, J. B. (1994). *Structured clinical interview for DSM-IV–Axis I disorders.* New York, NY: New York State Psychiatric Institute.

Frank, E., Kupfer, D. J., Perel, J. M., et al. (1990). Three-year outcomes for maintenance therapies in recurrent depression. *Archives of General Psychiatry, 47*, 1093–1099.

Frank, E., Swartz, H. A., & Kupfer, D. J. (2000). Interpersonal and social rhythm therapy: Managing the chaos of bipolar disorder. *Biological Psychiatry, 48*, 593–604.

Goodwin, D., & Jamison, K. (1990). *Manic-depressive illness.* New York, NY: Oxford University Press.

Isenberg, K. E., & Zorumski, C. F. (2000). Electroconvulsive therapy. In: B. J. Sadock & V. A. Sadock (Eds.), *Comprehensive textbook of psychiatry* (7th ed., pp. 2503–2515). New York, NY: Lippincott Williams & Wilkins.

Jamison, K. R. (1999). *Night falls fast: Understanding suicide.* New York, NY: Alfred A. Knopf.

Keitner, G. I. (1990). *Depression and families: Impact and treatment.* Washington, DC: American Psychiatric Press.

Kendall, P. C., Foster, S. L., Haaga, D. A., Lambert, M. J., & Smith, T. W. (1998). Empirically supported psychological therapies. *Journal of Consulting and Clinical Psychology, 66(1)*, 1–216.

Kessler, R. C., McGonagle, K. A., Zhao, S., et al. (1994). Lifetime and 12-month prevalence of DSM-III-R psychiatric disorders in the United States. Results from the National Comorbidity Survey. *Archives of General Psychiatry, 51*, 8–19.

Klerman, G. L., & Weissman, M. M. (1993). *New applications of interpersonal psychotherapy.* Washington, DC: American Psychiatric Press.

Kocsis, J. H., & Klein, D. N. (Eds.) (1995). *Diagnosis and treatment of chronic depression.* New York, NY: Guilford Press.

Kupfer, D. J. (1993). Management of recurrent depression. *Journal of Clinical Psychiatry, 54* (Suppl. 29–33), 34–35.

Kupfer, D. J., Frank, E., Perel, J. M., et al. (1992). Five-year outcome for maintenance therapies in recurrent depression. *Archives of General Psychiatry, 49*, 769–773.

Maj, M., Veltro, F., Pirozzi, R., Lobrace, S., & Magliano, L. (1992). Pattern of recurrence of illness after recovery from an episode of major depression: a prospective study. *American Journal of Psychiatry, 149*, 795–800.

Miklowitz, D. J., & Goldstein, M. J. (1997). *Bipolar disorder: A family-focused treatment approach.* New York, NY: Guilford Press.

Nathan, P. E., & Gorman, J. M. (Eds.) (1998). *A guide to treatments that work*. New York, NY: Oxford University Press.

Paykel, E. S. (Ed.) (1998). *Handbook of affective disorders* (3rd ed.). New York, NY: Guilford Press.

Rehm, L. P. (1981). *Behavior therapy for depression: Present status and future directions*. New York, NY: Academic Press.

Robins, L. N., & Regier, D. A. (Eds.) (1991). *Psychiatric disorders in America: The epidemiologic catchment area study*. New York, NY: The Free Press.

Rosen, L. E., & Amador, X. F. (1996). *When someone you love is depressed*. New York, NY: The Free Press.

Salloum, I. M., Mezzich, J. E., Cornelius, J. R., Day, N. L., Daley, D., & Kirisci, L. (1995). Clinical profile of comorbid major depression and alcohol use disorders in an initial psychiatric evaluation. *Comprehensive Psychiatry, 36,* 260–266.

Shea, S. C. (1999). *The practical art of suicide assessment*. New York, NY: John Wiley & Sons.

Thase, M. E. (1999). Long-term nature of depression. *Journal of Clinical Psychiatry, 60*(Suppl. 14), 3–9.

Weissman, M. M., Markowitz, J. C., & Klerman, G. L. (2000). *Comprehensive guide to interpersonal psychotherapy*. New York, NY: Basic Books.

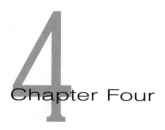

Chapter Four

The Anxiety Disorders

Mark Jones • Oommen Mammen

In this chapter we will discuss assessment and treatment of the anxiety disorders. The anxiety disorders are: generalized anxiety disorder, panic disorder and panic disorder with agoraphobia, obsessive–compulsive disorder, post-traumatic stress disorder, acute stress disorder, social phobia, and specific phobia.

Fear is the emotion that characterizes all of the anxiety disorders. Fear is not necessarily a bad emotion as it is a common human experience. One would be unprepared to deal optimally with life without fear. Fear is a signal of danger in the environment. It prepares a person to face the challenge and act to avoid perceived danger.

Anxiety can be adaptive as well as maladaptive. Without anxiety, one might not get to work on time, study hard for a test, or be "up for the game." However, excessive anxiety can be detrimental, causing severe distress, and impaired function. Avoidance may help reduce the distress of anxiety but will impair function by keeping the person from taking on tasks required for success. An example is someone with a teaching degree who avoids teaching because of a fear of talking in front of a group. She subsequently avoids the object of her fear, but feels frustrated at her inability to have the job she wants and is trained for.

Anxiety is experienced in three domains: cognitive, physical, and behavioral. In the cognitive realm, anxiety is experienced as worry or repetitive fearful catastrophic thoughts. Other cognitive manifestations are difficulty concentrating, trouble with recall, difficulty retaining new information, the mind going blank, and racing thoughts. Somatic, or physiological expression of anxiety, include restlessness, inability to relax, and feeling "keyed up." Anxiety can also be expressed in skin conditions such as hives, gastrointestinal difficulties such as diarrhea, excess stomach acid or "butterflies," muscular aches and tension, and headaches. People with anxiety disorders often encounter sleep disturbance. They may have trouble falling or staying asleep, or do not feel rested after sleeping through the night. Anxiety has been called "the great imitator," the mimic of many different physical problems. From ringing in the ears to blurred vision, anxiety can manifest in numerous ways often not associated with feeling nervous. Behavioral expressions of anxiety include movements such as repeatedly getting up and down, pacing, fidgeting, and tapping. Common defenses against feeling anxious are avoidance and escape. If the feared situation is either avoided through physically distancing from the object or situation or is experienced only briefly, the feeling of anxiety is diminished.

Assessment and intervention are necessary when anxiety symptoms occur frequently, cause significant levels of distress, or interfere with a person's quality of life or the ability to fulfill role responsibilities. When untreated, anxiety disorders usually do not improve and lead to loss of opportunities in interpersonal, social, and vocational realms.

Generalized Anxiety Disorder

■ DESCRIPTION

Generalized anxiety disorder (GAD) is a chronic condition comprised of daily symptoms of anxiety without a phobic focus that manifests with significant subjective distress and physiological symptoms. GAD is characterized by persistent feelings of tension, jitteriness, and being on edge. The person acts as if something terrible may happen at any minute. Feeling tense and jumpy, the GAD afflicted person has more trouble with normal activities than his peers, is sometimes hard to live with, but is usually not incapacitated (Goodwin, 1986). Researchers have questioned whether GAD is a separate disorder since its symptoms overlap with those of other anxiety disorders and depression (Barlow, Blanchard, Vermilyea, Vermilyea & Di Nardo, 1986). Generalized anxiety is a common symptom of major depression, but can exist independent of depressed mood. GAD is characterized by two or more areas of worry. Typical worries of GAD are: financial problems, relationships, health, the future, and work. Worries about these topics lead to frequent feelings of the primary symptom — apprehensive expectation. Individuals experience generalized anxiety according to both their transient states of mind and more stable individual anxiety trait variations. Those high in trait anxiety have more worries (Barlow, 1988). Other features of generalized anxiety include: inability to discontinue worry, frequent and intense worry, disruption of attention, and impairment with decisions. The reason for the worry changes as circumstances change (Rapee and Barlow, 1991).

■ DIAGNOSIS

The criteria for GAD, according to DSM-IV (APA, 1994) are as follows. *Excessive anxiety and worry about a number of events or activities occur more days than not for at least 6 months.* The 6-month requirement differentiates normal time-limited worries such as health or job security from the general anxiety syndrome which is a persistent worry with a single focus. *The person with GAD finds it difficult to control the worry.* Early diagnostic criteria differentiates the pathological nature of GAD from less severe presentations of worry where it is easier to switch off the emotion. *Anxiety and worry are associated with three (or more) of the following six symptoms (with at least some of the symptoms present for more days than not for the past six months): restlessness, feeling keyed up or on edge, fatigue, difficulty concentrating or mind going blank, irritability, muscle tension, and sleep disturbance.*

DSM-III-R's (APA, 1987) complete list of 18 symptoms of GAD was paired down to 6 in an attempt to capture what defines the disorder as separate from other anxiety presentations. The presence of multiple somatic symptoms continues to be common with GAD.

Also stipulated by DSM-IV (APA, 1994), the focus of anxiety cannot be the subject of another anxiety disorder (social anxiety, panic attacks, abandonment, or obsessional fears), eating disorder (anorexia, bulimia), or physical complaint (hypochondriasis or somatization). The persistent worry must be present for 6 months prior to the diagnosis of a mood disorder. GAD cannot be diagnosed as comorbid with a mood disorder given the symptom overlap and increased presence of anxiety within mood disorders, unless there is evidence for GAD pre-dating the mood disorder.

■ PREVALENCE

Prevalence of GAD is estimated to be approximately 3 percent. There is no clear genetic evidence for transmission of GAD, but the familial association of the trait of anxiety has been observed. Comorbid presentation of GAD with other anxiety, mood, and substance disorders is common. Onset is frequently reported in childhood but can occur later in life with the onset of adult responsibilities (parental, economic, and vocational) and exacerbated stress for persons in their 20s and 30s (APA, 1994).

■ TREATMENT

GAD can be treated and responds to treatment with cognitive behavioral therapy and certain medications. Cognitive behavioral therapy for GAD uses a reactive model for understanding anxiety. External circumstances of life do not trigger the feeling of anxiety, but rather the cognitions generated by the person. The patient is taught to observe thoughts preceding and sustaining anxious feelings and sensations. The person learns to identify cognitive distortions in anxiety-activating thoughts. They learn to analyze thoughts for evidence and facts as opposed to the distortions of emotional reasoning, catastrophizing, jumping to conclusions, and fortune telling (Burns, 1980).

Labeling the distortion and accepting that the thought is not rational is the first step to creating a more evidence-based perspective to decrease anxiety. The next step is to ask questions about the distorted thought in order to change a person's thinking. Questions might include, "How do I know for certain that. . ." and "Is there any other alternative way of looking at this that makes more sense?" This leads to formulation of rational thoughts replacing distorted ones. The patient records daily his/her distorted thoughts and rational counter thoughts.

A pattern of cognitions peculiar to GAD exists, in which the person thinks of himself/herself as vulnerable and threatened by life events, while also feeling unable to cope with adversity (Butler & Booth, in Rapee & Barlow, 1991). These thoughts are viewed as an hypothesis by the cognitive therapist. Patients are directed to monitor and record their worries daily. This helps them learn more about the situations that influence their worry and allows them to see their worries on paper. This encourages objective thought analysis. Here, the therapist directs the patient to think about his/her worries rather than trying to avoid or escape them. The patient is assigned a specific time period in which he/she is to focus on a particular worry instead of ruminating about the worries in a random, unstructured manner. The combination of thought countering and exposure changes the quality of the worry experience.

Relaxation exercises decrease physiological arousal and are assigned twice daily to create an alternative response to the anxiety. These exercises may be directed at the muscles as with systematic muscle relaxation, or breathing focused, with slow diaphragmatic breathing, or cognitive focused, using guided imagery to induce a different mental set and decrease anxiety. Therapy for GAD needs to focus on anxious cognitions, behavioral avoidance, and physical tension. Secondary symptoms of depression and demoralization can be targeted through reactivating areas of potential support and opportunities for social activity (Butler & Booth, in Rapee & Barlow, 1991). Targeting situational avoidance is recommended. It is necessary to decrease avoidance behavior if the cycle of GAD is to be broken. For the GAD client to succeed he/she must change from a passive to an active stance and learn how to become more responsible for his/her anxiety management.

■ MEDICATION TREATMENT

GAD pharmacological treatment trials lag behind those for other anxiety disorders (Connor & Davidson, 1998). The three groups of medications used in the treatment of GAD are antidepressants, benzodiazepines, and azapirones. (Buspirone is the only azapirone approved for clinical use.) Of the antidepressants, the selective serotonin reuptake inhibitors (SSRIs) are a reasonable choice to treat GAD (Rocca, Fonzo, Scotta, Zanalda & Ravizza, 1997). Also, a recent double-blind placebo-controlled trial showed the serotonin/norepinephrine reuptake inhibitor (SNRI) antidepressant venlfaxine to be effective in treating GAD (Davidson, DuPont, Hedges & Haskins, 1999). The benzodiazepines class of medications are clearly effective in reducing symptoms of GAD. They have the advantage of being rapidly effective, but compared to antidepressants they may be less helpful in reducing psychic symptoms of anxiety compared to somatic symptoms (Hoehn-Saric, McLeod & Zimmerli, 1988). Though questions have been raised about their long-term efficacy, clinical experience suggests that there are patients who benefit from these agents over prolonged periods (Schatzberg, Cole & DeBattista, 1997). Another concern about benzodiazepine use is the potential for addiction. In general, however, benzodiazepine misuse is uncommon among persons without a prior or current problem with substance abuse (Wesson, Smith, Ling & Seymour, 1997). Wesson et al. (1997) have also addressed the nosologic and legislative issues that have complicated discussions about the abuse potential of prescription benzodiazepines. Attempts are currently underway to develop agents related to benzodiazepines but without addiction liability (Connor & Davidson, 1999). Buspirone has the advantage of lacking abuse potential and the side effects of benzodiazepines such as sedation, and motor cognitive impairment. Like anti-depressants, it takes weeks to be effective. The drug hyroxyzine has also shown potential in treating GAD, based on the results of randomized double-blind placebo-controlled trial (Lader & Scotto, 1998). Many clients with GAD require extended medication treatment. Nevertheless, whichever agent is used for treatment, it is still worth attempting to taper off medications after 6–12 months.

Panic Disorder/Panic Disorder with Agoraphobia

■ DESCRIPTION

Panic disorder is very common with a prevalence rate of 3.5 percent of the population afflicted (Weisman et al., 1997). Epidemiological data indicate women are twice as likely to be affected as men (Piggot, 1999). Twin studies indicate a genetic contribution to the development of panic disorder. Relatives of people with panic disorder are 4–7 times as likely to have the disorder as persons in the general population (APA, 1994).

Panic disorder is characterized by panic attacks (not exclusively situation-specific), fear of further panic attacks and/or changes in behavior to avoid panic or deal with the panic attacks. Panic attacks can be present in any of the anxiety disorders. In other anxiety disorders, panic attacks are situationally bound or cued, meaning they are triggered by a specific situation.

In social phobia, panic attacks occur in response to the thinking about or engaging in the feared interpersonal or social situation or activity. In specific phobia, panic attacks are precipitated by the presence of the feared object or situation and are highly correlated to the proximity of the object. In obsessive–compulsive disorder, panic attacks are in response to thinking about the obsession or coming into contact with the feared situation or object. Panic attacks are present in post-traumatic stress disorder when an aspect of the original trauma is re-experienced or an association to it is encountered. In GAD, panic attacks, are a reaction to worries, and build gradually over a long period of time. In panic disorder, attacks are experienced as "out of the blue." Attacks suddenly begin in a public place or at home. The attacks peak within 10 minutes, with a rapidly escalating feeling of fear in combination with physical symptoms such as rapid breathing, pounding heart, feeling flushed, lightheadedness, and tremor. Feeling of foreboding, fear, and apprehension arise. Thoughts of being seriously ill or that life is in danger are common (Goodwin, 1986).

Panic attacks are frequently associated with the feeling of impending doom, dying, or "going crazy." The specific fears are often based on prior experience. If one's father had a heart attack one may fear having a heart attack as well. If an uncle was hospitalized for schizophrenia, one may fear becoming psychotic. Panic attacks are described as "overwhelming"—like standing in front on an oncoming train. Panic attacks can occur frequently throughout the day or only occasionally. They often start with an initial terrifying attack precipitating a visit to an emergency room. The individual becomes preoccupied with the idea that something of a physical (or mental) nature is wrong with them, causing a fear of further attacks. There is often then a progression towards hyperawareness of physical sensations and avoidance of feelings associated with the attacks. The body is closely monitored for physical symptoms felt during an attack (e.g., breathing, heart rate changes, and sweating). Any indication of these symptoms may precipitate an escalation of fear and worry which culminates in another panic attack. Multiple visits to emergency rooms and health care providers are common. Due to the numerous physical sensations and catastrophic fears associated with panic attacks, the person may focus on many different symptoms with the belief of being very ill. Physicians will explore possibilities of physical causation based on their specialties. Commonly, panic patients go to primary care providers, cardiologists, pulmonary specialists, and neurologists. This in turn may result in unnecessary assessment and medical treatment for conditions that are actually panic symptoms. The person is often concerned about having a panic attack in a social setting and worries that distress will be apparent to others. This often leads to avoidance of social events, leaving early, or not participating or interacting with others. Sometimes an additional diagnosis of social phobia may be warranted if the individual escalates in their ideation and restricted involvement.

■ ASSESSMENT OF PANIC ATTACKS AND PANIC DISORDERS

DSM-IV (APA, 1994) states that the diagnosis of panic disorder requires at least two full panic attacks. A panic attack is comprised of four or more symptoms, with a sudden onset and no precipitating event or trigger causing the attack. The unprovoked panic attacks of panic disorder are differentiated from panic attacks occurring within other anxiety disorders by the lack of an obvious trigger or predictability. A panic attack with less than four symptoms is a limited symptom panic attack or, less formally, a mini-panic.

The following are symptoms of a panic attack.

1. *Palpitations, pounding heart, or accelerated heart rate*: the person describes fears that their heart is pounding so loudly and with such a rapid beat that it must surely be damaged or will lead to a heart attack. There is no evidence that panic attacks have ever led to an actual heart attack.
2. *Sweating*: the person has feelings of being too hot or flushed and associates this with panic. Activities or events that lead to these feelings are avoided.
3. *Trembling or shaking*: this is described by many as an internal feeling which is rarely visible to onlookers.
4. *Sensations of shortness of breath or smothering*: this is associated with the feeling of needing to leave situations to get outside for air. Activities that increase the breathing rate are often limited or avoided.
5. *Choking*: this feels like the muscles of the throat are constricted.
6. *Chest pain or discomfort*: these are major contributors to the belief that a heart attack is occurring. The muscles of the

chest wall may become sore from rapid, shallow chest breathing.

7. *Nausea or abdominal distress*: the fear that one will need to void one's bowels is not uncommon and contributes to fears of embarrassing oneself if unable to find a bathroom.

8. *Feeling dizzy, unsteady, lightheaded or faint*: this often leads to the belief that one will pass out and embarrass oneself or even lose control of their vehicle.

9. *Derealization (feelings of unreality) or depersonalization (being detached from oneself)*: these feelings are associated with the belief that one is going crazy.

10. *Fear of losing control or going crazy*: these feelings may cause parents to be afraid of being alone with their young children for fear they will lose control and harm them.

11. *Fear of dying*: these frightening thoughts related to death are reactions to the powerful physical events of the panic attack. Misinterpretation of the physical sensations of the fight/flight system lead the person to jump to conclusions about medical problems.

12. *Paresthesias (numbness or tingling sensations)*: this is a common symptom associated with the fear of cardiac arrest.

13. *Chills or hot flashes*: feeling goosebumps and shivering or feeling hot, sweaty, and flushed.

Cognitive symptoms are common with panic attacks, but associated more frequently with panic disorder attacks. The fearful thoughts that one may lose control or "go crazy" or that one is dying define the panic disorder. Panic disorder has been called a "phobia of the body," the body going crazy and trying to take the mind with it. Panic disorder attacks are about fear of survival, either physical or mental. In the moment of the panic, the possibility of imminent death or loss of sanity appears very real for the patient. Panic disorder attacks are especially unnerving because they are unpredictable and leave the person unable to explain them. In turn, this allows for the imagination to create catastrophes of medical illness, psychosis, and loss of control as either present or imminent. The person experiences a feeling of intense fear and scans the environment for danger. When unable to perceive danger, the search turns inward to the probability of physical or mental malady.

DSM-IV lists the diagnostic requirements for panic disorder:

1. *Recurrent unexpected panic attacks*: these attacks are unexpected by the person at the beginning of the disorder. After having panic disorder for some time, the person is able to better predict the triggers for panic attacks, although some attacks may still be unexpected.

2. *At least one of the attacks has been followed by one month (or more) of one (or more) of the following symptoms (?)*:

   A. *Persistent concern about having additional attacks*: here inter-current anxiety is common. The person experiences worry about having another attack and not knowing when it will happen.

   B. *Worry about implications of the attack or its consequences (examples include, losing control, having a heart attack or "going crazy")*. The phrase "Worry about the implications" refers to worries that one has a serious illness or is developing mental instability.

   C. *A significant change in behavior related to the attacks*: the phrase "a significant change in behavior" refers to coping strategies that the person creates. These might include lifestyle changes such as discontinuing drinking coffee because the feeling of jitteriness from caffeine is associated with an attack.

Agoraphobia is the most prominent behavioral change associated with panic disorders. It stems from the Greek agora, the market place, or fear of public places. Agoraphobia is fear of places or situations in which panic attacks have occurred. Agoraphobic situations are generalized, meaning if a person has a panic attack in a restaurant, all restaurants may be avoided. The resulting panic disorder with agoraphobia is the distress associated with certain situations avoided. Related to this is the fear that one will develop an attack where help or medical attention may be unavailable. This feeling may arise when the person is away from facilities or caregivers believed to be necessary for potentially life-saving medical interventions.

Agoraphobia can be more crippling than the actual panic attacks because the person develops such a preoccupation to prevent panic attacks. He/she avoids places associated with panic or where he/she feels an attack is likely to occur. Again, this is due to the false belief that the panic attack is threatening to one's life and/or sanity. Due to agoraphobic fear, vacations or trips may be postponed, since panic attack victims feel uncomfortable leaving the house and stay at home to be safe. Other people feel the opposite, they fear more at risk if left alone. It is common for the person to develop "safe zones" where he/she is on familiar terrain and feels less threatened. Generally, this is the person's own neighborhood. Driving is one activity that may be curtailed to safe areas, or only for essential business such as going to work. The safe zone may be as small as one's own house or yard, or may extend to an hour drive from the house. Agoraphobics fear that they will become dysfunctional and become unable to continue with whatever they are engaged in, in the event of an attack, or become a danger to other people. Parents will worry that they cannot safely drive their children since they may cause a crash if they have a panic attack. Parents may also worry that they will inadvertently injure their children in the midst of an attack. Agoraphobics also fear that they will become lost and be unable to cope. There is no evidence that any of these fears are valid.

In an effort to cope with agoraphobia, people with panic disorder develop strategies in addition to the "safe areas" mentioned. The most common strategy is to have a companion along when leaving home or going outside the safe zone. Companions might include kids, spouse, parents, or a pet. A companion provides them with the feeling that they are not alone if a panic attack strikes. Busy places such as shopping malls, stores, and banks are avoided. Waiting in line causes stress while anxiety builds and physical symptoms occur. Shopping carts are often abandoned while fleeing from the situation. To avoid waiting in line, agoraphobics sometimes buy groceries in small quantities, at off peak times or at convenience stores. The urge to escape, to get out quickly, or to get some fresh air is common with panic attacks. Desirable seats at church or the movies are in the back near the door, and on the end of the row near the aisle. This way, a fast getaway can be insured, if necessary. Triggers for panic fears are situations where the person is trapped. Appointments with the dentist or hairstylist are postponed due to fear of feeling stuck and being unable to get up and leave. Similarly, restaurants can induce agoraphobic distress where one cannot leave after ordering a meal. Other triggers include tunnels, bridges, closed spaces, crowds, driving, being far from home, airplanes, buses, walking, and florescent lighting.

People with panic disorder employ various strategies to maintain their equilibrium and avoid panic attacks. They may avoid activities that create physical sensations associated with panic. Exercise routines are abandoned to avoid feeling out of breath, hot, sweaty, and experiencing an increased heart rate. Caffeine is reduced or avoided fearing that it may induce a panic attack. Alcohol may be avoided for fear of a difference in perception. These are related to fears of derealization and depersonalization or to feeling dizzy. Strong sunlight is avoided, as it is feared that one will become overheated and this will lead to panic. Strong emotions such as anger are suppressed to avoid panic associated with adrenaline or increased heart rate. Any activity that creates feelings similar to panic can cause fearful thoughts or lead to avoidant behavior.

■ COMORBIDITY

Comorbid with panic disorder is the presence of other anxiety disorders. Seventy percent of people with panic disorder seen in primary care settings are diagnosed with other psychiatric problems (Roy-Byrne et al., 1999), especially generalized anxiety disorder (GAD). GAD is thought to be a step in the development of a panic disorder. Social phobia, specific phobia, and major depressive disorder also frequently occur.

■ TREATMENT

Cognitive behavioral therapy (CBT) is the most efficacious treatment for panic disorder. While CBT is often used in combination with medication, it can be used as a first-line treatment for panic disorder. Panic control treatment (PCT) is a CBT treatment for panic disorder developed by Barlow and Craske (1989). PCT is a brief therapy combining psychoeducation about panic attacks as well as the physiological underpinnings of anxiety. The patient acquires skills including: relaxation training to decrease physiological arousal, interoceptive exposure to desensitize the panic sufferer to their fearful symptoms, and cognitive therapy to restructure "scary thoughts" and create a rational view of panic symptoms. Patients in PCT treatment are told to catalog the maladaptive strategies used to perpetuate a fundamental error in how they view panic attacks (e.g., thinking that panic attacks and the symptoms which comprise them are "dangerous"). Barlow categorizes these strategies as coping mechanisms, safety measures, distractions, and "hanging on for dear life." Safety measures protect the patient from anxious feelings and may include a cell phone (to never be out of reach in case of a medical or other emergency), water (in case of dry throat), medication, or even a good luck charm. Distractions, such as turning the TV on to avoid thinking about having a panic attack also serve to avoid anxiety. "Holding on for dear life" measures might include gripping the steering wheel tightly; or touching a wall while walking by. These strategies provide tangible reassurance to the anxious patient. Unfortunately, these maladaptive coping strategies prevent the patient from getting used to their anxiety and reinforce that anxiety is dangerous. Patients assume that the experience of anxiety is dangerous and must be avoided. Anxiety is perceived as a scary feeling (e.g., panic attacks). This is a central tenet of treatment for any of the anxiety disorders.

For humans, experience is defined as a combination of what we perceive through our senses, combined with how we react with thoughts. Anxiety is a reaction to what is happening to us, followed by our thoughts about it, our physical sensations, and then our behavior. If we learn to listen to our thoughts, understand the physiology of anxiety and pay attention to what we do, we can understand where our emotions originate. This allows additional control over what we experience emotionally as anxiety and provides tools for working through fear, rather than avoiding it.

Panic attacks are the activation of the body's fight/flight (alarm) system. This system is a part of the survival equipment and allows people to respond physically and mentally to a threat to their safety. When presented with danger, the autonomic nervous system responds in a variety of ways. It prepares the body for action by secreting adrenaline, which speeds up heart rate and breathing, and selectively directs blood to the muscles. This creates physical sensations, such as palpitations (feeling one's heart pounding), breathlessness, and lightheadedness. The body prepares for action; vision narrows to focus on the danger and the mind is hypervigilant, searching the surroundings for the threat. Panic attacks are a misinterpretation of events activating the body's survival system. The repetitive nature of panic attacks is a cycle of fear. It keeps the person anxious, hypervigilant, and fearing the next panic, thereby causing the next panic and additional fear and apprehension.

■ PANIC CONTROL TREATMENT (PCT)

PCT involves up to eleven patient sessions. Through the sessions, the patient learns to view panic attacks more objectively and in a context of a normal physiological process rather than as a dangerous event requiring "hanging on for dear life" or sanity. PCT is comprised of three interventions which target behavioral, cognitive, and physiological domains.

1. *Breathing retraining therapy* (BRT) provides the patient with a method to decrease physiological arousal and to create an atmosphere to examine faulty cognitions. The patient learns to breathe slowly and deeply using the diaphragm and focus on breathing. This reduces tension and slows down thoughts

and physical behavior. Ten minutes of BRT twice daily is assigned and self-assessed.

2. *Countering* these "scary" thoughts with more evidence based and logical thinking decreases the fear-inducing stimuli. The principal focus is the body. People with panic disorder are hyper-aware of their bodies, and misinterpret physical symptoms as an indication of danger. A pounding heart is perceived as a heart attack rather than the more likely explanation of feeling excited or anxious. Medication side effects are misinterpreted as a cause for alarm, instead of as a nuisance.

3. *Interoceptive exposure.* Symptoms are induced to desensitize the patient. Dizziness might be induced by spinning in a chair. Rapid heart beat and sweating occur while running in place. Symptoms of hyperventilation are induced by breathing very quickly for 2 minutes while standing. The patient monitors and records all data from these exercises and reviews them with the therapist, who then designs the next step. Induction exercises work by reducing the fear reaction to each relevant physical symptom through repetitive exposure to it. Initially, the exposure is conducted with the therapist, then as homework outside of the therapy session, until they habituate. The patient seeks out naturalistic situations that will induce symptoms. Using repetitive exposures, the patient learns to tolerate the physical symptoms associated with the anxious feelings. This leads to habituation to the anxiety and extinguishes the reaction to the physical symptom.

When panic symptoms are experienced, the patient's perspective on the context and the reaction to them are altered. The panic attack is gradually understood differently and consequently decreases in frequency and intensity. For patients with panic disorder with agoraphobia, formerly avoided agoraphobic situations are confronted with repetitive situational exposures in a hierarchical fashion. This helps the patient systematically develop increased tolerance for anxiety. The patient gradually habituates to the situation without using any coping strategy other than tolerating exposure to anxiety. Combined symptom induction and situational exposure exercises create the most challenging triggers. Patients gradually acclimate when performing repetitive exposure work without distractions, challenging anxious thoughts, and countering these thoughts.

Case Study

Janet started having panic attacks when she was in grade school. The panic continued daily through her childhood and adolescence. Janet saw many therapists and took a variety of medications without significant change in her symptoms and fears related to her attacks. Janet was hospitalized in her early 20s due to increasing frequency and severity of panic attacks after getting married and having a child. She developed severe agoraphobia and did not leave her home without her husband, family, or close friend for several years. The course of Janet's panic waxed and waned throughout the next 20 years, which is typical. It did not remit, however, other than for a few brief weeks. Rarely did Janet go through a day without panic attacks and significant fear of additional attacks. In spite of her panic attacks, Janet lived a fairly normal life. She raised her children and helped her husband with their landscape business. Life for Janet required many strategies for coping with panic and fear of panic. She never went anywhere without a cell phone, had a safe zone around her neighborhood and the route to work. Janet never left her husband's side when they traveled out-of-town, and always drove instead of flying, never rode on buses, avoided bright sunlight (unless in the pool), and never drove very far outside of her safe zone unless accompanied by a companion. Daily she experienced thoughts that she might die or go crazy with the next panic attack, which she felt, was inevitable, but tried to postpone for as long as she could.

Janet began PCT at age 35. In PCT she learned about panic and anxiety through her assigned weekly readings, and devoted herself to absorbing information that she found extremely relevant. Janet practiced her breathing retraining twice daily as assigned and consequently learned to decrease her physical arousal. Her therapist taught her to spot and then decatastrophize thoughts such as "I'll probably die of a heart attack or a stroke" when she was panicking. Janet learned how to remind herself that what she was learning about anxiety indicated that the symptoms were a normal part of her body's defenses, and not dangerous. She learned her "alarm system" was going off too frequently and inappropriately and it was not in any way harmful. Likewise she learned that the experience of panic was largely due to the various symptoms of hyperventilation. Other "scary symptoms" such as feeling breathless, were desensitized through interoceptive exposure to exercises such as holding her breath for 30 seconds and building up to longer times; running in place for 2 minutes, etc.

Janet's most scary symptoms, such as dizziness and light-headedness, were adapted to by no longer trying to avoid and fear them. The sensations were deliberately created and intensified through exercises, initially with the therapist. As homework, she spun in her office chair. After 2 weeks, Janet no longer felt fearful of feeling dizzy.

As she mastered the cognitive and physiological exposures, she began to work with her therapist on exposure to situations she had avoided all her life. A hierarchy ranking the situations in order of less to more anxiety/distress was created. Janet then worked on situations 3 times a week. These included riding buses, driving on highways by herself, and increasing the distance from her "safe zone." Janet gradually gave up her "safety" and distracting behaviors, left the cell phone at home, and faced her anxiety without having to distract herself with the radio. She learned that the experience of anxiety was uncomfortable until she got used to the situations, but that it didn't harm her.

Eleven sessions spread over about four months. At the conclusion, Janet reported occasional mini-panics. She seldom had full symptom panics and reported her fear of panic to be mild. She now had the ability to process her fearful thoughts and to create rational thoughts about her symptoms. In general, she reported an absence of fear due to physical sensations. She was able to experience many of the situations formerly avoided with varying degrees of anxiety, but generally without panic.

The goal of panic disorder treatment is reduction of the fear and avoidance of anxiety symptoms through exposure and cognitive countering of "scary thoughts," so that significant distress and interference is eliminated or significantly reduced. Anxiety symptoms continue to varying degrees due to normal symptom fluctuations and life stresses. How the person manages them creates the difference between relapse and successful treatment.

■ MEDICATION TREATMENT

Medication for panic attacks and panic disorder includes antidepressants, benzodiazepines, and other agents. Initially, the antidepressants used were tricyclic antidepressants (TCAs) and monoamine oxidase inhibitors (MAOIs). Though studies have shown these agents to be efficacious, their use has been supplanted by the more recently developed selective serotonin reuptake inhibitors (SSRI) antidepressants fluoxetine, sertraline, paroxetine, fluvoxamine, and citalopram. Concerns over TCA use are related to their lethality in overdose and side effects such as rapid heart beat and dizziness, which can mimic those of panic. The dietary restrictions needed with MAOI use limit their use. SSRIs have become first-line treatments because they are not associated with the problems of TCAs and MAOIs. Antidepressant efficacy in the short-term treatment of panic disorder has been demonstrated in randomized double-blind placebo-controlled trials. These studies suggest that the SSRIs are superior in efficacy to TCAs and benzodiazepines in short-term treatment (Boyer, 1995). Treatment is typically initiated at lower than standard doses in order to minimize panicked responses to medication side effects which include gastrointestinal symptoms, initial anxiety, sedation, and sexual dysfunction.

There are two approaches to benzodiazepine use in the context of SSRI treatment. Benzodiazepines may be used as a bridge during the 3–6 weeks required for antidepressants to take effect and then tapered off (Sheehan, 1999). Some patients find it hard to discontinue the benzodiazepine and stay on varying doses of the medication (Gorman, 1997). Concerns about addiction are typically not a problem for most persons who have not had trouble with other addictions (Wesson et al., 1997) and benzodiazepines can be used as a front line agent for acute and maintenance treatment of panic disorder (Ballenger et al., 1988; Schweizer, Rickels, Weiss & Zavodnick, 1993). Other agents that have been used to treat panic disorder include the antidepressants venlafaxine and nefazodone, and the anticonvulsants valproic acid and gabapentin (Sheehan, 1999).

Few studies have addressed the efficacy of longer-term treatment and the related question of the duration of medication required. The limited available data (Lecrubier & Judge, 1997; Michelson, Pollack, Lydiard, Tamura, Tepner & Tollefson, 1999) suggest continued benefits and reduced relapse with treatment up to 6–9 months. If medication is used, treatment is continued for about a year and tapered gradually over 4–6 months. If symptoms recur after discontinuation, the medication will need to be restarted.

Obsessive–Compulsive Disorder

Twenty years ago, OCD was believed to be a rare disorder. Today, it is recognized as the fourth most common psychiatric disorder with a prevalence rate estimated at 2–3 percent. OCD has been recognized for centuries with a degree of understanding. The catholic church labeled the condition "excessive scrupulosity" when rituals and compulsions were exhibited by priests and parishioners (Greist, 1994). Only recently have psychotherapy treatments with consistent successful outcome existed. Treatment of OCD requires specialized training in exposure with response prevention, a cognitive behavioral therapy (CBT). In the past decade, the CBT for OCD moved out of the research facilities and into the community. Unfortunately, many individuals receive inadequate treatment. On a positive note, the availability of outpatient therapists trained in exposure with response prevention is limited, but increasing.

■ DESCRIPTION

OCD is the presence of repetitive thoughts, impulses or images that create discomfort, usually experienced as moderate to intense by the patient. The person attempts to decrease this discomfort by doing something with their thoughts. He/she might say a prayer, reassure themselves or review the situation by checking to make sure nothing happened. They may do similar things behaviorally such as looking at the stove to make sure the pilot light is on or the switches are off, looking under the car to make sure there is not a body underneath, or watching the evening news to check on whether anyone was killed in the vicinity where they were that day. OCD involves doubting and hesitation; difficulty with decision-making to the degree that functioning is impaired (Neziroglu & Yaryura-Tobias, 1991).

Severe generalized anxiety, recurrent panic attacks, debilitating avoidance, and major depression are often present with OCD. Personality disorders are frequently diagnosed in OCD as well (Pigott, 1999). OCD is a difficult disorder to live with both for the afflicted and their families. The stress on the person and degree of impairment lead to behavioral changes that the family is asked to assist in. Frequently family members are entreated to help with checking, washing, and allowing the afflicted individual to avoid OCD triggers. OCD is difficult to diagnose, due to the various presentations of OCD.

■ ONSET AND COURSE

Most people with OCD report they had symptoms since childhood but experienced OCD as a serious problem beginning in their teens or twenties. Males typically experience an onset at ages 6–15 and females at ages 20–29 (APA, 1994). The course of the illness tends to be chronic with waxing and waning of symptoms. While remission and improvement have been reported without the treatment, the more usual course is maintaining or worsening of symptoms. Symptom exacerbation under stress is common, with a progressive deterioration of social, interpersonal, and vocational functioning.

■ ETIOLOGY

Neuro-imaging studies demonstrate the pathophysiology of OCD involves abnormal functioning along specific frontal-subcortical brain circuit. OCD symptoms are thought to be associated with increased activity in the areas of the orbitofrontal cortex, caudate nucleus, thalamus, and anterior cingulate gyrus (Saxena, Brody, Schwartz & Baxter, 1998). These areas of the brain's pre-frontal cortex exhibit increased activity in people with OCD compared to normal controls. Treatment with both serotonergic medications and cognitive-behavioral therapy decreases this overactivity. This circuit which connects the frontal lobes of the cerebral cortex is involved with judgment and planning and connects with the basal ganglia, which assists with filtering messages before passing them to the thalamus, then back to the cortex. Injuries to this system often are associated with obsessive and compulsive symptoms.

Some children infected with the streptococci bacteria develop obsessive–compulsive symptoms when the immune cells of the body attack the basal ganglia rather than the bacteria. Diseases of the basal ganglia such as Tourette's disorder and Sydenham's Chorea have a high prevalence of associated OCD symptoms. These findings contribute to understanding that damage to these regions disrupts the brain's functioning creating the symptoms of obsessive thoughts and rituals (Grinspoon, 1998). Three major pathways for the neurotransmitter serotonin pass through these areas and the only medications useful in treating OCD are those that increase brain concentrations of serotonin. Studies indicate relatives of OCD patients have higher rates of OCD and subthreshold OCD symptoms. An increased presence of tics (involuntary muscular movements of the body) has also been demonstrated among relatives of people with OCD (Pauls et al., 1995). There is a 10 percent chance of inheriting OCD from a diagnosed parent. Identical twins have a greater chance of both having OCD than fraternal twins. OCD can present postpartum when new mothers develop symptoms of OCD following delivery, as well as depression.

■ DIAGNOSIS

A person is diagnosed with OCD, according to DSM-IV (APA, 1994), with *obsessions and/or compulsions*, a departure from

DSM-III-R (APA, 1987) in which it was necessary to have both obsessions and compulsions to be diagnosed with OCD. Obsessions often are neutralized with a compulsion. Similarly, as compulsions are driven by obsessions, the presence of a compulsion without an obsession is unusual. Both obsessions and compulsions can be thoughts, and are not always observable. Examples of thought compulsions are counting, mentally reviewing, and praying. Obsessions are recurrent and persistent thoughts, impulses, or images, experienced as intrusive and inappropriate, which cause marked anxiety or distress. The person tries to ignore or suppress such thoughts or neutralize them with some other thought or action. The belief or feeling that the obsession must be responded to creates the compulsion. The emotional response to the obsession may give the message to the brain that this is an important thought and that it should therefore be attended to and repeatedly re-visited. Conversely, if the person is able to have a neutral response to the obsession, it often will decrease in the frequency of the repetition (Phillipson, 1991). The person recognizes that the obsessional thoughts, impulses or images are a product of his or her own mind.

Compulsions are defined by repetitive behaviors or mental acts that the person feels driven to perform in response to an obsession or according to rules that must be applied rigidly. The words chosen convey how controlling the disorder is for the patient. The rules are unique to the affected person but often follow a pattern, sometimes culturally based. The number 13 is sometimes felt to be a "bad" number, but so are 3 or 9 or any other number meaningful to the patient. Likewise, "good" numbers may then be utilized to neutralize the "bad" ones. The person formulates a set of rules that create intense anxiety if they are not rigidly applied. The behaviors or mental acts are aimed at preventing or reducing distress or preventing some dreaded event or situation from occurring. However, these behaviors or mental acts either are not connected in a realistic way with what they are designed to neutralize or prevent, or, they are clearly excessive. Sometimes there is a realistic, but exaggerated connection, for example, washing hands repeatedly to prevent illness. Frequently, the connection between the obsession and compulsion is irrational.

The person often recognizes that the obsessions or compulsions are excessive or unreasonable. The range of insight present in OCD extends from rational understanding, that the obsessions represent unrealistic or exaggerated concerns, to an overvalued ideation (a wavering belief in the rational with some belief in the obsession), to a delusional belief in the truth of the obsessions. In the latter case, the additional diagnosis of delusional disorder may be used. The obsessions or compulsions cause marked distress, are time-consuming (take more than one hour a day), or significantly interfere with the person's normal routine, occupational functioning, or usual social activities or relationships (DSM-IV, American Psychiatric Association, 1994). It is not abnormal to have occasional intrusive odd thoughts and to perform behaviors such as doubting and checking. For a diagnosis to be given, the symptoms must cause significant personal distress or interference with functioning.

■ SPECTRUM DISORDERS

Spectrum disorders of OCD are seemingly related such as eating disorders, body dysmorphic disorder, hypochondriasis, trichotillomania, and kleptomania. Others argue that impulse control disorders such as compulsive gambling should also be recognized as an obsessional disorder. Spectrum disorders share many features with OCD, including repetitive intrusive thoughts or behaviors, comorbidity, and response to serotonergic medications (Hollander, 1998). The diagnostic boundaries between OCD and other disorders may be clarified when the relationship of disorders with obsessional components is united under a new category. Recently, there has been discussion of creating a new category within Axis I for obsessive spectrum disorders and moving OCD from anxiety disorders to this new category. This would also allow for disorders such as schizophrenia that has OCD traits (estimated at 10 percent) to have a schizo-obsessive modifier. This might also be the modifier for those with OCD who do not have insight into their obsessive thoughts (Eisen, Phillips & Rasmussen, 1999).

■ OBSESSIONS

Obsessions often express the idea that one may harm others or oneself. Fears of sexually molesting someone, jumping out of a window, harming someone, or contracting a dreadful disease are typical. Obsessions of having left behind part of oneself or that one has become disconnected from oneself are more common with patients with schizotypal or schizophrenia disorders. In contrast to phobias, in OCD, the danger exists sometimes in the thought, which must be avoided in the same way a phobic avoids the feared object. Every time it is experienced, the obsession can have the same emotional impact as re-experiencing a trauma (Barlow, 1988).

Unfortunately, the obsessions repeat frequently and for some patients, are experienced almost continuously. To varying degrees, the obsession is resisted vigorously or is completely surrendered. Much time is spent thinking about obsessions. Others attempt to solve whatever puzzle the obsession presents. The following are examples of specific types of obsessions.

1. *Pure obsessive*: A man complained dwelling for hours each day on the ratio of the gears on his mountain bike, and whether they should be altered. In this case the obsession and the compulsion to think about it merge into what Baer (1993) terms the "pure obsessive." The ruminations may manifest as religious or moral concerns. Doubting obsessions are also common. The obsession may also manifest as an impulse or image. They are repetitive, intrusive, and demand a reaction that constitutes the OCD cycle.

2. *Contamination*: These fears generally pertain to fear of contact with bodily fluids, often with a specific fear, such as acquiring AIDS. Therefore, contact with blood may present itself as the worst fear. Associated triggers may develop such as fear of objects that are red, seeing anyone with a bandage, or sitting on spots on chairs that might be blood. For contamination obsessions, as with all forms of OCD, avoidance is a common defense. Contact with anything touched by others is

avoided. For example, one patient became panicky after having stepped on a band-aid. He simultaneously knew he could not logically be in danger from a band-aid on the sole of his shoe but then became worried about "what if there was a hole in my shoe?"

3. *Magical thinking*: The association of a chain of events linking the object, activity, or person with the obsession is common. The fear of something horrific happening at the end is a form of magical thinking associated with OCD. Innocuous objects or routine activities are experienced as causing panic level anxiety. If one picks up an object with the right hand rather than the left, it may lead to disaster.

4. *Aggressive*: The second most common form obsessions take are aggressive in nature, such as the fear of harming others through doing something or not having done something. These are not homicidal thoughts, as there is no intent to act on them. The thoughts are shocking and horrifying to the patient. For example, one patient was obsessed about running over someone with his car and frequently checked under the car for bodies or traces of blood. A woman compulsively checked every candle in the house, even ones in drawers that were never lit. Her obsessive concern that "the candles might be lit" necessitated the checking. The fearful consequence of not checking was not just that the house might burn down, but that a fireman would be killed fighting the fire.

5. *Responsibility*: An exaggerated feeling of responsibility is a common trait of obsessions. The incorrect amount of chlorine in one's swimming pool may become a source of obsessional concern such as possibly causing illness or injury. The seal on the microwave oven leaking radiation and contaminating the household, or turning a light off incorrectly could cause a short circuit and a fire. As a consequence, the person checks repetitively, or avoids the triggering object, or performs a safeguarding ritual, such as saying a prayer or tapping a set number of times.

6. *Perfection*: Exactness obsessions may be expressed through rituals involving such a need for perfection that tasks become

intolerable. For example, the person may take an hour to write a check exactly or he/she may avoid check writing altogether due to the inability to do it good enough or because it takes too long.

7. *Sexual*: Sexual obsessions are common with distress due to the repetition of sexual thoughts, impulses or images, which are often repugnant. These are not sexual fantasies; rather they are experienced as odd and upsetting. The person is confused about whether he or she acted on a sexual obsession and experiences much distress trying to decide what to believe.

8. *Slowing*: Obsessive slowing is an uncommon, but severely disabling symptom for a subgroup of OCD (Veale, 1993). People take an inordinate amount of time doing routine tasks such as taking an hour to shave. Obsessive slowing that is not clearly a consequence of an obsession may represent a related disorder.

9. *Hoarding*: Hoarders are overwhelmed with the belief that they cannot throw things away. They worry they may need the item or that it is irreplaceable. They have an excessive emotional attachment to objects and find it difficult to organize them.

10. *Scrupulosity*: Scrupulosity is the belief that one may have committed sacrilege over minor or non-existent transgressions. For example, a person worries they may not take communion because they have chewed a stick of gum or brushed their teeth. The direction is that they may not eat before communion, and the worry is that the gum or toothpaste may be a violation of this rule.

11. *Compulsions*: The compulsion may or may not follow logically from the obsession. The compulsion often reduces anxiety, but not always. The following are common compulsive behaviors of OCD patients.

12. *Checking*: Compulsive checking generally involves the prevention of harm, or the attempted resolution of doubt. Checking can be done mentally. It is common to mentally review all interactions for the presence of a feared event.

Repetitive reviewing can be due to doubts about what was said or heard. The most common forms of checking involve whether something was done related to potential danger. Checking can also involve whether a mistake was made.

13. *Cleaning*: Compulsive cleaning is done to decontaminate an object or oneself, usually to prevent harm to the person or to those whom they are trying to protect from being contaminated. Activities such as showering may be avoided and done very infrequently as they are too time-consuming, sometimes taking several hours or more.

14. *Repetition*: Compulsive repeating of thoughts and actions are frequent, with the times repeated often counted until the "right" number is reached. For example, a patient repetitively touched objects such as a table top, a required amount of times to prevent feeling anxious. Another example, a woman drives around her block a required number of times to prevent harm to her family. The repeating compulsion may be with or without magical thinking to prevent harm.

15. *Counting*: Compulsive counting is performed as a ritual or in order to know when to perform other rituals such as the number of steps to take or the number of times to wash one's hands. Counting can reveal when to start or stop something because of a good or bad number. For example, it might involve driving around the block a certain number of times in order to arrive on a lucky number.

16. *Comorbidity*: Up to 70 percent of people with OCD have a current or past history of major depressive disorder. Other common comorbid presentations are eating disorders, anxiety disorders, especially specific phobias, social phobia, panic disorder, substance abuse, and tic disorders. A high prevalence of Axis II disorders also present comorbid with OCD. Most common in OCD are obsessive–compulsive, dependent and avoidant personality disorders. Also present are histrionic, borderline, and schizotypal personalities (Hollander & Stein, 1997). There is evidence that the presence of a comorbid personality disorder is a poor prognostic indicator (Jenike, 1998).

■ TREATMENT

Two treatments for OCD have proven effective in treating OCD: serotonergic medications and a behavioral therapy combination of exposure with response prevention.

Exposure with Response Prevention

In this treatment, patients are asked to confront and remain in contact with the things or situations that they fear without doing anything to decrease their discomfort until their fear decreases (Greist, 1994). Treatment begins with a thorough behavioral analysis of the patient's obsessions and compulsions. Avoided objects or situations indicate obsessive triggers. After cataloging these symptoms, a hierarchy is created that lists the various activities (thoughts or behaviors) necessary to work on through exposure. Each item on the hierarchy is assigned a Subjective Units of Discomfort Scale (SUDS) rating (Foa & Wilson, 1991). The SUDS is a scale to measure the degree of OCD-related distress present if the activity is done without ritualizing or neutralizing. Neutralizing is anything the patient does to decrease anxiety and thereby interferes with the process of habituation. Patients are asked to monitor and record all compulsions they are unable to refrain from doing from their first day of treatment. This provides a baseline for beginning treatment. Exposures begin at a 40 on the 100-point hierarchy, then gradually move up the scale to confront the most highly feared exposures. It is necessary that the patient refrain from as many rituals as possible, or delay the ritual as long as possible. Participation in exposures makes the response, or ritual prevention (not performing compulsions in response to obsessive thoughts) easier.

The most difficult task of exposure and response prevention is when the patient, without the therapist, confronts the feared situation and does nothing to neutralize the fear. The therapist assigns the patient time alone during treatment sessions for exposures and response prevention in order to help the patient adjust to doing exposures without the help of the therapist. Assistance is helpful initially, but for the patient to be successful with stopping their rituals, they must be able to face their OCD triggers without the therapist.

Following the treatment session, the patient monitors and records his/her compliance with response prevention for homework. Exposure homework takes 1–2 hours daily.

Cognitive Interventions

Cognitive therapy with OCD patients provides understanding of the nature of OCD as a psycho-neurological illness that improves only with a change in behavior, neurochemistry, or both. A shared understanding of the treatment rationale and the concept of habituation are useful. Cognitive therapy helps the individual understand that obsessions do not mean anything about themselves personally. Whether obsessions are related to violence, sacrilege, or aberrant sex, this is not a reflection on the patient. This eases the patient's mind, while allowing them to let go of ruminations and emotional reactivity to the obsessions.

Cognitive models of OCD suggest a number of different variables that may play a role in the development and maintenance of obsessive compulsive symptoms (Freeston & Ladouceur, 1996). Perfectionistic beliefs cause patients to overestimate their responsibility for negative events. It also creates a greater belief in their being responsible (Bouchard, Rheaume & Ladouceur, 1999). Patients benefit from cognitive analysis and restructuring of their distorted thoughts of perfection and responsibility. This facilitates the efficacy of behavioral exposures.

OCD patients have higher than average beliefs in "thought action fusion," the belief that thinking something makes it more likely to happen or to be true. A propensity to thought action fusion increases both intrusive thoughts and the number of triggers for these thoughts. It leads to greater distress and more resistance to exposure work (Rassin, Merckel, Muris & Spaan, 1999). Attending to this belief and assisting the patient in moderating it will improve his/her ability to benefit from the treatment and to let go of overvalued or distorted thinking.

Problems with obsessive rumination are a consequence of the meaning attached to the content of the thought. Increased ritualizing is associated with attributing responsibility for the thought to the self (Salkovskis, Forrester & Richards, 1998). The cognitive intervention needs to target the distorted belief in responsibility, thereby reducing the distress experienced because of the thought. Decreased emotional response to the intrusive thought then allows for a more neutral stance and decreases the frequency of the thought.

■ MEDICATION TREATMENT

The two groups of medications found to be most effective in the treatment of OCD are the SSRIs and the highly serotonergic TCA clompiramine. Efficacy has been demonstrated in rigorous double-blind placebo-controlled trials (Goodman, 1999). The SSRIs are used as first line treatment because they are better tolerated by patients compared to the TCA clompiramine. Compared to depression and other anxiety disorders OCD requires higher doses of medication and a longer period of time for medication response. In contrast to treatment for depression, the initial response of OCD to antidepressants can take 4–8 weeks and progressive improvement can continue for months. Thus, a medication is tried for 10–12 weeks at therapeutic doses prior to switching agents for lack of efficacy. Some patients have a partial response to medication while others do not respond at all. If a first SSRI does not help, it is worth trying another from the same class as patients who do not respond to one may respond to another (Leonard, 1997). If a second SSRI does not help, then a trial of the TCA clomipramine is suggested. If there is partial response to the SSRI, clompiramine can be added to augment therapeutic effects. Given the tendency to partial treatment response, various other augmentation strategies can be used. These include agents such as buspirone, lithium, and both typical and atypical antipsychotics such as haloperidol and risperidone (Jenike, 1998). Experimental immunological treatments have been tried for a subtype of OCD, which is one of a group of disorders (e.g., rheumatic fever, Sydenham's chorea) that develops after streptococcal infection (Allen, Leonard & Swedo, 1995).

Post-traumatic Stress Disorder and
Acute Stress Disorder

Acute stress disorder (ASD) and post-traumatic stress disorder (PTSD) are symptoms of depression, anxiety, and physical symptoms that develop following a very upsetting experience. They relate to a traumatic event in which they were involved, witnessed, or have a relationship with the victim.

About 2.3 percent of the population will experience PTSD in their lifetime (Dupont, Rice, Shiraki & Rowland, 1994). PTSD can develop at any age and is more likely to occur in women then men. Thirty percent of men and women who have witnessed war, soldiers, or civilians, experience PTSD. PTSD is often accompanied by substance abuse, depression, and other anxiety disorders.

■ DIAGNOSIS

Diagnosis of both ASD or PTSD occurs after the person is exposed to a psychologically distressing event. Examples include: being robbed, sexually assaulted, experiencing domestic violence, witnessing an accident where people are killed, or being involved in a natural disaster, riot, or war. ASD is the development of anxiety and dissociative symptoms shortly after exposure to a traumatic stressor. Continuation of symptoms beyond one month is diagnosed as PTSD. ASD may precede the onset of PTSD, or may be gone within a week or two. It is uncertain to determine who will react to a given stressor and develop PTSD. Various factors affect the development of PTSD, including personality, availability of support, the patient's interpretation of the traumatic event, and the timeliness and quality of clinical intervention.

■ DIAGNOSTIC CRITERIA OF ACUTE STRESS DISORDER (ASD)

ASD occurs when the person has been exposed to a traumatic event in which he or she experienced, witnessed, or was confronted with an event or events that involved actual or threatened death or serious injury, or a threat to the physical integrity of themselves or others, and the response involves intense fear, helplessness, or horror. During or after the distressing event, the person has three (or more) of the following dissociative symptoms: (1) a subjective sense of numbing, (2) detachment or absence of emotional responsiveness, (3) a reduction in awareness of his/her surroundings, (4) derealization, and (5) dissociative amnesia. Symptoms must cause significant impairment or distress and last from 2 days to 4 weeks (APA, 1994).

■ DIAGNOSTIC CRITERIA OF PTSD

The person with PTSD has been exposed to a traumatic event in which he or she experienced, witnessed, or was confronted with an event or events that involved actual or threatened death or serious injury, or a threat to the physical integrity of self or others. The person's response involves intense fear, helplessness, or horror.

The traumatic event is persistently experienced in one (or more) of the following ways: (1) recurrent and intrusive distressing recollections of the event, (2) acting or feeling as if the traumatic event were recurring, (3) intense psychological distress at exposure to internal or external cues that symbolize or resemble an aspect of the traumatic event, and (4) physiological reactivity on exposure to internal or external cues that symbolize or resemble an aspect of the traumatic event. These cues may be memories, a song, a person's face, a smell, a situation. Any of these triggers may then lead to rapid changes in the person's mood, or to physical changes such as breathing, sweating, muscle tension, headaches, tremor, or palpitations.

Persistent avoidance of stimuli associated with the trauma and numbing of general responsiveness (not present before the trauma) are indicated by three (or more) of the following: (1) efforts to avoid thoughts, feelings, or conversations associated with the trauma, (2) efforts to avoid activities, places or people that arouse recollections of the trauma, (3) inability to recall an important aspect of the trauma, (4) markedly diminished interest or participation in significant activities, (5) feelings of detachment or estrangement from others, restricted range of affect, and (6) sense of a foreshortened future.

Persistent symptoms of increased arousal (not present before the trauma) are indicated by two (or more) of the following: (1) difficulty falling or staying asleep, (2) irritability or outbursts of anger, (3) difficulty concentrating, (4) hypervigilance, and (5) exaggerated startle response.

"Acute" is specified when the symptoms last less than 3 months and "chronic" for more than 6 months. "With Delayed Onset" is specified when the disorder does not manifest for more than 6 months after the trauma (APA, 1994).

ASP and PTSD are similar in diagnostic criteria. The duration of time inflicted is the principal difference. ASD places more emphasis on the presence of "three or more dissociative symptoms" while PTSD does not include derealization or depersonalization. The diagnostic criteria overlap, but are emphasized differently. ASP may or may not require treatment during the month's duration. Chances are better that it may not progress to PTSD with effective intervention. Lesser traumas not meeting the criteria of ASD or PTSD may be coded as adjustment disorders.

■ DESCRIPTION

The person with PTSD is in a fragile state. These traumatized patients lose their feeling of being safe in the world and within themselves. Alterations in thinking patterns, emotional equilibrium, and biochemistry follow the trauma. Psychological losses experienced are the ability to modulate or temper strong feelings, maintain connections with others, and maintain a positive self-identity (Matsakis, 1994). Anhedonia, increased irritability, loss of libido, alienation and withdrawal, and disrupted relationships with partners are common. Traumatized individuals often express negative feelings about themselves, self-blame, and negative feelings about their community. They suffer from feelings of anxiety and depression (Foa, Davidson & Frances, 1999).

■ CRITICAL INCIDENT STRESS DEBRIEFING (CISD)

Emergency services personnel experience daily trauma and ASD as a consequence of their jobs. So-called "first responders" to an emergency may suffer emotionally from this frequent barrage of human tragedy. CISD is designed to assist emergency personnel in coping with the frequent traumatic events involved in their job. Rapid intervention is used, usually within days of the trauma. It is not therapy, but rather an opportunity to talk with the others involved in the incident about what happened and how they feel about it. It allows for dissemination of information about normal reactions to stress and coping strategies (Mitchell & Everly, 1993).

■ TREATMENT

Trauma victims with PTSD have difficulty healing. They lack one of the basic healing mechanisms of the mind, reverie (defined as abstracted musing, daydreaming) (Davies, *American Heritage Dictionary*, 1976). This mechanism contributes to the resting of the healthy mind. Trauma victims will not allow their mind to wander as it gravitates to the painful and unresolved issues of the trauma. Instead, deprived of the ability to experience reverie, the mind is stuck, as if the film has frozen on the frame of the trauma, and cannot move on. One of the principal components of PTSD therapy is to assist in the integration of the trauma into normal experience, so that the person can then move on with life (van der Kolk, 1994).

Cognitive behavioral approaches have been designed specifically to desensitize and increase habituation to PTSD cases in the acute reactions of victims of crime and rape. This involves relaxation, cognitive training, and imaginal exposure to the trauma (Foa & Zoellner, 1998). Stimuli from the trauma become associated with normal life events, giving patients the capacity to produce strong feelings of fear and anxiety. Neutral stimuli, such as persons, situations or events present at the time of the trauma, produce conditioned responses such as fear and disorientation. Anxiety responses may generalize to stimuli similar to ones present during the trauma. The cognitions of the trauma victim acquire the same ability to generate anxiety due to the conditioning effect when they are associated with the trauma (Foa & Zoellner, 1998).

■ STRESS INOCULATION TRAINING

The PTSD patient is taught stress inoculation training (SIT). This intervention addresses the three domains of anxiety: physiological symptoms, behavior, and cognition. The combination of relaxation breathing, muscle relaxation, and cognitive restructuring of anxiety inducing distorted thoughts is taught. These skills, along with behavioral modeling and the provision of a model explaining what happened and how to recover, allow the individual to confront imaginal exposure to the trauma. The emotional response to the trauma is normalized as an understandable response to the fear of the trauma. Targeted symptoms in SIT are a sense of loss of control, flashbacks, difficulty concentrating, feelings of guilt, negative feelings about self and sadness or depression. After nine sessions of SIT skills the second stage of the treatment, prolonged exposure, begins.

■ PROLONGED EXPOSURE

Prolonged exposure allows trauma victims to habituate to the experience of the trauma through intensive re-enactments of the scene with the therapist, and on audio tape at home between sessions. The therapist directs the patient to close his or her eyes, remember the details of the trauma, and vividly describe it as if is happening now. The therapist is supportive but directive, and communicates understanding of the fear this creates (Foa & Zoellner, 1998). Through supported confrontation of the trauma memories, the patient is able to regain control of his/her life. He or she becomes able to integrate the trauma experience and recall it without emotions so intense as to cause disruption in life.

Exposure-based treatments designed to facilitate re-experiencing the trauma can have very dramatic results. After repeated systematic imagination of events associated with the trauma over a number of sessions, the full emotional experience may burst forth, resulting in a dramatic display of intense emotion. The object of therapy is to work through this emotion and prevent further avoidance of emotion-laden triggers. This emotional abreaction is encouraged rather than discouraged (Barlow, 1988).

■ MEDICATION TREATMENT

Medications can be used to treat the core symptoms of PTSD and also to treat comorbid psychiatric disorders. They are frequently added to treatment when psychotherapy alone has failed to provide satisfactory results. Also, medications may be used when treatment starts, especially if the disorder severity is moderate or severe, or if there is a comorbid psychiatric disorder. Antidepressants are typically used to treat PTSD, and have the additional advantage of treating comorbid mood and anxiety disorders. The SSRIs are considered as first-line treatment both because of their efficacy and their tolerability and ease of use (Davidson & Connor, 1999). In the event of partial response to treatment, a mood-stabilizing medication (e.g., valproic acid or lithium) or a tricyclic antidepressant (Foa et al., 1999) are added. If there is poor response to the first antidepressant, newer antidepressants such as nefazodone and venlafaxine can be used, or a mood stabilizer or second SSRI can be used (Foa et al., 1999). Mood stabilizers are an appropriate first-line treatment when there is comorbid bipolar disorder or if there are prominent problems with anger, aggression and impulsivity. Though useful, TCAs and MAOIs are not used early in treatment because of difficulties with their use (i.e., side effects, risk in overdose, and MAOI dietary restrictions). Also, some patients may benefit from beta adrenergic antagonists (such as propranolol) which may help reduce high levels of arousal and explosiveness.

Treatment is continued for at least a year. It may then be gradually tapered off, with relapse being an indication to restart treatment (Davidson & Connor, 1999). An alternate is to attempt a taper of medication after 6–12 months for acute PTSD and after

12–24 months for chronic PTSD (Foa et al., 1999). Some patients may require medication for much longer periods.

Social Phobia

■ DESCRIPTION

Social phobia is a fear of negative evaluation within an interpersonal context. Either specific types of interpersonal interactions (specific social phobia) or social settings in general (generalized social phobia) are seen as threatening to the self. The perceived possibility of social disapproval equates to a threat to the person's integrity. The social phobia carries a cognitive set comprised of a critical audience scrutinizing his or her performance, a rigid idea about what is acceptable and the belief that to fail is catastrophic and irreparable. Social phobia generally has onset following puberty peaking in the late teens (Marks, 1987). It rarely occurs after the age of 30. Shyness since childhood is frequently reported and seems to be genetically influenced. Anxiety consequent to this set of beliefs can vary with the person and within the social setting. As with the other anxiety disorders, avoidance, and escape are used extensively. Likewise, the failure to achieve cultural and personal goals due to the avoidance can be demoralizing and thus contribute to depression, which frequently coexists with social phobia.

■ SOCIAL DANGER

The perception of the social event as a conflict activates the body sympathetic system of defense (Beck, Emory & Greenburg, 1985). The sense of danger resides in the belief that one is in danger of embarrassment. The overt symptoms are somewhat less alarming than a panic attack, as there is not a fear of death or insanity. But, similar symptoms include feeling flushed, sweating profusely. The body's alarm system activates if one is faced with a predator and the ability to move and speak are frozen.

This reaction renders the person incapable of dealing with the social situation.

■ PHOBIC SITUATIONS

Social situations commonly reported by those with social phobias to be distressing include talking on the phone, talking with strangers, dealing with people in authority or someone attractive, initiating conversation, disagreeing, or talking to a group. Public speaking is anxiety arousing to the general public, and often at the top of the avoidance hierarchy for social phobia. Any performance situation may generate social phobic feelings; the larger the group, the greater the anxiety in most cases.

Males with social phobia often have problems using a public restroom to urinate due to the presence of others or the fear that others may walk in. If there is a bathroom stall to use they feel shielded from view and can urinate. However, in crowded public events such as sports or concerts, even this relatively private setting may be insufficient and trigger an inhibitory effect, and cause an inability to start the flow of their urine.

The hierarchical importance of the audience is also an issue. A teacher may feel confident lecturing to undergraduates, but feel very anxious addressing colleagues. This issue of confidence relates to the cognitive set, which underlies the formation of fear. The perception that the audience or evaluator is a superior to the socially anxious person increases the magnitude of the distress. As the person feels more vulnerable he or she feels less confident (Beck et al., 1985).

■ SHAME

Shame is consequent to the failure to perform according to personal and societal expectations and can feel devastating. If the affected persons believe their social image has been tainted, and care about the observer's opinion of them, shame is felt (Beck et al., 1985). Shame due to failing to meet expectations extends beyond the immediate social event. While the anxiety is experienced prior to and during the event, but ceases to be a problem following it. The shame can lead to depression as the individual continues to create negative beliefs related to the perceived substandard performance.

■ SOCIAL DEFICITS

Some markedly socially anxious people exhibit deficits in social skills. The defining characteristic is the absence of skills allowing social relationships. People with social skill deficits talk "at" rather than "with" people, and talk too much about themselves. They tend to be monotonous and lack eye contact (Bryant, Trower, Yardley, Urbieta & Letemendia, 1976). Patients who lack social skills training and have social anxiety benefit from treatment that addresses both problems. There is a continuum of social anxiety from discrete social phobias limited to one or more specific situations to generalized shyness in its extreme form with personality features. This generalized form is more pervasive and long lasting. Here, avoidant personality disorder is diagnosed along with social phobia (Barlow, 1988). The defining characteristic of avoidant personality disorder is hypersensitivity to rejection. Relationships cannot be risked without the guarantee of acceptance.

■ DIAGNOSIS

The following criteria is required for the DSM-IV diagnosis of social phobia.

1. A marked and persistent fear of one or more social or performance situations in which the person is exposed to unfamiliar people or to possible scrutiny by others.
2. The person fears that he/she will act in a way (or show anxiety symptoms) that will be humiliating or embarrassing. The notion that one must not appear to be anxious is a trait of social phobia. Phobic individuals are afraid that they will be seen as fearful due to their sweating, blushing, tremor, and

stammer. As physical symptoms escalate, this concern about being seen as being anxious adds to the fear, both in the moment and in anticipation of the event. Measures to prevent symptoms range from use of beta-blockers to running for hours before an event so as to "not be able to sweat." The person believes that the presence of anxiety symptoms is shaming, since it reveals to the onlooker that he/she is anxious.

3. Exposure to the feared social situation provokes anxiety.
4. Although the person recognizes that the fear is excessive or unreasonable, the feared social or performance situations are avoided or else are endured with intense anxiety or distress. Avoidance may take the form of using alcohol or other drugs to diminish the feelings or the insistence on being accompanied by another person to feared events. The duration spent in the feared event may be abbreviated by coming late and leaving early. Avoidance or distress in the feared social situation interferes significantly with the person's normal routine, occupational functioning, or social activities or relationships. People suffer from the curtailment of vocational aspirations or career choice due to avoidance of interpersonal situations. The inability to meet and talk with potential partners is frequently a limitation imposed by social phobia (APA, 1994).

■ ASSOCIATED FEATURES

Associated features of the disorder are hypersensitivity to criticism, difficulty being assertive, and low self-esteem. Co-morbid disorders associated with social phobia are panic disorder, obsessive–compulsive disorder, mood disorders, substance-related disorders and somatization disorders. Generalized social phobia is associated with avoidant personality disorder. Prevalence is estimated at 3–13 percent of the population (APA, 1994).

■ TREATMENT

Successful treatment of social phobia involves changing the cognitions or beliefs creating the fearful mindset and reducing the avoidant behavior. Cognitive behavioral therapy is the psychotherapy of choice. Cognitive interventions are similar to the treatments of other anxiety disorders. The patient must learn to view anxiety as a reaction to thoughts about the situation. This then triggers the body's fear reactions and inhibits the ability to function socially, which in turn is perceived as shameful. Patients learn to identify an exaggeration of the situation's threat and an under-estimation of their ability to cope. As with generalized anxiety disorder and panic disorder, formulating the problem then breaking it down to the various cognitive, physiological and behavioral components is very helpful for the patient.

Treatment helps the patient learn to identify automatic thoughts and understand the distorted nature of thinking as it pertains to interpersonal situations. The patient is taught to question the accuracy of distorted thoughts and re-formulate them as rational. This process decreases physiological arousal and enables the patient to interact socially without body paralysis.

The next step is to practice in a role-playing format combining cognitive countering with behavioral practice (rather than avoidance). Both in-session practice and homework is based on a hierarchy utilizing the Subjective Units of Discomfort Scale (SUDS), to identify and rank behavioral exposures according to distress (Foa & Wilson, 1991). For example, talking with a stranger might be rated a 60, talking with one's boss a 70 and talking with an attractive potential dating partner an 80. The scale allows the therapist and client to rate the various triggers/situations of social fears.

Case Study

Joe has a specific social fear of speaking with women, especially attractive ones. In the beginning of treatment, he was assigned the task of recording his automatic thoughts when he encountered women. He recorded both his thoughts and feelings. Joe noticed thoughts such as "she thinks I'm unattractive" or "she would never be interested in me." He learned to view these as examples of distorted thinking (mind reading and fortune telling). He asked himself "what evidence do I have for these thoughts?", "how do I know what she is thinking or how she may react to me?" Joe created a rational thought to replace the anxiety arousing distorted thought "I won't know how she will react unless I talk to her." In addition, his thought record included a section to prepare him for the possibility of rejection "even if she is not interested in me, at least I'll find out. If she rejects me, it doesn't mean that all women will do so. Rejection is painful but I can live with it if I don't engage in further distorted thoughts." Working in a group format is most effective as it allows for support from others with whom to practice exposures (Heimberg, 1997).

These group procedures can be adapted to individuals. It is useful for the therapist to accompany the person for the preliminary exposures since the patient gains practice utilizing his/her cognitive countering. For example, the therapist may accompany the patient to a public place, be available in between interactions for encouragement, and help process automatic thoughts immediately after encounters. If public speaking is the targeted behavior, the therapist may arrange to meet the patient at a Toastmasters group and discuss automatic thoughts before and after the patient's presentation while supporting his/her efforts to discontinue avoidance.

Relaxation methods such as progressive muscle relaxation, guided imagery, or diaphragmatic breathing reduce physiological arousal and associated symptoms. Due to the patient's fear of appearing anxious, it is important to address the appearance of symptoms with cognitive and exposure techniques. Regular assessment of the person's depression is recommended throughout treatment due to the frequent comorbidity of depression with social phobia. As the person confronts fear, he or she may feel the consequences of being overly critical of oneself.

■ MEDICATION TREATMENT

Medications used to treat social phobia are antidepressants, high-potency benzodiazepines, beta-blockers, and other agents. The SSRIs have become front-line medication for social phobia (Liebowitz, 1999) due to their efficacy and safety and ease of use compared to the MAOIs, which are the other class of antidepressant with documented efficacy in clinical trials (e.g., Liebowitz et al., 1992). The TCAs have not been shown to help with social phobia (Simpson et al., 1998). Another reason for the use of SSRIs is that they are effective in treating the frequently comorbid anxiety and depressive disorders. As with panic disorder, SSRIs are started at lower than standard doses and slowly increased to prevent anxiety over somatic symptoms. The short-term efficacy of SSRIs has been documented in controlled clinical trials (e.g., Stein, Fyer, Jonathan, Davidson, Pollack & Wiita, 1995). While dosage requirements are similar to those used to treat depression some patients benefit from higher doses. High-potency benzodiazepines such as alprazolam and clonazepam can be used to effectively treat social phobia. They, however, do not treat the frequently comorbid depression and anxiety disorders such as OCD and PTSD. More frequently, benzodiazepines are added to SSRIs to provide some symptomatic relief before the SSRI has taken effect. One advantage of benzodiazepines is that they rapidly decrease anxiety and can therefore be used on an "as needed" basis to cope with sudden anxiety in settings where the person needs to stay calm. Beta-blocker drugs block beta-adrenergic receptors that are stimulated by the stress hormone adrenaline. This hormone, released as anxiety, stimulates the adrenergic receptors to cause somatic manifestations of anxiety such as rapid heart beat, rapid breathing, and tremulousness. Beta-blockers such as propranolol and atenolol reduce the anxiety. They are effective in the treatment of nongeneralized forms of social phobia (e.g., public speaking or stage performance), but are less effective in treating generalized social phobia (Liebowitz et al., 1992). For nongeneralized social phobia, these medications are frequently used on as needed basis 1–2 hours prior to the event. When used like this, it is important for the patient to have tried the agent previously to ensure that there are no adverse medication side effects (e.g., low blood pressure and pulse with dizziness). Other agents that may help alone or as an augmentation strategy are the antidepressants venlafaxine and nefazodone, and the anticonvulsant gabapentin. Long-term medication data is limited. SSRIs can show continuing benefits and help prevent relapse even after acute treatment (Stein et al., 1996). At this point, it is recommended that treatment be continued for a year after substantial improvement. If symptoms recur after a slow taper of medication, long-term treatment may be necessary.

Specific Phobias

■ DESCRIPTION

Specific phobia is estimated to have a lifetime incidence of 5–10 percent making it the most common of psychiatric disorders. However, it is rarely the presenting problem at medical or psychiatric facilities. Types of specific phobia seen in psychiatric clinics are primarily claustrophobia, blood phobia, illness/injury phobia, injection phobia, dental phobia, and small animal phobia (Barlow, 1988). Specific phobia is a reaction of significant anxiety when confronted by, or when imagining a specific situation, object, animal, or activity. Panic level anxiety is common when faced with the phobic trigger. The proximity to the situation is correlated with the level of anxiety. The person has significant distress about having the disorder and it interferes with life when he/she is in contact with the phobic object/situation. Phobic patients seek treatment when the phobic-related behavior causes significant interference in their life and their coping techniques have failed. Changes in their environment may bring on an exacerbation of their phobia.

■ DIAGNOSIS

Diagnostic criteria for specific phobia include (APA, 1994):

1. Marked and persistent fear that is excessive, unreasonable, and cued by the presence or anticipation of a specific object or situation.
2. Exposure to the phobic stimulus almost invariably provokes an immediate anxiety response, which may take the form of a situationally bound or predisposed panic attack.
3. The person recognizes the fear is excessive or unreasonable.
4. The phobic situation is avoided or endured with intense anxiety or distress.
5. The avoidance, anxious anticipation, or distress in the feared situation interferes significantly with the person's normal routine, occupational functioning, social activities or relationships, and there is marked distress about having the phobia. For example, if the person has a fear of a phobic trigger object like snakes, but lives in a city and rarely if ever thinks about or encounters snakes, he or she will not be diagnosed with a phobia. DSM-IV stipulates this disorder must cause significant distress or interference.

■ ONSET AND COURSE

The etiology of specific phobia is usually in response to a traumatic event in childhood. It is a chronic condition with a less than 20 percent change of remitting without treatment. Blood and injury phobias, situational and animal phobias are likely family based in their transmission. There is a frequent co-occurrence between specific phobias and anxiety disorders, especially panic disorder with agoraphobia (APA, 1994).

■ TREATMENT

The recommended therapy for specific phobia is cognitive behavioral exposure based treatment. Systematic desensitization treatment for specific phobias was an early behavioral therapy intervention, and led to research into the behavioral treatment of other anxiety disorders like panic-disorder-related agoraphobia. Treatment involves behavioral analysis of the cognitions, behavior, and physical sensations involved in the phobia. The phobic triggers and situations are ranked according to a Subjective Units of Distress Scale (SUDs) as with OCD or social phobia treatment, and then an exposure treatment plan is formulated. After repetitive exposure for a sufficient time (1–2 hours) the individual habituates to the phobic trigger. The next item on the hierarchy becomes the next exposure task.

Case Example

Angela had a swallowing phobia that created the feeling that she had a great difficulty swallowing. Angela thought she couldn't eat anything requiring chewing, for fear she would choke and die. Maladaptive coping strategies were used to reduce the anxiety from exposure to the phobic activity of eating. Angela would only eat alone as she felt the need for absolute quiet. Most foods were avoided and she had reduced her intake to liquids and very soft foods or liquified-foods from the blender.

Treatment involved progressive exposure to food that was increasingly challenging to chew. Angela was taught to challenge scary thoughts about eating and to look for the evidence that corroborates her fear and create a more rational thought. For example, Angela was taught to ask herself, "What evidence do I have that I will choke on this meat?" She also asked, "Wasn't I able to chew things for many years and swallow them like everyone else?" She was taught to then formulate a rational thought, "If I chew it appropriately and allow myself to relax, it is likely that I will swallow as readily as most people." Also countered are over-estimations concerning the danger of dying if she should choke. "If I do choke, how likely is it that it will lead to my death? Have I ever choked and not died?" She was taught relaxation techniques in general with particular attention to her throat muscles. Angela was also taught to visualize the desired goal of swallowing the meat, or whatever challenging food she was working on. Angela habituated to the feared item on the hierarchy, then moved up to the next item.

Situations or proximity to feared objects are ordered and ranked according to the item's ability to create fear. As with Angela, graduated hierarchies for the progression of exposures are beneficial in that they allow patients to gradually acclimate to their fears. For Angela, a lower level exposure would be a banana, rated at 40, while peanut butter might be an 80, and a piece of steak a 90. If the higher level items are started first, the treatment can succeed. However, there is the danger that patients may prematurely stop treatment as the level of distress is less easily tolerated. The cognitive component combines the countering of distorted thoughts and the explanation of the treatment rationale and psychoeducation concerning the nature of phobias, avoidance and habituation. It is important that the patient remain in the feared situation until their anxiety diminishes to a significant degree. The exposure should be repetitive and frequent until the fear decreases. Patients with specific phobias respond readily to exposure treatment.

REFERENCES

Allen, A. J., Leonard, H. L., & Swedo, S. E. (1995). Case study: A new infection-triggered, autoimmune subtype of pediatric OCD and Tourette's syndrome. *Journal of the American Academy of Child & Adolescent Psychiatry, 34*(3), 307–311.

American Psychiatric Association (APA) (1987). *Diagnostic and statistical manual of mental disorders,* 3rd ed., revised. Washington, DC: American Psychiatric Association.

American Psychiatric Association (APA) (1994). *Diagnostic and statistical manual of mental disorders*, 4th ed. Washington, DC: American Psychiatric Association.

Baer, L. (1993). Behavior therapy for obsessive-compulsive disorder in the office-based practice. *Journal of Clinical Psychiatry, 54* (6 Suppl.), 10–15.

Ballenger, J. C., Burrows, G. D., DuPont, R. L., Jr., Lesser, I. M., Noyes, R., Jr., Pecknold, J. C., Rifkin, A., & Swinson, R. P. (1988). Alprazolam in panic disorder and agoraphobia: results from a multi-center trial. I. Efficacy in short-term treatment. *Archives of General Psychiatry, 45*(5), 413–422.

Barlow, D. H. (1988). *Anxiety and its disorders*. New York, NY: Guilford Press.

Barlow, D. H., Blanchard, E. B., Vermilyea, J. A., Vermilya, B. B., & Di Nardo, P. A. (1986). Generalized anxiety and generalized anxiety disorder: Description and reconceptualization. *American Journal of Psychiatry, 143*, 40–44.

Barlow, D. H., & Craske, M. (1989). *Mastery of your anxiety and panic*. Albany: Graywind.

Beck, A. T., Emory, G., & Greenburg, R. L. (1985) *Anxiety disorders and phobias*. New York: Basic Books.

Bouchard, C., Rheaume, J., & Ladouceur, R. (1999). Responsibility and perfectionism in OCD: An experimental study. *Behavior Research and Therapy, 37*(3), 239–248.

Boyer, W. (1995). Serotonin uptake inhibitors are superior to imipramine and alprazolam in alleviating panic attacks: A meta-analysis. *International Clinical Psychopharmacology, 10*(1), 45–49.

Bryant, B., Trower, P., Yardley, K., Urbieta, H., & Letemendia, F. (1976). Social inadequacy among psychiatric outpatients. *Psychological Medicine, 6*, 101–112.

Burns, D. (1980). *Feeling good: The new mood therapy*. New York: William Morrow Co.

Butler, G., & Booth, R. G. (1991). Developing psychological treatments for generalized anxiety disorder. In: R. M. Rapee & D. H. Barlow (Eds.), *Chronic anxiety, generalized anxiety disorder and mixed anxiety-depression*. New York, NY: Guilford Press.

Connor, K. M., & Davidson, J. R. (1998). Generalized anxiety disorder: neurobiological and pharmacotherapeutic perspectives. *Biological Psychiatry, 44*(12), 1286–1294.

Davies, P. (Ed.) (1976). *American Heritage Dictionary of the English Language*. New York: Dell Publishing.

Davidson, J. R., & Connor, K. M. (1999). Management of posttraumatic stress disorder: diagnostic and therapeutic issues. *Journal of Clinical Psychiatry, 60* (Suppl. 18), 33–38.

Davidson, J. R., DuPont, R. L., Hedges, D., & Haskins, J. T. (1999). Efficacy, safety, and tolerability of venlafaxine extended release and buspirone in outpatients with generalized anxiety disorder. *Journal of Clinical Psychiatry, 60*(8), 528–535.

Dupont, R. L., Rice, D. P., Shiraki, S., & Rowland, C. (1994) Economic costs of obsessive–compulsive disorder. Unpublished.

Eisen, J. L., Phillips, K. A., & Rasmussen, S. A.(1999). Obsessions and delusions: The relationship between obsessive-compulsive disorder and the psychotic disorders. *Psych Annals, 29*(9), 515–522.

Foa, E. B., Davidson, R. T., & Frances, A. (1999). The expert consensus guideline series: Treatment of posttraumatic stress disorder. *Journal of Clinical Psychiatry, 60* (Suppl. 16).

Foa, E. B., & Zoellner, L. A. (1998). Posttraumatic stress disorder in female victims of assault: Theory and treatment. In: E. Sanavio et al. (Eds.), *Behavior and cognitive therapy today: Essays in honor of Hans J. Eysenck*. Oxford, UK: Anonima Romana.

Foa, E. B., & Wilson, R. (1991). *Stop obsessing*. New York: Bantam Books.

Freeston, M. H., & Ladouceur, R. (1996). *The cognitive behavioral treatment of obsessions: A treatment manual*. Quebec: Université Laval.

Goodman, W. K. (1999). Obsessive-compulsive disorder: Diagnosis and treatment. *Journal of Clinical Psychiatry, 60* (Suppl. 18), 27–32.

Goodwin, D. (1986). *Anxiety*. New York/Oxford: Oxford University Press.

Gorman, J. M. (1997). The use of newer antidepressants for panic disorder. *Journal of Clinical Psychiatry, 58* (Suppl. 14), 54–58.

Greist, J. (1994). Behavior therapy for obsessive compulsive disorder. *Journal of Clinical Psychiatry, 55* (Suppl. 10), 60–68

Grinspoon, L. (Ed.) (1998). Obsessive–compulsive disorder Part II. *Harvard Mental Health Letter, 15*(5), November, 1–4.

Heimberg, R. G. (1997). A cognitive behavioral treatment package of social anxiety. In: W. T. Roth & I. D. Yalom (Eds.), *Treating anxiety disorders. The Jossey–Bass library of current clinical technique*. San Francisco, CA: Jossey- Bass Inc.

Hoehn-Saric, R., McLeod, D. R., & Zimmerli, W. D. (1988). Differential effects of alprazolam and imipramine in generalized anxiety disorder: somatic versus psychic symptoms. *Journal of Clinical Psychiatry, 49*(8), 293–301.

Hollander, E. (1998). Treatment of obsessive–compulsive spectrum disorders with SSRIs. *British Journal of Psychiatry Supplement, 35*, 7–12.

Hollander, E., & Stein, D. J. (1997). *Obsessive–compulsive disorders: Diagnosis–etiology–treatment*. New York: Marcel Dekker.

Jenike, M. A. (1998). Drug treatment of obsessive compulsive disorders. In: M. A. Jenike, L. Baer & W. E. Minichiello (Eds.), *Obsessive compulsive disorders: Practical management* (3rd ed., pp. 469–532). St. Louis: Mosby.

Lader, M., & Scotto, J. C. (1998). A multicentre double-blind comparison of hydroxyzine, buspirone and placebo in patients with generalized anxiety disorder. *Psychopharmacology, 139*(4), 402–406.

Lecrubier, Y., & Judge, R. (1997). Long-term evaluation of paroxetine, clomipramine and placebo in panic disorder. Collaborative Paroxetine Panic Study Investigators. *Acta Psychiatrica Scandinavica, 95*(2), 153–160.

Leonard, H. L. (1997). New developments in the treatment of obsessive-compulsive disorder. *Journal of Clinical Psychiatry, 58* (Suppl. 14), 39–45.

Liebowitz, M. R. (1999). Update on the diagnosis and treatment of social anxiety disorder. *Journal of Clinical Psychiatry, 60* (Suppl. 18), 22–26.

Liebowitz, M. R., Schneier, F., Campeas, R., Hollander, E., Hatterer, J., Fyer, A., Gorman, J., Papp, L., Davies, S., & Gully, R. (1992). Phenelzine vs atenolol in social phobia. A placebo-controlled comparison. *Archives of General Psychiatry, 49*(4), 290–300.

Marks, I. M. (1987) *Fears, phobias, and rituals: Panic, anxiety, and their disorders.* New York/Oxford: Oxford University Press.

Matsakis, A. (1994). *Post-traumatic stress disorder, a complete treatment guide.* Oakland: New Harbinger Publications.

Michelson, D., Pollack, M., Lydiard, R. B., Tamura, R., Tepner, R., & Tollefson, G. (1999). Continuing treatment of panic disorder after acute response: Randomized, placebo-controlled trial with fluoxetine. The Fluoxetine Panic Disorder Study Group. *British Journal of Psychiatry, 174,* 213–218.

Mitchell, J. T., & Everly, G. S. (1993). *Critical incident stress debriefing—An operations manual for the prevention of traumatic stress among emergency services and disaster workers.* Ellicott City: Chevron Publishing.

Neziroglu, F., & Yaryura-Tobias, J. A. (1991). *Over and over again.* San Francisco: Jossey-Bass Publishers.

Pauls, D.L., et al. (1995) A family study of OCD. *American Journal of Psychiatry, 152*(1), 76–84.

Phillipson, S. (1991). Thinking the unthinkable. *The Obsessive-Compulsive Newsletter, 5*(4), Obsessive-Compulsive Foundation.

Pigott, T. A. (1998). Obsessive-compulsive disorder: symptom overview and epidemiology. *Bulletin of the Menniger Clinic, 62* (4 Suppl.), 4–32.

Piggott, T. A. (1999a). Gender differences in the epidemiology and treatment of anxiety disorders. *Journal of Clinical Psychiatry Supplement, 18* (16), 4–15.

Pigott, T. A. (1999b). A review of the efficacy of selective serotonin reuptake inhibitors in obsessive-compulsive disorder. *Journal of Clinical Psychiatry, 60*(2), 101–106.

Rapee, R., & Barlow, D. (Eds.) (1991). *Chronic Anxiety.* New York: Guilford Press.

Rassin, E., Merckel, H., Muris, P., & Spaan, V. (1999). Thought-action fusion as a causal factor in the development of intrusions. *Behavioral Research and Therapy, 37*(3), 231–237.

Rocca, P., Fonzo, V., Scotta, M., Zanalda, E., & Ravizza, L. (1997). Paroxetine efficacy in the treatment of generalized anxiety disorder. *Acta Psychiatrica Scandinavica, 95*(5), 444–450.

Roy-Byrne, P., Stein, M., Russo, J., Mercier, E., Thomas, R., McQuaid, J., Katon, W., Craske, M., Bystritsky, A., & Sherbourne, C. (1999). Panic disorder in the primary care setting: comorbidity, disability, service utilization, and treatment. *Journal of Clinical Psychiatry, 60*(7), 492–499.

Salkovskis, P. M., Forrester, E., & Richards, C. (1998). Cognitive-behavioral approach to understanding obsessional thinking. *British Journal of Psychiatry Supplement, 35*, 53–63.

Saxena, S., Brody, A. L., Schwartz, J. M., & Baxter, L. R. (1998). Neuroimaging and frontal-subcortical circuitry in obsessive-compulsive disorder. *British Journal of Psychiatry Supplement, 35*, 26–37.

Schatzberg, A. F., Cole, J. O., & DeBattista, C. (1977) *Antianxiety agents, manual of clinical psychopharmacology* (3rd ed., pp. 223–259). Washington, DC: American Psychiatric Press.

Schweizer, E., Rickels, K., Weiss, S., & Zavodnick, S. (1993). Maintenance drug treatment of panic disorder. I. Results of a prospective, placebo-controlled comparison of alprazolam and imipramine. *Archives of General Psychiatry, 50*(1), 51–60.

Sheehan, D. V. (1999). Current concepts in the treatment of panic disorder. *Journal of Clinical Psychiatry, 60* (Suppl. 18), 16–21.

Simpson, H. B., Schneier, F. R., Campeas, R. B., Marshall, R. D., Fallon, B. A., Davies, S., Klein, D. F., & Liebowitz, M. R. (1998). Imipramine in the treatment of social phobia. *Journal of Clinical Psychopharmacology, 18*(2), 132–135.

Stein, M. B., Chartier, M. J., Hazen, A. L., Kroft, C. D., Chale, R. A., Cote, D., & Walker, J. R. (1996). Paroxetine in the treatment of generalized social phobia: open-label treatment and double-blind placebo-controlled discontinuation. *Journal of Clinical Psychopharmacology, 16*(3), 218–222.

Stein, M. B., Fyer, A. J., Jonathan, R., Davidson, T., Pollack, M. H., & Wiita, B. (1999). Fluvoxamine treatment of social phobia (social anxiety disorder): A double-blind, placebo-controlled study. *American Journal of Psychiatry, 156*, 756–760.

Veale, D. (1993). Classification and treatment of obsessional slowness. *British Journal of Psychiatry, 162*, 198–203.

van der Kolk, B. (1994). The body keeps the score: Memory and the evolving psychobiology of posttraumatic stress. *Harvard Review of Psychiatry, 1*(5), 253–262.

Weisman, M. W., et al. (1997). The cross national epidemiology of panic disorder. *Archives of General Psychiatry, 54*(4), 305–309.

Wesson, D. R., Smith, D. E., Ling, W., & Seymour, R. (1997). Sedative-hypnotics and tricyclics. In: J. H. Lowinson, P. Ruiz, R. B. Millman, & J. G. Langrod (Eds.), *Substance abuse: A comprehensive textbook* (pp. 223–230). Baltimore, MD: Williams & Wilkins.

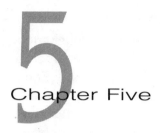

Chapter Five

Schizophrenia

Jason Rosenstock • Noreen Fredrick • Rohan Ganguli

Introduction

The first clearly described case of schizophrenia in English literature probably dates back to 1810, when Bethlem Hospital's John
Haslam described the case of James Tilly Matthews, who became
convinced that an "infernal machine" was torturing and controlling him. In a series of illustrations, Matthews showed how the
machine undertook "lobster-cracking, bomb-bursting, and brain
lengthening" in an effort to subdue him (in Stone, 1997).

Certainly patients who suffer from such delusions and hallucinations have long fascinated our society. One of the hallmarks of
humanity is the proper functioning of the mind's higher order cognitive and perceptual processes; it is in large part what separates
human beings from animals. Patients who develop schizophrenia
lose core cognitive functioning and usually show quite dramatic
behavioral symptoms and social decline. How can the mind
become so "unglued" in some patients? What happens to such
people over time? Can patients with these problems be restored
to sanity?

One of the major obstacles to answering these questions has
been the heterogeneity of schizophrenia. In fact, illnesses as
diverse as catatonia, hebephrenia, and paranoia started out as

separate diagnostic entities, at least until Emil Kraepelin lumped them together in 1899 under the rubric of dementia praecox, based on a common longitudinal course and prognosis. Eugen Bleuler renamed the disorder "schizophrenia," or "split mind," in 1911, extending the "lumping" to the "group of schizophrenias." Even today, DSM-IV (American Psychiatric Association, 1994) continues to utilize neo-Kraepelinian criteria to describe schizophrenia, encompassing a wide variety of clinical presentations: from the agitated patient who fears that aliens have inserted recording devices in the hospital vents to the amotivated and expressionless patient who denies hallucinations but has little to say about anything else anyway. Heterogeneity, therefore, hampers research efforts and challenges our classification schema.

But schizophrenia in general challenges psychiatry on a variety of other fronts. Almost mockingly, the origin of the illness defies explanation—despite massive neuroscientific research and the devoted pursuits of the finest psychiatrists of previous and current generations. Moreover, even though we know a great deal about rehabilitation and recovery from this disorder, schizophrenia continues to exact a devastating toll on patients, families, and society as a whole. Most recently, schizophrenia has come to serve as an "outlier" in the managed care revolution: a chronic illness that does not fit neatly into short-term, episode-based, cure-oriented, and resource-rationed care models.

The most essential paradox of schizophrenia is its clear status as a biologically based disorder, but with environmental and psychosocial factors significantly influencing its course. As such, physicians alone cannot adequately treat this illness. Therapy requires the collaboration of a variety of mental health professionals and community resources.

These challenges and paradoxes make schizophrenia all the more important to study, learn from, and understand. To that end, we present a brief overview of the illness, with special attention to the epidemiology, etiology, assessment, comorbidity, and treatment of schizophrenia. Family issues, self-help, and outcome measurement will also be addressed. We hope this chapter provides a basic summary of the current thinking on schizophrenia; readers interested in more in-depth discussions of issues we raise are encouraged to pursue sources listed in the reference section.

Prevalence

Roughly 2 million Americans suffer from schizophrenia. Schizophrenia is an illness without boundaries. It occurs in all cultures and in all socioeconomic groups. The National Institute of Mental Health's Epidemiologic Catchment Area Study used the DSM-III criteria for schizophrenia and found the lifetime prevalence ranged from 0.6 to 1.9 percent of the population, slightly less than 1 case per 100 persons in the population (Robins, Helzer, Weissman et al., 1984). Schizophrenia can occur to anyone at any time but the risk is greater if an individual has a relative with schizophrenia. The probability of an individual developing schizophrenia if neither parents nor brothers nor sisters has the illness is about 1 percent. If a parent or sibling has the illness the chances of developing schizophrenia go up to 10 percent. If both parents have schizophrenia chances go up to 40 percent. Onset of schizophrenia tends to be late adolescence or early adulthood. Onset of the illness is somewhat different by sex: schizophrenia affects more men than women in the 16–25-year age group and affects more women in the 25–30-year age group (Weiden, Scheifler, McEvoy et al., 1999).

Profiles

Case Study 1

Joe was a good student all through high school. He was a member of the football team, maintained good grades, and made honor roll each semester. He was outgoing and popular. Toward the end of his first semester of college, everything began to change. Joe no longer ate meals with his friends; in fact he began to isolate in his room. He began to ignore his personal hygiene and stopped attending classes. Joe had difficulty concentrating and had to read the same sentence over and over. He began to believe that the words in his textbook had special meaning for him and somehow were giving him a message for a secret mission. Joe began to suspect that his roommates were tampering with his phone and his computer, that they were monitoring his activities. Joe became afraid that his roommates knew about the messages in his textbook and were now trying to manipulate him. Joe began to believe his roommates could read his thoughts, in fact anyone he passed in the hall or on the street could tell what he was thinking. When Joe was alone in his room he could hear the whispers of those he believed were monitoring him. He couldn't quite make out what they were saying but he was convinced they were talking about him.

Case Study 2

Roger is a 36-year old male who has a long history of hearing a voice that tells him to hurt himself and others. He has responded to this voice in the past and spent time in prison for assaulting an individual with a knife. He also fears being hurt by his enemies resulting in his not sleeping in order to protect himself. Roger actively uses alcohol, cannabis and cocaine to manage his symptoms. Roger has a long history of stopping his medications due to the discomfort he experiences from side effects: He reports that he feels so restless and can't stop pacing. He initially experienced relief when using drugs and alcohol but soon found that the more he used the more paranoid and guarded he became and his symptoms would return with a vengeance. Roger's constant worry of hurting others and fear of being harmed has resulted in occasional suicidal ideation with plan. He is not able to recognize the connection of medication and drug use with symptom control and exacerbation, respectively. Roger also struggles with diabetes and fluctuating blood sugars due to poor nutrition and alcohol use.

Case Study 3

Edward spends all day in bed, if he can. Before he got sick, he used to enjoy spending time with his family, or working. Sometimes he thinks about working, and sometimes he makes plans, but he simply cannot seem to get to interviews or vocational rehabilitation appointments. When he visits his parents, they try to draw him out, talking about family issues, or politics; Edward doesn't have much to say. Although he denies feeling depressed, and he expresses hope about the future, he hardly ever smiles and hates to do the dishes or make his bed. Psychiatrists have asked him about voices—but Edward insists he has never heard any. When he was hospitalized initially, he remembers, he had a hard time keeping his thoughts straight, and he knows he was acting strangely because the police picked him up wandering the streets at night in a scuba-diving suit. But Edward can't remember why, and it doesn't seem important to him anymore anyway.

Causes

The actual cause of schizophrenia has eluded psychiatry for years, in large part due to the fact that there is no single cause for the illness. Schizophrenia, as these cases illustrate, represents a heterogeneous group of disease states, with several etiological pathways leading to similar outcomes, but with important differences in clinical presentation. Nevertheless, we can divide these pathways into two major routes: biological and psychosocial/environmental. Both domains carry relevance for schizophrenia pathogenesis, and for most patients with this illness, the etiology must be considered as multifactorial.

Biological factors certainly must be involved in the development of schizophrenia. Twin studies have shown that the concordance rate for monozygotic sibling pairs approaches 45 percent, while concordance for dizygotic pairings drops to 20 percent. If a person has a first-degree relative with schizophrenia, their relative risk of developing the disorder themselves is 10 percent; for second-degree relatives, the relative risk drops to 3 percent.

Therefore, a genetic contribution to the etiology of schizophrenia clearly exists, and much effort is currently underway to elucidate this link (Kendler, McGuire, Gruenberg et al., 1994).

The exact method of inheritance, however, has long been elusive to researchers. The genetic transmission is probably non-Mendelian. A single locus with incomplete penetrance or variable phenotypic expressivity is possible, and linkage and association studies have suggested some possible "hot spots" for schizophrenia transmission—chromosomes 6, 8, and 22 have been flagged. However, findings have either been contradicted or confirmed only in select subpopulations (e.g., African-American women). Given the multifactorial nature of the etiology, the heterogeneous clinical presentation, sampling problems, and other methodological issues, it will probably be impossible to localize and isolate one chromosome or gene that causes schizophrenia in all patients (Nimgaonkar, Rudert, Zhang et al., 1997).

Working backward, treatment strategy itself has led researchers to speculate on other biological factors that may lead to schizophrenia—particularly biochemical causes. Because the efficacy of antipsychotic medication correlates with dopamine receptor blockade (especially the D2 receptor), Carlsson, Hansson, Waters, and Carlsson (1997) have postulated that schizophrenia may be caused by either a relative excess of dopamine in the brain or an overexcitation of post-synaptic dopamine receptors. The so-called dopamine hypothesis (Willner, 1997) is also supported by a variety of other evidence, but the relationship between dopamine and psychotic symptoms is nonspecific and does not explain negative symptoms (Schwartz, Diaz, Borodet et al., 1998). The recent development of "atypical" antipsychotics has spurred research into serotonin, with evidence suggesting a correlation between negative symptom improvement and serotonin receptor antagonism, as well as feedback relationships between serotonergic and dopaminergic neurons in the frontal lobe (Meltzer, 1995). Glutamate and other excitatory amino acids like aspartate have attracted the most recent attention as possible offenders in schizophrenia, with particular focus on NMDA receptors in temporal and limbic regions of the brain (Olney & Farber, 1995; Mohn, Gainetdinov, Cron & Koller, 1999).

Neuroimaging and neuropathological investigations have supplemented biochemical work, as scientists hope to clarify structural/neuroanatomical and functional/neurophysiological factors that may lead to schizophrenia. The single best-documented finding from such studies is the presence of cortical atrophy in the brains of schizophrenia patients. However, the difference is small (perhaps a 6 percent reduction in total brain volume) and rather nonspecific (Raz & Raz, 1990; Harvey, Run, DuBoulay et al., 1993; Gur, Mozley, Resnick et al., 1991; Buckley, 1998a).

Specific brain regions of interest have included the striatum, the temporal lobe and associated limbic structures, the prefrontal cortex, and the thalamus. Findings have been somewhat inconsistent, frequently confounded by the effects of antipsychotics and patient selection. Nevertheless, many patients with schizophrenia seem to have larger basal ganglia volumes (especially the caudate), with asymmetries in superior temporal gyrus and hippocampal volumes (smaller on the left) (Gur & Pearlson, 1993).

Negative symptoms have been specifically linked with "hypofrontality"—lower blood flow or glucose metabolism in frontal lobe structures (Andreasen, Rezai, Alliger et al., 1992). Neuropsychological deficits are consistent with prefrontal lobe dysfunction, especially the dorsolateral prefrontal cortex, an area of the brain intimately involved with abstract thinking and mental planning (Weickert & Kleinman, 1998).

A wide variety of other biologically based theories of schizophrenia have been proposed, ranging from abnormalities in phospholipid metabolism and cell membrane structure (Horrobin, 1998), to immunological abnormalities either in cytokines or autoantibodies (Rothermudnt, Arolt, Weitzsch et al., 1998). One of the oldest etiological theories posits infectious agents, especially viruses, as a cause of the illness; however, the evidence remains inconclusive and the vector, even if it exists, could only account for a small proportion of cases (Mednick, Machon, Huttunen et al., 1988).

Infections provide a useful segue to discussing environmental causes of schizophrenia. Second-trimester viral infections are but one kind of in utero insult that may predispose a person to developing schizophrenia. Other insults include malnutrition, birth trauma, and hypoxia, although most patients do not have such perinatal complications (McNeil, 1995; Cannon, Mednick, Parnas et al., 1993; Sacker, Done, & Crow, 1996).

Another environmental factor that may contribute to schizophrenia is the patient's family life, particularly communication styles. Ambiguous use of language—such as inconsistent references or partial disqualifications—may confuse and distract growing children, interfering with the development of efficient information processing. Although theories about "schizophrenogenic mothers" have been rejected, an interactive effect between genetic risk and "communication deviance" seems to exist, suggesting that environmental factors may indeed increase a person's risk for developing the disorder (Wahlberg, Wynne, Oja et al., 1997).

These multitudinous threads of possible etiologies come together in the neurodevelopmental model of schizophrenia. Over the past decade or so, this explanatory model has gained momentum as Daniel Weinberger (1987) and others have tried to marshal evidence from neuroanatomy, neuroimaging, genetics, immunochemistry, epidemiology, animal studies, and a variety of other sources. The model seeks to address the long-standing mystery of why and how patients come to have this disorder—and in particular, why the symptoms begin in late adolescence or early adulthood. Neurodevelopmentalists suggest that schizophrenia grows out of abnormal brain development beginning in utero, a kind of "doom from the womb," based on genetic susceptibility and in many cases environmental insults. Age of symptom onset can then be explained by adolescence-related developmental changes in the central nervous system, especially synaptic pruning (Keshavan, Anderson, Pettegrew et al., 1994); the illness has a fairly static picture thereafter. This theory has been supported by a wealth of neurobiological studies which particularly explore the crucial period early in the course of the illness, or even before the recognition of the disorder itself.

Despite a wider acceptance of the neurodevelopmental model, there are many aspects of the disorder that cannot be explained, and the competing neurodegenerative model (with its roots in Kraepelinian conceptions of dementia praecox) cannot be completely refuted. For example, Rapoport, Giedd, Blumenthal et al. (1999) have recently published outstanding longitudinal studies in adolescents with schizophrenia showing progressive ventricular enlargement years after a first diagnosis of schizophrenia. Perhaps etiologic heterogeneity can explain some of the conflicting evidence; methodological inconsistencies have certainly hampered research in this area; and some have argued that the models may be more complementary than anti-thetical (Waddington, Lane, Scully et al., 1998). Nevertheless, the growth of and challenges to the neurodevelopmental model have made the past few years a very exciting time for clinicians and researchers alike, and the model sets the agenda for etiological speculation and research into the 21st century.

Common Effects

Schizophrenia, like other severe and persistent mental illnesses, has a representative natural history that includes: (1) onset at a young age; (2) a relapsing and remitting course over years; and (3) remissions that are characterized by incomplete symptom resolution or residual functional deficits. The disorder can have profound effects on the patient, the family, and society as a whole.

The worst outcome in schizophrenia is suicide. About 20 percent of patients with the illness attempt to kill themselves, and 10 percent complete the act. Most patients who suicide do so shortly after a hospitalization—50 percent within 6 months—and the attempts are associated with increased levels of insight and hopelessness. Such patients usually have higher premorbid functioning and suicide early in the course of illness. Other risk factors include:

low-dose medication, abrupt disruptions in pharmacotherapy, social isolation, male gender (75 percent of suicides), and non-supportive families (Drake, Gates, Whitaker, & Cotton, 1985; Weiden et al., 1999).

For patients who survive with schizophrenia, the symptom burden alone is often overwhelming. Positive symptoms such as hallucinations or thought disorganization can severely impair functioning and cause significant distress. Negative symptoms such as avolition and poverty of thought, along with cognitive dysfunction (particularly in attention and working memory), greatly hamper quality-of-life and may be more closely linked with ultimate functional attainment (Ho, Nopoulos, Flaum et al., 1998).

Other effects can be grouped into basic functioning domains:

- *Educational.* With an illness onset in late adolescence or early adulthood, educational impairment is common. Many patients drop out of high school or college. Functional illiteracy occurs frequently.
- *Occupational.* Occupational disability is also common for patients with schizophrenia. At least 80 percent of such patients lack employment, and many qualify for permanent disability.
- *Socioeconomic.* Not surprisingly, many of these patients suffer from poverty and homelessness. Perhaps one-quarter to one-third of the homeless have schizophrenia, and patients with the disorder are at nearly 20 times higher risk of becoming homeless (Mobray, 1985). The low socioeconomic class of patients with this disorder, previously thought to represent a risk factor ("social causation" theory), is now acknowledged to reflect the "downward drift" of patients who cannot achieve in society because of the illness itself.
- *Legal/Violence.* Although the general population fears that people with schizophrenia will commit violent crimes at a high rate, most studies of legal involvement suggest that any increase in arrests is due to misdemeanors like disorderly conduct rather than felonies. In fact,

patients with schizophrenia are far more likely to be victimized by crime than the general public (Maxmen & Ward, 1995). Violent acts are usually committed by patients with active paranoia, not on any medication, and abusing substances (Steadman, Mulvey, Monahan et al., 1998).

- *Medical.* Patients with schizophrenia may have poor self-care and general medical follow-up, predisposing them to greater medical illness, decreased physical functioning, and a shortened life span.
- *Emotional.* Emotional effects of such an illness and its consequences may include guilt, shame, hopelessness, and anger.
- *Family/Interpersonal.* The symptoms and disabilities can severely impair family and interpersonal relations. Social disruptions are common, and patients may need to cope with much isolation and conflict. Most find it hard to attain developmental milestones, especially independence, identity, and intimacy. Patients with schizophrenia are less likely to marry, more likely to divorce or separate, less likely to be sexually active, and have fewer children (Maxmen & Ward, 1995).

Meanwhile, parents of such patients suffer uncertainty, guilt, anger, financial burden, and hopelessness, siblings may progress through stages of resentment, guilt, and anxiety about their own vulnerability for schizophrenia.

Assessment

For patients suspected of having schizophrenia, the assessment consists mostly of the history and mental status examination, supplemented by a physical examination and relevant testing. Unfortunately, there is no single test or finding that discriminates between those with and without the illness; diagnosis remains based on the overall clinical presentation. Diagnostic criteria as outlined in the DSM-IV (American Psychiatric Association, 1994) include:

A. *Characteristic symptoms*: Two (or more) of the following, each present for a significant portion of time during a one-month period (or less if successfully treated):

1. delusions
2. hallucinations
3. disorganized speech (e.g., frequent derailment or incoherence)
4. grossly disorganized or catatonic behavior
5. negative symptoms, i.e., affective flattening, alogia, or avolition

Note: Only one Criterion A symptom is required if delusions are bizarre or hallucinations consist of a voice keeping a running commentary on the person's behavior or thoughts, or two or more voices conversing with each other.

B. *Social/occupational dysfunction*: For a significant portion of the time since the onset of the disturbance, one or more major areas of functioning such as work, interpersonal relations, or self-care are markedly below the level achieved prior to the onset (or when the onset is in childhood or adolescence, failure to achieve expected level of interpersonal, academic, or occupational achievement).

C. *Duration*: Continuous signs of the disturbance persist for at least 6 months. This 6-month period must include at least 1 month of symptoms (or less if successfully treated) that met Criterion A (i.e., active-phase symptoms) and may include periods of prodromal or residual symptoms. During these prodromal or residual periods, the signs of the disturbance may be manifested by only negative symptoms or two or more symptoms listed in Criterion A present in an attenuated form (e.g., odd beliefs, unusual perceptual experiences).

D. *Schizoaffective and Mood Disorder exclusion:* Schizoaffective Disorder and Mood Disorder with Psychotic Features have been ruled out because either (1) no major depressive, manic, or mixed episodes have occurred concurrently with the active-phase symptoms; or (2) if mood episodes have occurred during active-phase symptoms, their total duration has been brief relative to the duration of the active and residual periods.

E. *Substance/general medical condition exclusion:* The disturbance is not due to the direct physiological effects of a substance (e.g., a drug of abuse, a medication) or a general medical condition.

F. *Relationship to a Pervasive Developmental Disorder:* If there is a history of Autistic Disorder or another Pervasive Developmental disorder, the additional diagnosis of Schizophrenia is made only if prominent delusions or hallucinations are also present for at least a month (or less if successfully treated).

To determine if patients meet these criteria, clinicians should begin with a thorough history of the present illness. How long have the psychotic symptoms been going on? Was there a trigger or precipitant? Are there comorbid or confounding symptoms—depression, anxiety, mania, or recent substance abuse? What is the temporal relationship between psychosis and these other symptoms?

Past psychiatric history is obviously crucial, and social history in particular may help uncover prodromal signs and symptoms of the disorder. Family history of psychotic or non-psychotic psychiatric illnesses is very relevant, as is screening for substance use and abuse. Past medical history may reveal head injuries, seizures, or other general medical problems that may affect diagnosis and treatment.

Collateral history is usually essential in clarifying the diagnosis in cases of suspected schizophrenia. Sources of information might include family, teachers, friends, employers, or any other observers who may have interacted with the patient at some point. Medical records often provide crucial information about past symptoms or work-up.

■ MENTAL STATUS EXAMINATION

Many kinds of psychiatric disorders will present with psychosis or related symptoms, and these must be differentiated from schizophrenia:

- *Mood disorders*
  - bipolar disorder with psychotic features
  - major depression with psychotic features
- *Other psychotic disorders*
  - schizoaffective disorder
  - brief psychotic disorder
  - schizophreniform disorder
  - delusional disorder
- *Substance use*
  - cannabis
  - hallucinogens (LSD, PCP)
  - amphetamines
  - alcohol (withdrawal or intoxication)
- *Personality disorders*
  - borderline
  - schizotypal
  - schizoid
  - paranoid
- *Anxiety disorders*
  - obsessive–compulsive disorder (OCD)
  - post-traumatic stress disorder (PTSD)
- *Other*
  - delirium
  - dementia
  - malingering
  - factitious disorder
  - pervasive developmental disorder (PDD, especially autistic disorder)

— postpartum psychosis
— culture-bound syndromes (amok, koro, etc.)

Several formal screening tests, scales, and inventories have some utility in the clinical assessment of schizophrenia. The Brief Psychiatric Rating Scale (BPRS) contains 18 items of positive, negative, and other associated symptoms—useful for both assessment and monitoring of progress (Overall, 1988). Similar ratings of core symptoms include the SANS and SAPS (Scale for the Assessment of Negative and Positive Symptoms, respectively) and the Positive and Negative Symptoms Scale (PANSS) (Kay, Fiszbein, & Opler, 1987).

Overall levels of functioning and health can be recorded either through DSM-IV's Axis V or GAF score (American Psychiatric Association, 1994), Clinical Global Inventories (CGI), or SF12 rankings. Comorbidity can be measured through standard assessment tools such as the Beck or Hamilton Rating Scales for depression and anxiety, the Addiction Severity Index (ASI), or the Yale–Brown Obsessive–Compulsive Scale (Y-BOCS). Assessment for neurological abnormalities can be conducted with the Simpson-Angus Rating Scale or the Abnormal Involuntary Movement Scale (AIMS).

■ PHYSICAL EXAMINATION

A wide variety of general medical conditions may mimic the symptoms of schizophrenia:

- *Neurological*
  - cerebrovascular accident
  - complex partial epilepsy (especially temporal lobe)
  - brain tumor (especially frontal or limbic)
  - Parkinson's disease
  - Huntington's disease
- *Endocrine*
  - thyroid disorders

- — parathyroid disorders
- — Cushing's disease
- *Metabolic*
  - — B$_{12}$ deficiency
  - — folate deficiency
  - — thiamine deficiency
- *Infectious*
  - — HIV
  - — neurosyphilis
  - — herpes encephalitis
- *Other*
  - — systemic lupus erythematosus
  - — Wilson's disease
  - — medications (antihypertensives, anticholinergics, disulfiram, etc.)
  - — hepatic encephalopathy
  - — acute intermittent porphyria

A thorough physical examination, focusing on the neurological exam, is a necessary component in the assessment of those suspected of having schizophrenia. So-called "soft" neurological signs—such as incoordination, abnormal cerebellar signs, increased blink rate, and eye-tracking abnormalities—should be carefully screened for. Any evidence for general medical conditions—such as an enlarged thyroid gland, or abdominal pain—needs to be fully evaluated.

Similarly, medical testing and laboratory work should be performed to rule out general medical causes of psychotic symptoms. For "first-break" patients, such testing should include:

- Neuroimaging, preferably magnetic resonance imaging (MRI).
- Electroencephalography (EEG).
- Complete blood count with differential.
- Urine drug screen.
- Electrolytes, including calcium, magnesium, and phosphorus.

- RPR or other tests for syphilis.
- Thyroid function tests.
- As indicated: ceruloplasmin/urinary copper, HIV, porphyrins, cortisol, other.

■ SUPPORT

If a diagnosis of schizophrenia is suspected, the information should be communicated carefully but honestly to the patient and family. Often, uncertainty exists as to the final diagnosis. First-episode patients may have psychosis for less than 6 months, for instance; substance use, mood symptoms, or other factors may make it impossible to say absolutely that a patient has schizophrenia rather than a different psychosis-related condition.

Families benefit from as much support as possible following a diagnosis of schizophrenia. Family meetings with members of the treatment team, preprinted literature, articles and videos for patients and families may help in the process. Psychoeducation is the most important goal initially, but families (and patients) do better with continued support over time—perhaps through a referral to the Alliance for the Mentally Ill, a multifamily support group, or other peer/family advocacy efforts.

For both patients and families, it is important to watch for and guard against hopelessness. The diagnosis of schizophrenia does not mean that the patient's life is over, although expectations may need to be adapted. The focus for patients and families (and for providers) should not be on disability and deficits, but on recovery and rehabilitation. The sooner this process begins, the better the prognosis.

Comorbidity

Substance abuse may be the most important comorbidity in schizophrenia. Anywhere from one-third to two-thirds of patients with schizophrenia abuse at least one substance, most commonly alcohol, cannabis, and cocaine (in that order). Although some patients report self-medicating specific symptoms (e.g., using stimulants to relieve negative symptoms), most present with a variable temporal course that suggests two independently originating primary disorders: true dual diagnosis (Salloum, Moss, & Daley, 1991; Schneier & Siris, 1987; Hien, 1993; Mueser, Yarnold, Levinson et al., 1990).

The co-existence of substance abuse with schizophrenia has crucial implications for diagnosis, prognosis, and treatment. The effects of substance abuse (for example, alcoholic hallucinosis) can in many cases mimic the symptoms of schizophrenia, and clinicians must be mindful to distinguish clearly between the disorders. Substance abuse can certainly exacerbate symptoms of schizophrenia, and the presence of substance abuse serves as a profound negative prognostic sign: greater symptom burden; probably greater neurocognitive deficits; lower quality of life and medical health status; greater service utilization and treatment costs; and higher risks for violence, arrests, noncompliance, rehospitalization, and relapse (Bartels, Teague, Drake et al., 1993; Tracy, Josiassen, & Bellack, 1995). In order to treat these dually diagnosed patients, therapists must address substance use concurrently with schizophrenia, using an integrated, flexible format (Montrose & Daley, 1995).

Although research in this area has focused on alcohol, cannabis, and cocaine, the most commonly abused substance by patients with schizophrenia is actually nicotine. Greater than 70 percent (and probably closer to 90 percent) of patients smoke, much higher than the general population. Negative effects of nicotine include its role as a "gateway" drug to other substances of abuse, and the major general medical effects of smoking (especially cancer, cerebrovascular disease, and cardiovascular disease). On the other hand, smoking may play a role in reducing medication side effects (through induction of liver enzymes), and recent work on nicotinic receptors in schizophrenia suggests that nicotine may serve as a sensory gating aid, helping to improve the processing of auditory stimuli (Adler, Olincy, Waldo et al., 1998).

Psychiatric comorbidity is also important to recognize, especially depression. Although often difficult to distinguish from negative symptoms, depressive symptoms may occur concurrently with or more commonly immediately following an acute psychotic episode. Perhaps 50 percent of patients with schizophrenia will experience significant depressive symptoms, and such symptoms can dramatically impair quality of life, contribute to physical illness, and increase the risk for suicide (Siris, 1991).

Anxiety symptoms frequently develop in patients with schizophrenia, and many carry a full anxiety disorder in addition to schizophrenia. Obsessive–compulsive disorder (OCD) or significant obsessive–compulsive symptoms may occur in one-third of patients, enough to make some observers describe a separate illness: schizo-obsessive disorder (Tibbo & Warneke, 1999).

Treatment Approaches

For all patients with schizophrenia, the goal of treatment is symptom control and functional improvement. No cure has been found, so a disease management approach predominates. The mainstay of treatment continues to be antipsychotic medication, although pharmacotherapy remains a necessary but not sufficient approach: psychosocial treatments such as family therapy, cognitive remediation, social skills training, and psychosocial rehabilitation significantly improve outcome for patients with this illness, when combined with medication. It is important to note, moreover, that different treatment strategies may be best at different stages of the illness: acute episode versus post-discharge versus longitudinal/maintenance.

■ PSYCHOSOCIAL TREATMENTS

Supportive therapy has clearly been shown to be an effective psychosocial treatment, especially around the time of inpatient hospitalization, when patients are feeling overwhelmed and have shorter attention spans. Therapists focus on brief contacts, reassurance, stressor identification, and discharge planning. However, supportive therapy probably works best for patients already on medication, with psychosis resolving (Hogarty, Goldberg, Schooler, & Ulrich, 1974).

Probably the most important initial psychosocial intervention is *psychoeducation* (see below). Psychoeducation can serve to identify the illness, establish a collaborative relationship, and address guilt and dashed hopes. This work is best done as a continuous process rather than a one-time intervention, which will only have a limited effect on outcome and attitudes. Psychoeducation for families is as essential as for patients; the introduction of issues such as expressed emotion usually begins here (Anderson, Hogarty & Reiss, 1980).

For continuing treatment, *cognitive behavior therapy* (CBT) may yield important gains in symptom reduction. CBT methods may help a patient understand and recognize precipitants to psychotic decompensations; reality testing may help to "chip away" at even systematized delusions. A variety of behavioral approaches can help with hallucinations as well: distraction techniques, coping skills, and checking/clarifying. CBT as a whole can help a patient develop rational rather than emotional reactions to symptoms; the techniques also foster greater insight, reduce symptom burden and subjective distress, and shorten or prevent hospitalizations (Perris & Skagerlind, 1994; Kingdon & Turkington, 1998)

More broadly, *cognitive remediation* approaches can help reverse core cognitive deficits found in patients with schizophrenia. Neuropsychological deficits in attention, memory, or information processing are targeted, with interventions such as thought exercises and computer tests used to correct impairments. Although such strategies have been shown to improve performance on neuropsychiatric testing, cognitive remediation has to-date produced less dramatic amelioration of overall clinical symptoms or generalized behavior (Spaulding, Reed, Storzbach et al., 1998).

The psychosocial intervention with the oldest and strongest pedigree—and the widest implementation—is *social skills training*. Such treatment can help to address deficits in interpersonal skills, which lead to social isolation and subjective distress. Skills such as eye contact, assertiveness, body language, expressing interest, initiating social contact, and maintaining relationships can be learned through individual or group therapy, via discussion, a training manual, audiovisual material, facilitator guidance, and role playing. Outcome studies suggest clear gains in self-efficacy and confidence, with a more modest degree of skill generalization to the community, and a mild to moderate reduction in relapse or rehospitalization rates (Brenner & Pfammatter, 1998; Wirshing, Marder, Eckman et al., 1992).

Two other psychosocial treatments that have been discussed in schizophrenia are family therapy and insight-oriented individual psychotherapy. *Family therapy*, delivered either per family or with multiple families in attendance, has clear benefits in decreasing embarrassment, isolation, and guilt; when levels of expressed emotion are reduced, relapse and rehospitalization rates clearly improve (McFarlane, Lutens, Link et al., 1995). On the other hand, traditional *psychodynamic psychotherapy* probably does not help patients with schizophrenia, and may actually make some patients worse (May, 1968).

Combining elements of effective psychosocial treatments may yield synergistic outcomes. Hogarty, Greenwald, Ulrich, et al. (1997) developed "personal therapy" for patients, a long-term, semi-structured intervention featuring elements of cognitive and skills-based therapy—seeking to enhance social adjustment by identifying and managing intolerable emotions, with a treatment methodology focused on internal coping in stressful situations. Their recently completed 3-year study of personal therapy revealed that the intervention may be very helpful in reducing relapse and rehospitalization rates, as well as improving social adjustment and role performance for patients with schizophrenia. Interestingly, Hogarty and colleagues found that subpopulations may have differential responses, with those currently living with family faring better with personal therapy, and those living alone doing better with supportive therapy.

■ **SOMATIC TREATMENTS**

All psychosocial treatments should be provided with concurrent pharmacotherapy (see Table 5-1). Indeed, ever since the clinical release of chlorpromazine in 1952, medication has been the bulwark of schizophrenia management. Of the 15 or so antipsychotics available today, all—with the possible exception of clozapine— have similar positive symptom efficacy (70–80 percent) and time to response (2–8 weeks). However, atypical antipsychotics have clearly taken the place of typical neuroleptics as first-line treatment in this disorder, for two simple reasons: (1) superior efficacy in the treatment of negative and cognitive symptoms clusters; and (2) enhanced tolerability, with an almost negligible risk of extrapyramidal side effects (EPS), tardive dyskinesia (TD), and

TABLE 5-1. ANTIPSYCHOTIC MEDICATIONS

Class	Brand name	Generic name	Potency	Dose range (mg/day)	Cost
Phenothiazines	Mellaril	Thioridazine	95	40–800	$
	Prolixin	Fluphenazine	2	1–60	$$
	Serentil	Mesoridazine	30–50	30–400	$$
	Stelazine	Trifluoperazine	5	2–80	$$
	Thorazine	Chlorpromazine	100	25–2000	$
	Trilafon	Perphenazine	8	4–64	$$
Other typicals	Haldol	Haloperidol	2–3	1–100	$$
	Loxitane	Loxapine	10	30–250	$$
	Moban	Molindone	10	50–100	$$$
	Navane	Thiothixene	5	6–60	$$
	Orap	Pimozide	1	2–10	$$
Atypicals	Clozaril	Clozapine	50-80	75–900	$$$$
	Risperdal	Risperidone	1–2	1–10	$$$$
	Seroquel	Quetiapine	100	150–750	$$$$
	Zyprexa	Olanzapine	5–10	2.5–20	$$$$
Upcoming agents	Zeldox	Ziprasidone			

other major complications of typical antipsychotics (Andersson, Chakos, Mailman, & Lieberman, 1998).

When a patient presents with schizophrenia, the chosen pharmacotherapy should be based on several important factors:

- *Past response.* If a patient has tolerated and responded well to a particular antipsychotic in the past, all other factors being equal, that medication should be prescribed again.
- *Target symptoms.* Catatonia, for instance, should best be treated with aggressive benzodiazepine usage or electroconvulsive therapy. And as noted, atypical antipsychotics appear to have superior efficacy in the treatment of negative and cognitive symptom clusters. Furthermore, in patients with TD, atypical antipsychotics may help not only with symptom control but also by reducing the burden of dyskinetic movements.
- *Comorbidity.* Medical issues may affect the choice of antipsychotic (e.g., a patient with epilepsy may do better on fluphenazine, which has less of an effect on seizure threshold than chlorpromazine). Psychiatric comorbidity also may play a role: some evidence suggests that clozapine and perhaps other atypical antipsychotics may reduce substance abuse in patients with schizophrenia (Buckley, 1998b).
- *Side-effect profile.* For some patients, avoiding certain side effects (such as sexual dysfunction, weight gain, dystonia risk, or anticholinergic effects) may make particular medications less attractive choices. For other patients, some side effects (such as sedation) may be especially helpful.
- *Patient adherence potential.* Only fluphenazine and haloperidol are available in long-acting, depot (or decanoate) preparations. If a patient cannot or prefers not to take medication by mouth on a daily basis, administering injections every 2–4 weeks may be ideal.
- *Treatment-refractoriness.* Clozapine is the gold standard for patients who have failed two prior antipsychotic trials of

good duration (6 weeks) and sufficient dosage (300–1000 chlorpromazine equivalents).

- *Pharmacokinetics.* An antipsychotic with a half-life of greater than 24 hours, such as pimozide, may be useful for patients who are irregularly compliant but who refuse decanoate medication. Antipsychotics with a rapid time to onset, that can be administered intramuscularly (such as droperidol), may be ideal for agitated psychotic patients in the emergency room setting. Drug–drug interactions may also be relevant, although do not usually limit the choice of an antipsychotic.
- *Cost.* Cost may certainly be a factor in choosing a pharmacotherapy; certainly the newer atypical antipsychotics are quite expensive ($200 or more for a one-month supply). However, several pharmacoeconomic studies have suggested that reduced hospital costs and improved quality-of-life may compensate for these medication costs (Zito, 1998). Even for patients who cannot afford the medication, pharmaceutical companies have made samples and patient assistance programs readily available.

For the uncomplicated first-episode patient, an atypical antipsychotic may be the best option, initiated as soon as possible. If a typical antipsychotic is required, consider using prophylactic antiparkinsonian agents such as biperiden or benztropine; if a standing dose of an anticholinergic is not selected, at least make an antiparkinsonian available as needed, and monitor closely for extrapyramidal side effects. Other "prn" medication, especially lorazepam for anxiety or agitation, may be particularly useful in the acute setting. Massive loading dose or "rapid neuroleptization" risks significant adverse outcomes and is not recommended (Lehman, Steinwachs, & Co-Investigators, 1998).

If the initial pharmacotherapy does not help resolve symptoms, first confirm that the patient is actually taking the medication. Pill counts, mouth checks, and blood levels may help confirm adherence; if the patient refuses to take pills, consider elixir, decanoate, or forced medication. Secondly, if a therapeutic threshold exists for an antipsychotic blood level (for instance, haloperidol), check it and adjust dosing as needed. Finally, reconsider the diagnosis: does the patient really have schizophrenia? Are there unrecognized comorbidities that may be interfering in the treatment? Certainly, comorbidities such as depression, anxiety, or substance abuse should be treated aggressively. A variety of augmentation strategies exist to target such symptoms, as well as agitation in general (e.g., beta-blockers).

If psychosis still has not resolved despite a therapeutic dose and duration, compliance confirmation, and treated comorbidity, consider switching to a different antipsychotic—either an atypical or an antipsychotic from a different class. In patients regarded as treatment-refractory (having failed two therapeutic trials of antipsychotics), clozapine would be the next choice for treatment (Marder, 1996). And if the patient does not respond to these interventions, especially if significant mood symptoms are present, consider electroconvulsive therapy.

Once a patient responds to a medication regimen, the medication should be continued at the same dose after discharge. However, to avoid side effects and increase the odds of patient compliance, treating physicians should aim for the minimum effective dose: just enough for symptom reduction but not too much to risk side effects. Once an acutely ill patient is stabilized as an outpatient, it may even be possible to reduce the medication dose further. Some patients, especially first-episode patients who have been in complete remission for at least 1 year, may be able to discontinue antipsychotic medication entirely. If tapering off an antipsychotic, aim for 10 percent reductions every 6 weeks. However, due to high relapse rates, intermittent dosing is not recommended (Lehman et al., 1998).

Consistent medication is no guarantee of symptom-free survival outside the hospital. Even patients taking pharmacotherapy religiously may have a 2-year recurrence rate between 30 and 50 percent. However, these patients clearly do better than patients who do not take maintenance medication, over 70 percent of whom will suffer a recurrence within 2 years of the index episode.

Treatment Issues

Treatment of the individual with schizophrenia requires a comprehensive, biopsychosocial approach, maximizing symptom reduction, enhancement of functioning, and improvement in the quality of life.

Newer antipsychotics have played a tremendous role in the reduction and management of psychotic symptom. They do not, however, address the significant skill and social functioning deficits necessary to navigate throughout the daily routines of life. Difficulty recognizing and coping with difficult situations, stressors, and symptoms play a role in relapse.

The psychiatric rehabilitation/recovery model provides an overall framework to organize care. Psychiatric rehabilitation assists persons with long-term psychiatric disabilities increase their functioning so they are successful and satisfied in the environments of their choice with the least amount of ongoing professional intervention (Anthony, Cohen, & Cohen, 1983). The rehabilitation/recovery model embraces the need for treatment and symptom reduction and management while focusing on improving functioning and providing patients with the critical skills they need to live in the community. The overall goal is to help people function "despite" their disability. Psychiatric rehabilitation focuses on eliminating or overcoming barriers created by the disability and on promoting independent living, socialization, and effective life management. Perceived deficits tend to be daily living skills, social functioning, problem solving, housing, and vocational needs (Anthony, Cohen, & Farkas, 1990).

The basic assumptions set forth by the International Association of Psychosocial Rehabilitation Services are:

- Individuals with schizophrenia have the capacity to learn, compensate, adapt, and work toward their optimum level.
- Support is needed to reach this optimum level.
- Interventions should be based on the needs of the individual and this may vary at any given point in time.

Organizing care in a manner that addresses symptom management as well as increased functioning, quality of life, and ability to function in the community is compatible with the aims of managed care. This model strives to reduce the utilization of costly resources while promoting health and satisfaction (Jacobs & Malroy, 1994).

■ PSYCHOEDUCATION AND SKILL-BASED TRAINING

Psychosocial education and skill training build on strengths to help the patient identify and cope with problem areas, stressors, and daily life situations that others may take for granted. Skill training also provides an opportunity to practice new skills in a safe environment and allows the patient to comprehend the responses of those around him. Skill training can occur during one-to-one counseling or in a group setting.

Topics for Psychoeducation and Skills Training

Illness management — provide information about the symptoms of schizophrenia as experienced by each individual and validates their experience. Review specific and concrete examples of how to cope with persistent symptoms. Also review relapse prevention by helping patients identify specific experiences they have had related to relapse and creating a crisis plan.

Medication education — provide information about medication, effects, and side-effect profile. Educate about specific side effects such as dry mouth, akathisia, akinesia, weight gain, blurred vision, tremors, sensitivity to the sun, sexual dysfunction and tardive dyskinesia, along with specific tips on managing and reporting these to the physician.

It is also important to review:

- The nuts and bolts of getting prescriptions filled.
- Accessing pharmacy services and insurance issues.
- Keeping track of medicine and anticipating time for refills to avoid periods without medications and potential relapse.

- Assessing an individual's ability to manage their medicine, ability to read, handle the pill bottle, follow directions on label.

Stress management/Anger management—focus on specific skills and activities to identify and anticipate stressful situations; teach stress management skills; teach relaxation exercises and skills for distraction.

Problem-solving skills—review basic skills and process of problem solving; allow the patients opportunity to practice identifying problem; identify alternatives, selecting and trying out solutions and evaluating outcomes.

Social skills—focus on interpersonal effectiveness. Help the patient begin to notice what is happening to others around them, provide "coaching" on appropriate responses, role play a variety of situations to help individual begin to generalize some of the skills introduced.

Independent living skills—provide instruction and coaching for specific daily tasks such as creating a budget, paying bills, writing checks, using a bank card. These are skills often taken for granted but for many can result in significant stress and potential loss in living situations when bills and rent go unpaid. Assess the patient's ability to cook and shop.

Education about community resources—educate yourself and the patient to the community resources that are available. Resources may include the local church that the patient attends, drop-in centers, clubhouses. This process helps the patient begin to expand his network of support.

■ PROMOTING MEDICATION COMPLIANCE

Promotion of medication compliance occurs as part of the education process. It is important for all patients to understand what they are taking and why. It is also important to review side effects and how to manage them. This prepares the patient so they do not stop taking their medications when caught off guard or frightened. Disabling side effects are the most often cited reason for patients stopping their medications. Often this is under-recognized and underestimated by the physician (Tandon, Jebson, & DeQuardo, 1990). The occurrence of extrapyramidal side effects is associated with poor response to treatment. Extrapyramidal side effects adversely impact the already compromised level of functioning and quality-of-life patients with schizophrenia experience.

Tandon et al. (1990) have summarized the impact of extrapyramidal side effects on treatment outcomes. Akathisia is characterized by an uncomfortable feeling of restlessness and is subjectively very distressing. Reduced facial expression, decreased spontaneity, apathy and loss of expressive gestures characterize akinesia. These negative symptoms as a result of medications can be quite disabling. Additionally, the subjective feelings of extrapyramidal side effects include feeling a dullness and apathy in addition to the restlessness already mentioned. The appearance of side effects can be easily mistaken for symptoms of schizophrenia resulting with increased dosing of the very same medication that has caused the problem to begin with.

When suspecting that patients are not taking their medication, it is helpful to use an open, nonjudgmental approach to investigate what is getting in the way of their taking medications and how the clinician/MD can assist them. It is important to understand the patient's point of view, exploring the roadblocks and assisting the patient with problem solving. Common reasons for noncompliance include side effects, apathy, forgetfulness, denial, suspiciousness, substance abuse, inability to read, and complex medication regime.

To promote compliance:

- Educate about medication, effects, and side effects.
- Take the patient's discomfort seriously and actively manage side effects or consider changing medication.
- Simplify the medication regimen to once a day or twice daily dosing.
- Consider depot medications for those who have difficulty remembering to take their medication.

- Help the patient build in medication time as part of their normal daily routine.
- Use pill boxes.
- Assess ability to read.
- Assess ability to remove childproof caps.

■ SUBSTANCE ABUSE AND THE TREATMENT OF SCHIZOPHRENIA

Results form the NIMH Epidemiological Catchment Area (ECA) study on 20,000 individuals showed that 45 percent of all individuals with a lifetime diagnosis of schizophrenia (1.5 percent of the United States population) have met criteria for some form of substance abuse (Reiger, Farmer, Rae et al., 1990). Substance use complicates the treatment picture. It is often hard to tell when a patient is abusing a substance initially, as the typical behaviors you may associate with substance abuse are already present. The use of drugs and alcohol can worsen symptoms, even in small amounts. Substance abuse has negative effects on relationships, ability to manage living situations, and work; it often has legal implications as well. The schizophrenic patient is particularly vulnerable because of the tendency to stop medications in favor of their substance of choice. Individuals may abuse substances in order to be accepted as part of a group; to self medicate for management of symptoms or medication side effects; or because they like the way it makes them feel.

Individuals with schizophrenia and substance abuse are suffering from two very serious illnesses at the same time. Schizophrenic patients will often complain of the degree of difficulty, confrontation, and abstract concepts in the more traditional substance abuse treatment/rehabilitation centers. Minkoff (1991) has proposed different approaches to treating mental illness and substance abuse including sequential, parallel, and integrated treatment models. For the schizophrenic patient, integrated treatment makes sense, whenever possible it focuses on both the psychiatric and substance abuse issues. The same clinician continues to work with the patient on both problems. Integrated treatment decreases the potential chaos and mixed messages that could occur if services were provided in separate facilities (Montrose & Daley, 1995).

■ MANAGING CRISIS SITUATIONS

Prevention is always the goal when it comes to crisis situations. There will be times, however, despite the best planning and attempts to anticipate all likely situations that a crisis will occur. Assessment of safety is essential. Violence, suicide attempts, threats of hurting oneself or others are all crises that require immediate attention. Create a list of all emergency numbers to access help during a crisis and have them readily available. Be aware of the local commitment laws and available emergency services such as mobile crisis teams. While waiting for help, keep everyone safe. If there is property damage but no one is being hurt then wait for help. During periods of crisis all individuals experience a decreased capacity to problem-solve, take on new information, and process information. When attempting to talk with a patient who is in crisis speak clearly and concisely, with respect and dignity. Repeating yourself may be necessary. Take intimidation seriously. Respect the potential for violence in any individual. Consider your goal of the situation and avoid sounding threatening or punitive; this approach tends to escalate the situation. Listen to what the individual has to say and attend to the affect that is associated with it. Remember to treat the individual with respect and dignity at all times and to offer choices when at all possible. When the crisis is over use it as an opportunity to learn. Evaluate what was done, issues that led up to the crisis, and how or whether they were resolved.

■ MEDICAL ISSUES

Patients with psychiatric illness may also have medical illnesses. For those that do, daily management of physical symptoms can create a great deal of stress for the patient. Assess the patient's ability to manage their medical illness. Provide assistance with accessing appropriate medical care and coach the patient in regard to asking questions. Communication with the primary care physician can enhance treatment and minimize chaos for the patient.

■ CASE MANAGEMENT

Case management encompasses a wide range of services with the goal of minimizing the problems of poor service coordination and fragmentation. The essential focus is to attempt to assure the orderly, uninterrupted movement of an individual across a continuum of services (Craig, 1998). There are a variety of approaches to case management. In "Models of Case Management and Their Impact" (1998), Craig summarizes four types of case management services:

- Expanded broker models provide linkage and coordination of services. Professionals conduct treatment and the main function of case management services is to facilitate contacts for the right services.
- Personal strengths model is based on advocacy. Interventions are aimed at facilitating healthy behaviors.
- The rehabilitation approach focuses on improving living skills and is based on theory and practice of psychiatric rehabilitation.
- Assertive community treatment (ACT). The assertive community treatment approach is more directive in nature and is a multidisciplinary team organized as an accountable, mobile mental health team to provide treatment, rehabilitation, and support services for the individual where he lives (NAMI, 1996).

Each model of case management service supports a long-term relationship with the patient. As a clinician make yourself aware of the type of case management service provided in your area. It is important to understand the type of services that are provided and to discuss expectation and limitations up front. This will eliminate unnecessary frustration and problems. Patients must agree to case management services. They cannot be forced or court ordered.

Family Issues

As caregivers we cannot forget that families are a tremendous resource. They are literally on the "front line" and often are the main support for their family members. The experience of schizophrenia affects the entire family. Families are often the first to deal with bizarre behaviors and thinking. They may be as equally frightened and frustrated as the patient. Families want practical advice and information (Hatfield, 1993). Professionals are often not aware of the resources in their own communities nor are they aware of how to navigate through the bureaucracy of entitlements or insurance aware of the resources. Families want to be heard by the treatment and treated with respect. Remember that we are all on the same side.

Anderson, Hogarty, & Reiss (1980) have stated that the initial contact with the family can have a positive impact for the ongoing treatment relationship. They recommend "connecting" with family immediately, meeting with and assessing the strengths and needs of the family continuing this process over several sessions. They further identified key goals to facilitate the connecting process:

- Establish a relationship with genuine working alliance, a partnership that aims to help the patient.
- Understand the family issues and stresses that could contribute to the stress of the patient and family.
- Get an understanding of the family's resources and past attempts to cope.

- Emphasize family strengths.
- Establish a treatment contract with family and patient.

Families are a tremendous source of information that can help clinicians take care of their family member. They come to us with much experience and our key job is to listen to what they have to tell us. Professionals need to share power with families, especially related to areas that affect the lives of families and their family member (Spaniol, Zipple, & Fitzgerald, 1994).

Spaniol et al. (1994) have gone on to identify 15 strategies for sharing power with families:

- Clarify mutual goals
- Learn rehabilitation/educational approaches
- Don't force families to fit your model
- Acknowledge your own limitations
- Work as a team
- Point out family strengths
- Learn to respond to the intense feelings of family members
- Encourage family enrichment
- Learn about psychiatric illness and medications
- Give practical advice
- Learn community resources
- Meet local family support groups
- Make a personal commitment
- Acknowledge diverse beliefs
- Develop your own supports.

Family education can be done individually or within a group. The survival skills group model introduced by Anderson et al. (1986) provides a structured format for psychoeducation for families. This workshop model continues to be an effective means for family education today. The survival skills workshop provides for a full day seminar with a specific agenda related to schizophrenia; course of treatment; family issues; common problems that can be expected; what the family can do to help; and an opportunity for questions. This workshop model provides an opportunity for education as well as support and sharing of information between family members. Topics can be changed as the group continues to grow. Guest speakers such as physicians, pharmacists, NAMI representatives offer a variety of viewpoints that are helpful to families.

The National Alliance for the Mentally Ill is a tremendous resource for those suffering from schizophrenia and their families. NAMI groups offer publications and toll free hotlines, as well as providing a means to advocate for change.

Relapse Issues

Schizophrenia is, for most patients, a chronic illness with waxing and waning of symptoms, and with a risk of full-blown relapse or recurrence. As in other chronic medical conditions such as diabetes, congestive heart failure, and emphysema, patients, providers, and families need to be aware of this risk and prepare accordingly. Some patients are at higher risk of relapse than others. A variety of interventions may reduce the risk; early recognition of relapse may also help to limit morbidity.

Several negative prognostic signs at the earliest stages of schizophrenia may herald a chronic, relapsing and remitting course (Goldstein, 1988; Lieberman, Koreen, Chakos et al., 1996):

- Subacute onset without clear precipitant.
- Non-systematized delusions.
- Negative symptoms.
- Unmarried, minimal family support, and poor premorbid functioning.
- Family history of psychotic disorder.
- Male gender.

Relapses usually are preceded by prodromal signs and symptoms—perhaps sleep disruption, worsening social isolation, or an increase in auditory hallucinations. Patients and families should be encouraged to recognize these hallmarks of relapse, and work with caregivers to intervene as rapidly as possible. Unfortunately, clinicians and patients often do poorly at recognizing such signs and symptoms, making relapse prediction very difficult (Jorgensen, 1998).

Certain triggers exist to heighten the risk for relapse (Caton, 1984):

- *Non-adherence to pharmacotherapy.* Clearly the most important risk factor for relapse, medication noncompliance is unfortunately common. Anywhere between one-quarter to two-thirds of patients take less medication than prescribed. Side effects and poor insight are major contributors to this problem (McEvoy, Freter, Everett et al., 1989; Fenton, Blyler, & Heinssen, 1997).
- *Non-adherence to psychotherapy.* The dropout rate at some clinics approaches 75 percent, and the transition from inpatient to outpatient is a particularly risky time. Discharge planning, staff continuity, early appointments, and transportation assistance may all help.
- *Inadequate life support.* A variety of environmental stressors may contribute to relapse risk, especially housing problems, poverty, and poor hygiene and physical health. Lack of support makes it difficult for any patient to weather such stressful situations (Leavy, 1983; Norman & Malla, 1993).
- *Inadequate socialization/recreation.* Life support and socialization may certainly be related, but social skills deficits make it even harder for patients to develop social networks for life support. Skills training, weekend planning, recreation, and leisure therapy groups may be very helpful in mitigating these problems.
- *High levels of expressed emotion (EE) in families.* Patients who live in high EE families have a 56 percent relapse rate at 6 months following initial hospitalization; patients who live in low EE families have only a 21 percent relapse rate.

EE, incidentally, is co-factored with medication compliance in one study, such that the 9-month relapse rate for high EE/medication noncompliant patients is an astounding 92 percent, while low EE/med compliant patients have only a 12 percent rate—a staggering differential (Brown, 1959; Vaughn & Leff, 1976). Interventions include psychoeducation, both for illness and treatment; communication training and facilitation; containing outbursts, criticisms, and judgments; problem-solving training; and as a last resort limiting patient/family contact if high EE seems irreversible.

The other major trigger for relapse—loading on all these factors—is comorbidity, especially substance abuse. Continued marijuana use makes it almost 100 percent likely that a patient will have a relapse of schizophrenia; psychotic relapses are often preceded by substance relapses in otherwise stable, abstinent patients.

■ SELF-HELP GROUPS

Skill groups provide education but do not provide the opportunity to establish relationships outside of the caregiving setting. Self-help groups provide an opportunity for patients and their families to meet others who are in similar situations. Self-help groups offer an opportunity for sharing, support, problem solving, and growth by others who have similar experiences. It shifts the focus from being sick and needing treatment to that of being an individual who is contributing. Scharzer and Leppin (1989) conducted an analysis of 80 studies. They found a relationship between social support and psychological well being. Social supports can "buffer" the impact of physical and emotional stresses. People with schizophrenia tend to under-utilize their social supports. As relationships are lost people with psychiatric disabilities begin to rely on mental health professionals for support (Wilson, Flanagan, & Rynders, 1993). The beauty of the support group is that each individual brings with them the knowledge of their own life experience that can be shared and helpful to another.

Finding self-help groups and support is rather easy. Information about almost any support group imaginable is available by using the Internet. There are national self-help clearing-houses that can guide the user to specific information. Information about self-help groups is also available in local newspapers and government pages of the phone book, book stores and newsletters. Some of the types of self-help groups available are: Alcoholics Anonymous; Recovery Inc.; Survivors of Suicide; Emotions Anonymous; and Families of the Mentally Ill. The National Alliance for the Mentally Ill is a major resource for patients and families with web sites and local phone numbers.

Aftercare and Measuring Outcome

Because schizophrenia begins at such an early age the overall cost of care is quite high. It is estimated that schizophrenia costs the nation $32.5 billion dollars to treat ("Practical Information," *Psychiatric Times*, 1999). Measuring the outcome of the service makes sense to provide treatment that works and to assure appropriate reimbursement. Outcome data allow for objective measurement of service provision—not only what is done but how well it is done. Nationally accepted instruments allow providers to compare with other facilities working with similar populations. Home-grown tools are helpful and often provide very specific information about programs, but they generally cannot be used for comparison with other programs due to the level of specificity. State and county regulatory agencies require clinical outcomes, as do accreditation bodies such as JCAHO and CARF. Managed care companies use clinical outcomes to help make decisions as to where to allocate funding for services.

There are many instruments published that have demonstrated reliability and validity. What to measure and how much to measure is an issue worth considering carefully. Many people make the mistake of wanting to measure every aspect of the care they render. While the intent is noble the likelihood of following through with too many areas to measure results in nothing being measured. The recommendation is to select three or perhaps four areas to measure and follow through. The challenge is selecting the area of functioning. Dickerson (1997) reviewed instruments that measured two or more domains of community functioning and for which validity and reliability had been established. She identified the challenges to be identifying what domains to measure length of measure and limitations of self-report data. The areas typically measured included self-care and social relationships. Other areas to consider monitoring outcomes for are efficacy of medications; compliance with medication and satisfaction with treatment.

Other Issues

■ TARDIVE DYSKINESIA AND NEUROLEPTIC MALIGNANT SYNDROME

Although atypical antipsychotics have become the most frequently prescribed medication for schizophrenia, typical antipsychotics remain in wide use, and side effects—especially neurological—pose a challenge for patients and clinicians. The most common forms of extrapyramidal side effects (EPS), although treatable, may significantly impair quality of life and reduce medication adherence; the most serious forms may cause significant morbidity or even permanent disability. The two most serious adverse neurological effects are tardive dyskinesia (TD) and neuroleptic malignant syndrome (NMS).

TD results from chronic exposure to typical antipsychotics, although symptoms can develop as early as one month. Patients with TD most commonly experience mouth or tongue movements such as sucking, grimacing, puckering, or protrusions; other body parts may similarly be affected by slow, involuntary, irregular movements. More than 20 percent of patients exposed to typical antipsychotics will develop TD; risk factors besides duration of treatment include age, comorbid substance abuse (especially cannabis), and probably negative symptoms and organic brain syndromes (van Os, Fahy, Jones et al., 1997).

Prevention is obviously the best approach to TD: using an atypical antipsychotic first, using the minimum effective dose, and discontinuing an antipsychotic when it is no longer indicated. Informed consent should include TD, so patients are aware of the risk. Patients should be monitored regularly for signs and symptoms of TD, using rating scales like the AIMS exam every 6 months. If patients develop TD, management options include switching to an atypical antipsychotic or lowering the dose (although this intervention may initially worsen the movements). If neither of these options is possible, treating the patient with vitamin E, buspirone, benzodiazepines, or perhaps gabapentin (Hardoy, Hardoy, Carta & Cabras, 1999) may help some patients. Although previously thought to be progressive and irreversible, TD "levels off" for most patients—and some, especially those who switch to an atypical antipsychotic, may see the symptoms disappear entirely.

NMS is a serious, acute illness—less common than TD but potentially lethal. Symptoms include motor rigidity, autonomic instability, and altered mental status, most often accompanied by elevated levels of creatine kinase. Between 20 and 30 percent of patients who develop severe NMS may die, although most cases of NMS are fortunately mild or moderate. Risk factors include the use of high-potency typical antipsychotics, young, male, and organic brain syndromes. Management should start with the immediate discontinuation of the offending medication, and rapid provision of supportive care (hydration, managing electrolyte disturbances, and so forth). Treatment with dopamine agonists such as bromocriptine or dantrolene may be helpful in some cases. If a patient needs an antipsychotic after an NMS episode, clozapine may be the safest choice, although few cases have been reported with any of the other atypical antipsychotics.

■ MEDICATION IN PREGNANCY

All antipsychotics cross the placenta and are secreted in breast milk. However, there is no evidence of any major developmental abnormalities in the offspring of mothers who have taken antipsychotics during pregnancy. Potential risks of an antipsychotic to both mother and fetus must be balanced with the potential benefits. Chlorpromazine has been best studied, with no apparent teratogenicity from first-trimester use. Third-trimester use, however, has been associated with an increased risk of neonatal jaundice and EPS—perhaps related to impaired fetal clearance around the time of birth. Haloperidol may be the safest choice, although if possible any antipsychotic should be discontinued a few weeks prior to delivery (Hyman, Arana, & Rosenbaum, 1995).

REFERENCES

Adler, L.E., Olincy, A., Waldo, M., et al. (1998). Schizophrenia, sensory gating, and nicotinic receptors. *Schizophrenia Bulletin, 24*, 189–202.

American Psychiatric Association (1994). *Diagnostic and Statistical Manual of Mental Disorders*, 4th ed. Washington, DC: American Psychiatric Association.

Anderson, C.M., Hogarty, G., & Reiss, D.J. (1980). Family treatment of adult schizophrenic patients: A psycho-educational approach. *Schizophrenia Bulletin, 6*, 490–505.

Andersson, C., Chakos, M., Mailman, R., & Lieberman, J. (1998). Emerging roles for novel antipsychotic medications in the treatment of schizophrenia. *Psychiatric Clinics of North America, 21*, 151–179.

Andreasen, N.C., Rezai, K., Alliger, R., et al. (1992). Hypofrontality in neuroleptic-naïve patients and in patients with chronic schizophrenia: Assessment with xenon 133 single-photon emission computed tomography and the Tower of London. *Archives of General Psychiatry, 49*, 943–958.

Anthony, W., Cohen, M.R., & Cohen, P.F. (1983). Philosophy, treatment process, and principles of the psychiatric rehabilitation approach. In L.L. Bachrach (Ed.), *Deinstitutionalization: New directions for mental health services*, Vol. 17 (pp. 67–69). San Fransisco: Jossey-Bass.

Anthony, W., Cohen, M., & Farkas, M. (1990). *Psychiatric rehabilitation.* Boston: Center for Psychiatric Rehabilitation.

Bartels, S.J., Teague, G.B., Drake, R.E., et al. (1993). Substance abuse in schizophrenia: Service utilization and costs. *Journal of Nervous and Mental Diseases, 181,* 227–232.

Brenner, H.D., & Pfammatter, M. (1998). Outcome and costs of therapies. In T. Wykes, N. Tarrier, and S. Lewis (Eds.), *Outcome and innovation in psychological treatment of schizophrenia.* New York: Wiley and Sons.

Brown, G.W. (1959). Experiences of discharged chronic schizophrenic mental hospital patients in various types of living group. *Millbank Memorial Fund Quarterly, 37,* 105–131.

Buckley, P.F. (1998a). Structural brain imaging in schizophrenia. *Psychiatric Clinics of North America, 21,* 77–92.

Buckley, P.F. (1998b). Substance abuse in schizophrenia: a review. *Journal of Clinical Psychiatry, 59* (Suppl. 1), 26–30.

Cannon, T.D., Mednick, S.A., Parnas, J., et al. (1993). Developmental brain abnormalities in the offspring of schizophrenic mothers. I. Contributions of genetic and perinatal factors. *Archives of General Psychiatry, 50,* 551–564.

Carlsson, A., Hansson, L.O., Waters, N., & Carlsson, M. L. (1997). Neurotransmitter aberrations in schizophrenia: new perspectives and therapeutic implications. *Life Sciences, 61,* 75–94.

Craig, T. (1998). Models of case management and their impact on social outcomes of severe mental illness. In K. Mueser & N. Tarrier, (Eds.), *Handbook of social functioning in schizophrenia* (pp. 361–363). Boston: Allyn and Bacon.

Dickerson, F. (1997). Assessing clinical outcomes: the community functioning of persons with serious mental illness. *Psychiatric Services, 48,* 897–902.

Drake, R.E., Gates, C., Whitaker, A., & Cotton, P.G. (1985). Suicide among schizophrenics: A review. *Comprehensive Psychiatry, 26,* 90–100.

Fenton, W.S., Blyler, C.R., & Heinssen, R.K. (1997). Determinants of medication compliance in schizophrenia: empirical and clincial findings. *Schizophrenia Bulletin, 23,* 637-652.

Goldstein, J.M. (1988). Gender differences in the course of schizophrenia. *American Journal of Psychiatry, 145,* 684–689.

Gur, R.E., Mozley, P.D., Resnick, S.M., et al. (1991). Magnetic resonance imaging in schizophrenia. I. Volumetric analysis of brain and cerebrospinal fluid. *Archives of General Psychiatry, 48,* 407–412.

Gur, R.E., & Pearlson, G. (1993). Neuroimaging in schizophrenia research. *Schizophrenia Bulletin, 19,* 337–353.

Hatfield, A. (1993). *Dual diagnosis: Substance abuse and mental disorder.* Schizophrenia Homepage at www.schizophrenia.com.

Hardoy, M.C., Hardoy, M.J., Carta, M.G., & Cabras, P.L. (1999). Gabapentin as a promising treatment for antipsychotic-induced movement disorders in schizoaffective and bipolar patients. *Journal of Affect Disorders, 54,* 315–317.

Harvey, I., Ron, M.A., Du Boulay, G., et al. (1993). Reduction of cortical volume in schizophrenia on magnetic resonance imaging. *Psychologic Medicine, 23,* 591–604.

Hien, D. (1993). Special considerations for dually diagnosed schizophrenics and their families. In J. Solomon, S. Zimberg, & E. Shollar (Eds.), *Dual diagnosis: Evaluation, treatment, training, and program development* (Chapter 10). New York: Plenum Publishing.

Ho, B.C., Nopoulos, P., Flaum, M., et al. (1998). Two-year outcome in first-episode schizophrenia: predictive value of symptoms for quality of life. *American Journal of Psychiatry, 155,* 1196–1201.

Hogarty, G.E., Goldberg, S.C., Schooler, N.R., & Ulrich, R.P. (1974). Drugs and sociotherapy in the aftercare of schizophrenic patients: II. Two-year relapse rates. *Archives of General Psychiatry, 31,* 603–608.

Hogarty, G.E., Greenwald, D., Ulrich, R.S., et al. (1997). Three-year trials of personal therapy among schizophrenic patients living with or independent of family: II. Effects on adjustment of patients. *American Journal of Psychiatry, 154,* 1514–1524.

Horrobin, D.F. (1998). The membrane phospholipid hypothesis as a biochemical basis for the neurodevelopmental concept of schizophrenia. *Schizophrenia Research, 30,* 193–208.

Hyman, S.E., Arana, G.W. & Rosenbaum, J.F. (1995). *Handbook of psychiatric drug therapy,* 3rd ed. New York: Little, Brown and Co.

Jacobs, D., & Malroy, D. (1994). Anticipating managed mental health care: implications for psychosocial rehabilitation agencies. In: W. Anthony & L. Spaniol (Eds.), *Readings in psychiatric rehabilitation* (pp. 481–503). Boston: Center for Psychiatric Rehabilitation.

Jorgensen, P. (1998). Early signs of psychotic relapse in schizophrenia. *British Journal of Psychiatry, 172,* 327–330.

Kay, S.R., Fiszbein, A. & Opler, L.A. (1987). The positive and negative syndrome scale (PANSS) for schizophrenia. *Schizophrenia Bulletin, 13,* 261–276.

Kendler, K.S., McGuire, M., Gruenberg, A.M., et al. (1994). Clinical heterogeneity in schizophrenia and the pattern of psychopathology in relatives: results from an epidemiologically based family study. *Acta Psychiatrica Scandinavica, 89,* 294–300.

Keshavan, M.S., Anderson, S., Pettegrew, J.W., et al. (1994). Is schizophrenia due to excessive synaptic pruning in the prefrontal cortex? The Feinberg hypothesis revisted. *Journal of Psychiatry Research, 28,* 239–265.

Kingdon, D., & Turkington, D. (1998). Cognitive behaviour therapy of schizophrenia. Chapter 4 In T. Wykes, N. Tarrier, & S. Lewis (Eds.), *Outcome and innovation in psychological treatment of schizophrenia.* New York: Wiley and Sons.

Leavy, R.J. (1983). Social support and psychological disorder: a review. *Journal of Community Psychology, 11,* 3–21.

Lehman, A.F., Steinwachs, D.M., and the Co-Investigators of the PORT Project (1998). At issue: Translating research into practice: The Schizophrenia Patient Outcomes Research Team (PORT) treatment recommendations. *Schizophrenia Bulletin, 24,* 1–10.

Lieberman, J.A., Koreen, A. R., Chakos, M., et al. (1996). Factors influencing treatment response and outcomes of first-episode schizophrenia: implications for understanding the pathophysiology of schizophrenia. *Journal of Clinical Psychiatry, 57* (Suppl. 9), 5–9.

Marder, S.R. (1996). Management of treatment-resistant patients with schizophrenia. *Journal of Clinical Psychiatry, 57* (Suppl. 11), 26–30.

Maxmen, J.S., & Ward, N.G. (1995). *Essential psychopathology and its treatment,* 2nd ed. New York: W.W. Norton.

May, P.R.A. (1968). *Treatment of schizophrenia: A comparative study of five treatment methods.* New York: Science House.

McEvoy, J.P., Freter, S., & Everett, G., et al. (1989). Insight and the clinical outcome of schizophrenic patients. *Journal of Nervous and Mental Disease, 177,* 145–151.

McFarlane, W.R., Lukens, E., Link, B., et al. (1995). Multiple-family groups and psychoeducation in the treatment of schizophrenia. *Archives of General Psychiatry, 52,* 679–687.

McNeil, T.F. (1995). Perinatal risk factors and schizophrenia: Selective review and methodological concerns. *Epidemiology Review, 17*, 107–112.

Mednick, S.A., Machon, R.A., Huttunen, M.O., et al. (1988). Adult schizophrenia following prenatal exposure to an influenza epidemic. *Archives of General Psychiatry, 45*, 189–192.

Meltzer, H.Y. (1995). The role of serotonin in schizophrenia and the place of serotonin–dopamine antagonist antipsychotics. *Journal of Clinical Psychopharmacology, 15*, 2S–3S.

Minkoff, K. (1991). Program components of a comprehensive integrated care system for seriously mentally ill patients with substance abuse. *New Directions of Mental Health Services, 50*, 13–27.

Mobray, C.T. (1985). Homelessness in America: Myths and realities. *American Journal of Orthopsychiatry, 55*, 4–8.

Mohn, A.R., Gainetdinov, R.R., Cron, M.G., & Koller, B.H. (1999). Mice with reduced NMDA receptor expression display behaviors related to schizophrenia. *Cell, 98*, 427–436.

Montrose, K. & Daley, D. (1995). *Celebrating small victories: a primer of approaches and attitudes for helping clients with dual disorders.* Center City, MN: Hazelden.

Mueser, K.T., Yarnold, P.R., Levinson, D.F., et al. (1990). Prevalence of substance abuse in schizophrenia: Demographic and clinical correlates. *Schizophrenia Bulletin, 16*, 31–56.

Nimgaonkar, V.L., Rudert, W.A., Zhang, X., et al. (1997). Negative association of schizophrenia with HLA DQB1*0602: Evidence from a second African-American cohort. *Schizophrenia Research, 23*, 81–86.

Norman, R.M., & Malla, A.K. (1993). Stressful life events and schizophrenia. I: A review of the research. *British Journal of Psychiatry, 162*, 161–166.

Olney, J.W., & Farber, N.B. (1995). Glutamate receptor dysfunction and schizophrenia. *Archives of General Psychiatry, 52*, 998–1007.

Overall, J.E. (1988). The Brief Psychiatric Rating Scale (BPRS): Recent developments in ascertainment and scaling. *Psychopharmacology Bulletin, 24*, 97–99.

Perris, C., & Skagerlind, L. (1994). Cognitive therapy with schizophrenic patients. *Acta Psychiatrica Scandanavica Suppl., 382*, 65–70.

Practical information for health care professionals, schizophrenia and other psychotic disorders. Schizophrenia fact sheet (1999). *Psychiatric Times* at www.mhsource.com.

Rapoport, J.L., Giedd, J.N., Blumenthal, J., et al. (1999). Progressive cortical change during adolescence in childhood-onset schizophrenia. A longitudinal magnetic resonance imaging study. *Archives of General Psychiatry, 56,* 649–654.

Raz, S., & Raz, N. (1990). Structural brain abnormalities in the major psychoses: a quantitative review of the evidence from computerized imaging. *Psychology Bulletin, 108,* 93–108.

Reiger, D. A., Farmer, M.E., Rae, D.S., et al. (1990). Co-morbidity of mental disorders with alcohol and other drug abuse: results from the Epidemiologic Catchment Area Study (ECA). *Journal of the American Medical Association, 264,* 2511–2518.

Rothermundt, M., Arolt, V., Weitzsch, C., et al. (1998). Immunological dysfunction in schizophrenia: a systematic approach. *Neuropsychobiology, 37,* 186–193.

Robins, L.N., Helzer, J.E., Weissman, M.M., et al. (1984). Lifetime prevalence of specific psychiatric disorders in three sites. *Archives of General Psychiatry, 41,* 949–958.

Sacker, A., Done, D.J., & Crow, T.J. (1996). Obstetric complications in children born to parents with schizophrenia: A meta-analysis of case-control studies. *Psychologic Medicine 26,* 279–287.

Salloum, I.M., Moss, H.B., & Daley, D.C. (1991). Substance abuse and schizophrenia: Impediments to optimal care. *American Journal of Drug and Alcohol Abuse, 17,* 321–336.

Scharzer, L., & Leppin, A. (1989). Social supports and health: A meta-analysis. *Psychology and Health, 3,* 1–15.

Schneier, F.R., & Siris, S.G. (1987). A review of psychoactive substance use and abuse in schizophrenia: Patterns of drug choice. *Journal of Nervous and Mental Disease, 175,* 641–652.

Schwartz, J.C., Diaz, J., Bordet, R., et al. (1998). Functional implications of multiple dopamine receptor subtypes: the D1/D3 receptor coexistence. *Brain Research and Brain Research Review, 26,* 236–242.

Siris, S.G. (1991). Diagnosis of secondary depression in schizophrenia: implications for DSM-IV. *Schizophrenia Bulletin, 17,* 75–98.

Spaniol, L., Zikpple, A., & Fitzgerald, S. (1994). How professionals can share power with families of the mentally ill. In W. Anthony & L.

Spaniol (Eds.), *Readings in psychiatric rehabilitation* (pp. 308–318). Boston: Center for Psychiatric Rehabilitation.

Spaulding, W., Reed, D., Storzbach, D., et al. (1998). The effects of a remediational approach to cognitive therapy for schizophrenia. In T. Wykes, N. Tarrier, & S. Lewis (Eds.), *Outcome and innovation in psychological treatment of schizophrenia*, Chapter 8. New York: Wiley and Sons.

Steadman, H.J., Mulvey, E.P., Monahan, J., et al. (1998). Violence by people discharged from acute psychiatric inpatient facilities and by others in the same neighborhoods. *Archives of General Psychiatry*, *55*, 393–401.

Stone, M.H. (1997). *Healing the mind: A history of psychiatry from antiquity to the present.* New York: W.W. Norton and Co.

Tandon, R., Jebson, M., & DeQuardo, J. (1990). EPS: Subjective and mental aspects and their impact on outcome. *Clear Perspectives*, *2*, 13–17.

Tibbo, P., & Warneke, L. (1999). Obsessive-compulsive disorder in schizophrenia: Epidemiologic and biologic overlap. *Journal of Psychiatry and Neuroscience, 24*, 15–24.

Tracy, J.I., Josiassen, R.C., & Bellack, A.S. (1995). Neuropsychology of dual diagnosis: Understanding the combined effects of schizophrenia and substance use disorders. *Clinical Psychology Reviews*, *15*, 67–97.

van Os, J., Fahy, T., Jones, P., et al. (1997). Tardive dyskinesia: Who is at risk? *Acta Psychiatrica Scandanavica*, *95*, 206–216.

Vaughn, C.E., & Leff, J.P. (1976). The influence of family and social factors on the course of psychiatric illness: A comparison of schizophrenic with depressed neurotic patients. *British Journal of Psychiatry*, *129*, 125–137.

Waddington, J.L., Lane, A., Scully, P.J., et al. (1998). Neurodevelopmental and neuroprogressive processes in schizophrenia. *Psychiatric Clinics of North American, 21*, 123–149.

Wahlberg, K.E., Wynne, L.C., Oja, H., et al. (1997). Gene-environment interaction in vulnerability to schizophrenia: findings from the Finnish Adoptive Family Study of Schizophrenia. *American Journal of Psychiatry, 154*, 355–362.

Weickert, C.S., & Kleinman, J.E. (1998). The neuroanatomy and neurochemistry of schizophrenia. *Psychiatric Clinics of North America 21*, 57–75.

Weinberger, D.R., (1987). Implications of normal brain development for the pathogenesis of schizophrenia. *Archives of General Psychiatry, 44*, 660–669.

Weiden, P.J., Scheifler, P., McEvoy, J., et al. (1999). Expert consensus treatment guidelines for schizophrenia: A guide for patients and families. *Journal of Clinical Psychiatry, 10* (Suppl. 11), 73–74.

Willner, P. (1997). The dopamine hypothesis of schizophrenia: current status, future prospects. *International Clinics in Psychopharmacology, 12*, 297–308.

Wilson, M., Flanagan, S. & Rynders, C. (1993). The friends program: A peer support group model for individuals with a psychiatric disability. *Psychiatric Rehabilitation Journal, 22*, 239–247.

Wirshing, W.C., Marder, S.R., Eckman, T., et al. (1992). Acquisition and retention of skills training methods in chronic schizophrenic outpatients. *Psychopharmacology Bulletin, 28*, 241–245.

Zito, J.M. (1998). Pharmacoeconomcis of the new antipsychotics for the treatment of schizophrenia. *Psychiatric Clinics of North America, 21*, 181–202.

Suggested Patient and Family Educational Materials

Patient Videos
"Critical Connections: A Schizophrenia Awareness Video" (APA/ Zeneca, 1997)
"I'm Still Here: The Truth About Schizophrenia" (Janssen, 1997)

Handouts/Pamphlets
"Understanding Schizophrenia: A Guide for People with Schizophrenia and Their Families" (NARSAD/Janssen, 1996)
"You've Taken Your First Step" (Janssen, 1997)
"The Value of Clozaril Therapy" (Novartis, 1998)
"Schizophrenia: Help is available" (Channing Bete, 1996)

Websites
www.mentalwellness.com
www.mentalhealth.com
www.schizophrenia.com
www.nami.org

Monographs
Andreasen, N.C. (1984). *The broken brain: The biological revolution in psychiatry.* New York: Harper & Row.
Bernheim, K.F., Lewine, R.R.J, and Beale, C.T. (1982). *The caring family: Living with chronic mental illness.* New York: Random House.
Jeffries, J.J., Plummer, E., Seeman, M.V., and Thornton, J.F. (1990). *Living and working with schizophrenia,* 2nd ed. Toronto: University of Toronto Press.
Torrey, E.F. (1995). *Surviving schizophrenia: A family manual,* 3rd ed. New York: Harper & Row.
Walsh, M (1985). *Schizophrenia: Straight talk for families and friends.* New York: William Morrow and Co.

Chapter Six

Eating Disorders

Maria La Via ● Marsha Marcus

Eating disorders are psychiatric syndromes characterized by aberrant eating patterns and associated psychological characteristics related to eating, body shape, and weight. There are three categories of eating disorders included in the DSM IV: anorexia nervosa, bulimia nervosa, and eating disorders not otherwise specified. Binge eating disorder, although not officially listed as an eating disorder, has been included in the appendix under "criteria sets and axes provided for further study." This chapter will aim to describe each of these disorders separately, discuss their prevalence and causes, assessment, comorbidity, effects on the people with it, their families and society, and lastly, to discuss treatment issues such as relapse prevention.

Anorexia Nervosa

■ DIAGNOSIS

According to the DSM IV, anorexia nervosa is characterized by a refusal to maintain body weight at or above a minimally normal weight for age and height, an intense fear of gaining weight or becoming fat even though underweight, a disturbance in the way in which one's body weight or shape is experienced, and, in post-menarchal females, amenorrhea. The hallmark feature is a morbid fear of body fat, which does not lessen but instead increases with starvation and weight loss. The dietary restriction is willful, ego syntonic, and not accounted for by any known illness. The weight loss and body image distortion are often associated with excessive exercise, vomiting and/or laxative and diuretic abuse. Binge eating episodes develop in approximately 40 percent of patients over time. There are two subtypes of anorexia nervosa, restrictor and binge purge. The person with restricting type does not regularly engage in binge eating or purging behavior while the opposite is true for the person with binge eating/purge type. Purging behaviors include self-induced vomiting or the misuse of laxatives, diuretics, or enemas. The DSM IV diagnostic criteria (APA, 1994) for anorexia nervosa are shown in Table 6-1. DaCosta and Halmi (1992) found those people with anorexia nervosa who binge and/ or purge are likely to be more impulsive, socially involved, sexually active, and have more family dysfunction. They also tend to be older at the time of presentation for treatment and have had the illness longer (DaCosta & Halmi, 1992). In addition, they are somewhat heavier. People with restricting type of anorexia nervosa are more likely to be obsessional in style and more socially isolated and awkward.

TABLE 6-1. DIAGNOSTIC CRITERIA FOR ANOREXIA NERVOSA

1. Refusal to maintain body weight at or above a minimally normal weight for age and height (e.g., weight loss leading to maintenance of body weight less than 85 percent of that expected; or failure to make expected weight gain during period of growth, leading to body weight less than 85 percent of expected.)
2. Intense fear of gaining weight or becoming fat, even though underweight.
3. Disturbance in the way in which one's body weight or shape is experienced; undue influence of body weight or shape on self-evaluation, or denial of the seriousness of the current low body weight.
4. In post-menarchal females, amenorrhea. This is defined as the absence of at least three consecutive menstrual cycles. (A woman is considered to have amenorrhea if her periods occur only following hormone, e.g., estrogen administration.)

Specify type:
    Restricting type: During the current episode of anorexia nervosa, the person has not regularly engaged in binge eating or purging behavior (i.e., self-induced vomiting or the misuse of laxatives, diuretics, or enemas).
    Binge eating/purging type: During the current episode of anorexia nervosa, the person has regularly engaged in binge eating or purging behavior (i.e., self-induced vomiting or the misuse of laxatives, diuretics, or enemas).

Available evidence has suggested that the DSM IV criteria are applicable to children and adolescents. However, there are some problems with these diagnostic criteria for this age group. First, the absence of at least three consecutive menstrual cycles, either primary or secondary, can be difficult to ascertain, especially in young children. Second, the refusal to maintain body weight requires that weight be at least 15 percent below that expected for height and age. Starvation directly affects linear growth in children and adolescents thus making the calculation of expected weight difficult. Based on this, Bryan Lask and colleagues developed the Great Ormond Street checklist for use in children and adolescents. These are based on criteria originally proposed by Gerald Russell in 1970 and are listed in Table 6-2 (Lask & Bryant-Waugh, 1993).

■ PREVALENCE

The estimated prevalence of anorexia nervosa is 0.5–one percent of females and it is 10–20 times more common in females than in males (Garfinkel et al., 1996; Walters & Kendler, 1995). There is some evidence to suggest that in the prepubertal population, males represent a greater proportion (25 percent) than in adult populations (Lask & Bryant-Waugh, 1993). The onset of anorexia nervosa is typically between ages 10 and 30. The modal age of onset is at 17–18 with approximately 85 percent of patients having the onset of the illness in the adolescent years, between ages 13

TABLE 6-2. THE GREAT ORMOND STREET CHECKLIST

1. Determined food avoidance
2. Weight loss or failure to gain weight during the period of preadolescent growth (age 10–14) in the absence of any physical or other mental illness
3. Any two or more of the following:
   1. Preoccupation with body weight
   2. Preoccupation with energy intake
   3. Distorted body image
   4. Fear of fatness
   5. Self-induced vomiting
   6. Extensive exercising
   7. Purging (laxative abuse)

and 20. Studies have shown that the prevalence of anorexia nervosa in adolescence has increased during the past 50 years making this the third most frequent chronic illness among adolescent girls after obesity and asthma (Lucas et al., 1991). Eating disorders continue to be more prevalent in the Western industrialized nations, in Caucasians and in middle- and upper-class females. However, there is a trend towards an increasing diversity of ethnic and socioeconomic groups (Lacey & Dolan, 1988). A study by Lucas and colleagues showed a constant incidence rate for women over age 25 and for men in general. A significant increase was shown in incidence rates for females aged 15–24. Since the 1960s an increase was shown in females aged 10–14 (Lucas, Beard, O'Fallon & Kurland, 1991). This study further suggested that the incidence of the more severe and unremitting form of anorexia nervosa has remained constant. Today, teenagers may be more vulnerable to cultural pressures and may develop a milder form of the illness in the context of these pressures.

■ COURSE AND OUTCOME

Anorexia nervosa is a potentially fatal disorder with a high potential for relapse. Studies have shown a mortality rate of 0.5 percent per year, which is cumulative. This is the highest mortality rate of any psychiatric disorder (Sullivan, 1995). Clinicians report that early age of onset is associated with good outcome, but there is insufficient evidence in the literature to support this. It is likely that the prognosis in this younger group is no worse than that for older anorexics.

Recently, Strober and colleagues (Strober, Freeman & Morrell, 1997) completed a study looking at the long-term course of anorexia nervosa in adolescents treated in an urban specialty care setting. This study demonstrated that the course of anorexia nervosa is protracted, ranging from 5 to $6\frac{1}{2}$ years and that predictors of outcome are relatively few. Specifically, they found that although almost 30 percent of patients had relapses following discharge from the hospital, almost 76 percent met criteria for full recovery at the end of follow-up and relapse after recovery was relatively uncommon. There were no deaths in this series of patients. Conversely, Bryant-Waugh and colleagues (Bryant-Waugh, Knibbs, Fosson, Kaminski & Lask, 1988) looked at long-term outcome in early onset anorexia nervosa and although they found that about 60 percent of these patients did well, one-third of the children remained moderately to severely impaired and there were two reported deaths. Poor prognostic factors included onset at less than age 11, depression, and several family issues including a disturbed family life, one-parent families, and families in which one or both parents had been married before.

■ ETIOLOGY

The etiology of anorexia nervosa is not known; however numerous factors have been implicated in the cascade of events resulting in the illness. In the past, emphasis has been placed on the psychosocial factors associated with eating disorders including issues of individual development, family dynamics, social pressure to be thin, and the struggle to achieve identity. There is increasing evidence that suggests that genetic factors also may play a role in the etiology of anorexia nervosa. Family history and twin studies have yielded strong evidence that anorexia nervosa runs in families, particularly those with a history of depression and anxiety disorders. Identical twin siblings of patients with anorexia nervosa have higher rates of anorexia nervosa and bulimia nervosa with monozygotic twins having higher concordance than dizygotic twins (Walters & Kendler, 1995).

Biologically, we know that serotonin affects feeding behavior, mood, impulsivity, anxiety, and other species-specific behaviors. Several studies (Kaye, Gwirtsman, George & Ebert, 1991; Brewerton and Jimerson, 1996; Kaye, 1997) have documented differences in serotonin levels in acutely ill and recovered patients. In patients with anorexia nervosa, serotonin alterations are largely state-dependent but may play an important role in the maintenance of symptoms. In low-weight anorexic patients, research evidence has suggested reduced serotonin synthesis, uptake, and turnover, and reduced post-synaptic serotonin receptor sensitivity. Kaye and colleagues (Kaye et al., 1991) showed enhanced serotonin turnover in long-term weight-recovered restrictor anorexic patients. Levels of the primary metabolite of serotonin, 5-HIAA (5-hydroxyindoleacetic acid), as measured in cerebrospinal fluid are low in underweight anorexic patients, but rise to levels higher than normal after recovery.

From the social perspective, there are numerous risk factors that contribute to the development of an eating disorder. These risk factors include personal and sociocultural factors. Society's emphasis on thinness and exercise may support the anorexic patient's drive for thinness. The rising pressure to be thin and societal biases against obesity may contribute to body dissatisfaction, low self-esteem, and pathological dieting behavior in patients with anorexia nervosa. Numerous studies have shown a relationship between dieting and eating disorder behaviors (Polivy & Herman, 1985; Hetherton & Polivy, 1992). Often a period of severely restrictive dieting precedes the onset of anorexia nervosa as well as bulimia nervosa (Polivy & Herman, 1985). Some girls even report dieting starting as early as the third grade (Thelan, Powell, Lawrence, & Kuhnert, 1992).

Psychological and psychodynamic factors include theories about the patient, as well as the family. Bruch (1962, 1973, 1978) proposed that the self-starvation in anorexia nervosa represents a struggle for autonomy, competence, control, and self-respect. Crisp (1980) has described anorexia nervosa as an attempt to cope with fears and conflicts associated with psycho-biological maturity. The dieting and weight loss thus become ways in which the patient regresses to a prepubertal shape, hormonal status, and experience. The eating disorder can serve to draw members of a family away from focusing on developmental expectations that are potentially threatening to the child as the child transitions to puberty. It can also serve as a maladaptive way for a child to achieve autonomy in a family in which independence is seen as a threat to the family. Lastly, the eating disorder can be a diversion from other important issues such as parental conflict.

■ MEDICAL COMORBIDITY

Anorexia nervosa, like the other eating disorders, has multiple physical consequences in addition to its psychological, economic, vocational, legal, and spiritual sequelae. Serious medical complications are common. In some instances, these consequences are irreversible, indicating the need for early and aggressive treatments. It has been estimated that up to 55 percent of patients with anorexia have been found to require hospitalization for medical complications (Palla & Litt, 1988). The majority of physical findings are manifestations of starvation and dehydration.

The key medical and physical consequences can be described by the particular organ system affected. First, there are cardiovascular changes. Electrocardiogram changes can include, but are not limited to, a low voltage, T-wave inversion, and ST depression. Arrhythmias (abnormal heart rhythms) can be associated with hypokalemia (low potassium). There can be significant sinus bradycardia (slow heart rate), which is caused by starvation and does not reflect fitness secondary to compulsive exercise. There may also be hypotension (low blood pressure), congestive heart failure, and cardiomyopathy. Gastrointestinal changes are common and may include delayed gastric motility, pancreatitis with an elevated serum amylase, elevated liver function tests with occasional hepatitis, and acute vascular compression with intestinal obstruction. Hematologic changes may include mild anemia, leukopenia (low white blood cell count), and thrombocytopenia (low platelet count). Renal abnormalities may include an elevated blood urea nitrogen (BUN), decreased concentrating abilities of the kidney and partial diabetes insipidus. Skeletal abnormalities include osteoporosis (bone loss) and osteopenia (decreased bone density), small or decreased stature and myopathy (disorder of muscle tissue). Osteopenia is of particular concern as this is an illness that strikes during the adolescent years when bone formation is at its peak. Also, there is a brief period of accelerated growth early in the second decade of life that ends by the conclusion of the second decade of life. Starvation during early adolescence thus adversely affects ultimate height. Attempts to recover this "lost" height through adequate intake are generally unsuccessful after 13.5 years in females and 16 years in males (Lask & Bryant-Waugh, 1993).

Metabolic abnormalities can include hypercholesterolemia (high cholesterol), hypercarotenemia (high carotene levels often causing a pale yellow–red pigmentation of the skin), and low plasma zinc. Endocrine changes include amenorrhea, hypoestrogenemia (low estrogen levels), decreased follicle-stimulating hormone, decreased leutinizing hormone, ovarian cysts, a hypothyroid-like state with decreased thyroid stimulating hormone (TSH), and T3, hypercortisolism and increased corticotropin-releasing hormone, abnormal vasopressin response and in males, hypotestosteronemia (low testosterone levels). The thyroid abnormalities are reversible with weight restoration and in general, should not be treated with hormone replacement. The normal course of sexual maturation is disturbed as a result of malnutrition. There can be a failure to develop, or a loss of secondary sexual characteristics. Outcome studies of fertility in children with anorexia nervosa show that 31 percent continue to have amenorrhea, 14 percent have irregular menstruation, and 55 percent have regular menstruation after returning to a normal weight (Bryant-Waugh et al., 1988).

Brain changes have demonstrated (Lambe, Katzman, Mikulis, Kennedy & Zipursky, 1997; Katzman, Zipursky, Lambe & Mikulis, 1997) significant gray matter volume deficits and increased cerebrospinal fluid volumes, even in weight recovered patients. This may mean that the brain changes in anorexia nervosa are irreversible. Theoretically, reversible decreases in cognitive function are evident at low body weights and may lead to legal dilemmas such as whether a patient is competent to make decisions about treatment.

■ **PSYCHOSOCIAL COMORBIDITY**

People with anorexia nervosa often experience comorbid depression and anxiety, which along with the eating disorder symptoms can lead to social withdrawal and the loss of significant relationships. Families are often dramatically affected by this illness as well. As noted, this illness typically has its onset in the adolescent years when children are still living with the family. The illness may force the family, especially the parents, to focus much of their attention on the affected child leaving other children with less attention and often less supervision. These other children often become angry and resentful of the ill child. Parents may feel responsible for the onset of the illness as well as for making sure that the child eats adequately. Therefore, meal times often become battlegrounds. Families are devastated by the lack of productivity from ill children as the disease progresses, especially in the late stages. These are often very high achieving children of whom the parents expected much. This lack of productivity can be seen in society when these people require social services and support rather than becoming productive members of society.

■ ASSESSMENT

Assessment of anorexia nervosa is multidimensional and includes determining whether the patient has another medical illness or other psychiatric disorder that can account for their weight loss. There are multiple medical illnesses that result in weight loss including cancer, hyperthyroidism, and gastrointestinal problems, to name a few. Depressive disorders are often associated with a loss of appetite and subsequent weight loss. Schizophrenic or psychotic patients may have delusions about food that can lead to decreased caloric intake with resulting weight loss. Moreover, there are no simple laboratory tests or physical examination findings that can determine if the weight loss is secondary to anorexia nervosa. The initial assessment must include a thorough physical examination performed by the psychiatrist or another physician involved in the patient's care. Initial laboratory tests should include serum electrolytes, renal functions and glucose, a complete blood count with platelets and differential, liver functions, thyroid-stimulating hormone, serum calcium and phosphate as well as an electrocardiogram.

Next, an in depth clinical interview focusing on the symptoms of anorexia nervosa is needed. Anorexic patients are often anxious and secretive about their illness, which may make it difficult to obtain complete and accurate information about symptoms. It is more typical for these patients to be open in discussing their restrictive behaviors than bingeing or purging behaviors. It is extremely important to attempt to form a trusting relationship with the anorexic person. It is also often helpful to gather collateral information from family members and friends.

In addition, there are several structured interviews and self-report measures that may be utilized, but these are not necessary to make a diagnosis. The structured interviews include the eating disorder examination (EDE; Cooper & Fairburn, 1987; Fairburn & Cooper, 1993), the Structured Interview for Anorexia and Bulimia Nervosa (SIAB; Fichter et al., 1991), the Diagnostic Survey for Eating Disorders (DSED; Johnson, 1987), and the Yale–Brown–Cornell Eating Disorders Scale (YBC-EDS; Mazure, Halmi, Sunday, Rumano & Einhorn, 1994; Sunday, Halmi & Einhorn, 1995) all of which can be used to establish a diagnosis. The DSED can be used both as a self-report measure and as a semi-structured interview. Of these, the EDE has been the most researched; it is also available in both parent and child versions (Cooper & Fairburn, 1987).

The self-report questionnaires include the Eating Attitudes Test (EAT; Garner & Garfinkel, 1979), an abbreviated version, the EAT-26 (Garner, Olmsted, Bohr, & Garfinkel, 1982), the Kids Eating Disorders Survey (KEDS; Childress, Brewerton, Hodges & Jarrell, 1993), the Eating Disorders Inventory Symptom Check-list (EDI; Garner, Olmsted & Polivy, 1983) and the EDI-2 (Garner, 1991), and the Bulimia Test revised (BULIT-R; Thelan, Farmer, Wonderlich & Smith, 1991). The EAT has a version for school-age children (Maloney, McGuire & Daniels, 1988), the KEDS is applicable to middle-school children (Childress et al., 1993) and the EDI has normative data down to age 14 (Shore & Porter, 1990). The BULIT-R can be used to discriminate people with bulimia nervosa from those with anorexia nervosa and those without an eating disorder, although it is best used as a measure of the severity of bulimic symptoms (Smith & Thelan, 1984; Thelan et al., 1991; Thelan, Mann, Pruitt & Smith, 1987; Welch, Thompson & Hall, 1993). These self-report questionnaires may be most valuable when used as screening measures or as measures of treatment progress and outcome. Again, none of these can replace the interview in terms of making the diagnosis.

■ PSYCHIATRIC COMORBIDITY

Eating disorders are commonly associated with a history of other psychiatric disorders. Comorbid major depression has been reported in 50–75 percent of patients with anorexia nervosa (Halmi, Eckert, Marchi, Sampugnaro, Apple & Cohen, 1991). The lifetime prevalence of obsessive compulsive disorder among patients with anorexia nervosa has been estimated to be as high as 25 percent (Halmi et al., 1991). Comorbid anxiety disorders are common among patients with anorexia nervosa. There has been less evidence linking anorexia nervosa to substance abuse, but there is evidence that substance abuse is more common in the binge/purge subtype of anorexia nervosa (Halmi et al., 1991; Herzog, Keller, Sacks, Yeh & Lavori, 1992). Anorexia nervosa has also been associated with avoidant personality disorder and obsessive-compulsive personality disorder.

■ TREATMENT

Because anorexia nervosa is ego-syntonic, patients often resist treatment or efforts of family members and friends to engage them in treatment. The pros and cons of putting someone in treatment without their consent must be weighed. Treatment involves multiple modalities including medical and psychological treatment that can include individual, family and group therapy, as well as hospitalization. The APA has recently revised their guidelines for the treatment of both anorexia nervosa and bulimia nervosa (Yager et al., 2000).

The first treatment consideration is the medical stability of the patient, again underscoring the importance of a thorough physical examination in addition to the laboratory tests as described above. Some patients are so malnourished and medically unstable that medical hospitalization and stabilization are necessary prior to any psychiatric treatment. This often includes stabilization of electrolyte imbalances cardiac arrhythmias, and severe dehydration. The promotion of weight gain in the medical hospital is very difficult and should be reserved for psychiatric hospitalization, where a more structured program is usually possible. Nutritional management and psychoeducation alone can be effective in the least symptomatic patients.

Individual outpatient treatment is indicated for those who are experiencing less severe symptoms or for those who have successfully gained weight in other modes of treatment. It may be the first option of treatment in less severe cases and is often used to help patients continue on the road to recovery after hospitalization or more intensive outpatient treatment. Numerous reports have indicated that cognitive behavior therapy is efficacious in the treatment of anorexia nervosa (Garner, Vitousek & Pike, 1997; Vitousek & Hollon, 1990; Garner & Bemis, 1982). The focus of this type of therapy is on self-monitoring of food intake, bingeing and purging, and thoughts and feelings. It includes regular weighing, normalizing eating, identifying cognitive distortions, cognitive restructuring, and preventing relapse. Interpersonal therapy has not yet been studied. There are no controlled comparisons between long-term psychodynamic psychotherapy and other forms of treatment. Dialectical behavior therapy is also being used, but again, there are no controlled studies in anorexia nervosa.

One of the most important aspects of treating an eating disorder patient is to determine how often and who will weigh the patient. For the anorexic patient, weights should be obtained at least once weekly for outpatients or more often for those in more intensive treatment. Normal weight bulimic patients can be weighed much less frequently. Patients can choose whether to look or not and the weighing should be done at the beginning of the session. Anorexic patients often attempt to manipulate their weight through layering clothing, water loading, and attaching various different kinds of weight to the body. This must be carefully monitored.

Family therapy is indicated for all adolescent patients with anorexia nervosa in all levels of treatment and in some adult patients. In adolescent anorexia nervosa, research points to the efficacy of family therapy versus individual therapy. Russell and colleagues treated patients age 18 or younger with an illness duration of less than 3 years with family therapy for 1 year. When compared to individual therapy, the outcomes at 1 and 5 year follow-up showed the superiority of family therapy for the younger patient (age 18 or younger) and of individual therapy for the older patient (Russell et al., 1987; Eisler et al., 1997).

Intensive outpatient treatment is indicated for those who are not making progress in individual treatment or as a step down from partial hospitalization. Intensive outpatient treatment programs are inconsistently available across the US, especially those that are eating disorders specific. They typically involve 3 hours of programming per day an average of 3 days per week. They are behaviorally based, include a treatment team very similar if not identical to the inpatient treatment team. They include most of the modalities available in inpatient treatment only at much less intensity. These programs are typically not successful at promoting significant weight gain, for all of the reasons mentioned above, but can be used to step-down treatment from more intensive treatment or to step-up treatment in order to decrease the likelihood that more intensive treatment will be needed.

When available, a partial hospitalization is indicated for patients who do not yet need inpatient treatment but have been unable to gain weight in outpatient or intensive outpatient treatment. Others may have completed an inpatient hospitalization and continue to need intensive treatment. Partial hospitalization programs are inconsistently available across the country and should preferably be eating disorders specific. They typically involve 5–12 hours of programming per day from 3 to 7 days per week. These programs are behaviorally based, include a treatment team very similar if not identical to the inpatient treatment team and include most of the modalities available in inpatient treatment except that they are not typically as intense or available 24 hours a day. These programs are not as successful at attaining weight gain goals and the average weight gain has been estimated to be between 0.5 and 1 pound per week. It is more difficult to restrict exercising and purging behaviors, as these patients are not in the program 24 hours a day. It is also more difficult to reach the daily caloric goals that are set in an inpatient setting because behavioral consequences can not be enforced.

Psychiatric hospitalization is often necessary when the patient's weight is at or below 75 percent of ideal body weight or there has been a significant weight loss over a short period of time. In adolescents, this may be considered when weight is at or below 80 percent of ideal weight. Inpatient treatment is also warranted if there are significant medical or psychiatric consequences including suicidal ideation. Inpatient hospitalization can be used in two very different ways. Brief hospitalization may be used to treat the physical complications of the illness, to interrupt bingeing, vomiting or laxative abuse that pose medical risks or complications, or to manage and treat other associated conditions such as severe depression, risk of self-harm, or substance abuse.

Prolonged hospitalization can be used for weight gain in the severely underweight anorexic patient. Weight gain is best accomplished in an eating disorders specific, highly structured psychiatric hospital. This typically consists of a specialized multi-disciplinary treatment team that optimally includes a psychiatrist, internist, family physician or pediatrician, psychologist, social worker, dietitian, nurse practitioner, bachelor's level nurses, and bachelor's level therapists. These programs typically use a behavioral management approach, which relies mainly on a cognitive behavioral model (Anderson, Bowers & Evans, 1997). A combination of group therapy, family education and therapy, nutritional rehabilitation and education and medications, which may include psychotropic medications are used. Individual therapy is not typically a part of this treatment stage, as cognitive abilities are often significantly impaired at these low weights and patients are subsequently unable to benefit from individual therapy.

There must be some flexibility in the program so that individual patient's needs can be met, but at the same time there must be consistency and firm limit setting. Typically, medically stable patients are started on 35 cal/kg and are expected to eat 100 percent of meals. These calories are divided into 5 or 6 meals throughout the day and patients are under close staff observation during these meals. If they are unable to eat 100 percent, they are typically given a liquid supplement. Some programs will use a nasogastric tube if the patient is unwilling to drink the liquid supplement and is severely malnourished. At this point, behavioral consequences are also used to elicit positive behaviors. Calories are typically increased by 200–300 calories every 3–5 days in order to achieve an average weight gain of 2.5 pounds per week. Weight gain typically ranges from 2–5 pounds per week. There can be medical complications related to refeeding, but these are relatively rare if using oral food feedings. Common complaints include mild edema, constipation, bloating, shortness of breath, abdominal pain, sweating, and heat intolerance. Significant edema is relatively rare. It is most likely if the patient has been purging, receives intravenous alimentation or hydration, is significantly below normal weight or is medically compromised. Patients are restricted from exercising and lose privileges if they are found exercising. They are also typically restricted from purging by locking bathroom doors and are observed by staff during and after meals and at all times while using the bathroom.

Residential treatment, when available, should be considered in patients who are medically stable but continue to be in need of significant weight gain. Again, this is typically only successful if the treatment is in an eating disorders specific program. This treatment provides an opportunity for an extended period of intensive treatment and supervision for patients who do not require the close medical monitoring given in an acute care setting. Unfortunately, in the US, this level of treatment is difficult to find.

Outpatient medical management alone should be reserved for chronic patients who have participated in various forms of competently delivered treatment over the course of many years with no plans to work towards recovery. For these patients, continued psychotherapy, which is aimed at recovery, can be futile both for the patient and the therapist. It is often very difficult to make a decision as to when and with whom to terminate therapy. The goal of this type of treatment is aimed at maintaining medical and psychological stability. If at some point the patient wishes to restart psychotherapy aimed at recovery then this can be considered.

Pharmacotherapy should not be the primary method of treatment but may supplement the effectiveness of other appropriate psychotherapeutic or behavioral treatment modalities. Psychotropic medications have been studied over the years, initially with the aim to increase the rate and amount of weight gain, this met with little success. Antipsychotic medications were studied and demonstrated no significant difference compared to controls while significant side effects were found including hypotension, gastrointestinal (GI) side effects, and chronic neurological sequelae. Antidepressants have been widely studied because of the well-recognized association between anorexia nervosa and depression. Malnutrition can produce a psychological profile, which is indistinguishable from that seen in mild to moderate depression. These symptoms often resolve with improvement in nutrition. Initial studies involving antidepressants claimed success based on short-term weight gain and some reduction in the levels of depression. More recent studies have aimed to help patients to maintain weight already gained and to alleviate any comorbid symptoms. These studies have produced evidence for the efficacy of serotonin selective reuptake inhibitors in the reduction of depressive symptoms as well as weight maintenance but only after nutritional restoration (Kaye, Gwirtsman, George & Ebert, 1991; Ferguson, La Via, Crossan & Kaye, 1999). Recently, low-dose atypical neuroleptics have been used to address the severe obsessional thinking, anxiety, and psychotic-like thinking in anorexics with some success (La Via, Gray & Kaye, 2000). Anxiolytics may be used short term to address the anxiety related to refeeding. Appetite-enhancing agents such as cyproheptadine have demonstrated no enhancement of appetite or weight gain in controlled trials. Some studies involving prokinetic agents have shown an improvement in gastric emptying. These agents may be used for anorexia nervosa when there is significant distress associated with meals and when there is evidence of delayed gastric emptying. Estrogen has demonstrated no significant impact on bone density in women with anorexia nervosa. Calcium supplements are used to minimize the incidence of osteopenia and osteoporosis.

Bulimia Nervosa

■ DIAGNOSIS

Russell first described bulimia nervosa as a variant of anorexia nervosa in 1979, although bulimic-like behaviors had been documented in the literature much earlier. Before 1970, bulimia nervosa was rare. According to the DSM IV, bulimia nervosa is characterized by recurrent episodes of eating large amounts of food and feeling out of control followed by recurrent compensatory behaviors such as purging, fasting, or excessive exercise in order to prevent weight gain. The binge eating and compensatory behaviors must both occur an average of at least twice a week for 3 months. Aberrant eating patterns in bulimia nervosa are accompanied by an overconcern with shape and weight causing patients to evaluate themselves predominantly on the basis of body shape and weight. The person with bulimia nervosa typically maintains a normal weight although there can be a history of obesity, as well. There is no evidence of overt starvation although semi-starvation plays an important role in the onset and maintenance of this illness. These patients are less introverted and obsessive than the restrictor anorexic patients and more impulsive. There are two subtypes of bulimia nervosa, purging, and non-purging. The purging type regularly engages in self-induced vomiting or the misuse of laxatives, diuretics, or enemas. The non-purging type uses other inappropriate compensatory behaviors, such as fasting or excessive exercise, but does not regularly use self-induced vomiting, laxatives, diuretics, or enemas. There is evidence to suggest that the same criteria are applicable to adolescents. The DSM IV diagnostic criteria for bulimia nervosa are shown in Table 6-3.

■ PREVALENCE

The incidence of bulimia nervosa increased in the 1980s and now exceeds that of anorexia nervosa (Fairburn & Beglin, 1990; Hoek, 1991; Hall & Hay, 1991). The prevalence of bulimia nervosa is estimated to be between 1 and 3 percent of the female population (Garfinkel et al., 1995). Although the full syndrome is not common, the individual symptoms of bulimia nervosa, such as isolated episodes of binge eating and purging, occur in up to 40 percent of college women. Bulimia nervosa is more common in females than in males, approximately 10 times more common (DSM IV). There is a modal age of onset between mid-adolescence and the late 20s, which is later than that for anorexia nervosa. There is greater diversity in the typical socioeconomic class background than with anorexia nervosa. There is no data concerning sex differences in course or associated psychopathology. Preliminary stu-

---

TABLE 6-3. DIAGNOSTIC CRITERIA FOR BULIMIA NERVOSA

A. Recurrent episodes of binge eating. Binge eating is characterized by both of the following:
 1. Eating in a discrete period of time (e.g., within any 2 hour period), an amount of food that is definitely larger than most people would eat during a similar period of time and under similar circumstances.
 2. A sense of lack of control over eating during the episode (e.g., a feeling that one could not stop eating or control what or how much one is eating).
B. Recurrent inappropriate compensatory behavior in order to prevent weight gain, such as self-induced vomiting; misuse of laxatives, diuretics, enemas or other medications; fasting; or excessive exercise.
C. The binge eating and inappropriate compensatory behaviors both occur, on average, at least twice a week for 3 months.
D. Self-evaluation is unduly influenced by body shape and weight.
E. The disturbance does not occur exclusively during episodes of anorexia nervosa.

Specify type:
 Purging type: during the current episode of bulimia nervosa, the person has regularly engaged in self-induced vomiting or the misuse of laxatives, diuretics or enemas.
 Non-purging type: during the current episode of bulimia nervosa, the person has used other inappropriate compensatory behaviors, such as fasting or excessive exercise, but has not regularly engaged in self-induced vomiting or the misuse of laxatives, diuretics, or enemas.

---

dies suggest that there is an excess rate of homosexuality among male patients. The full syndrome of bulimia nervosa is rare in the first decade of life although there may be significant symptoms present in prepubertal children.

■ COURSE AND OUTCOME

The short-term course of bulimia is marked by fluctuating symptoms, with varying cycles of remissions and exacerbations. A seasonal component, similar to that of seasonal affective disorder, has been identified in a subset of patients (Brewerton, Krahn, Hardin, Wehr & Rosenthal, 1994). Recently, Keel and colleagues (Keel, Mitchell, Miller, Davis & Crow, 1999) published data suggesting that the number of women who continue to meet full criteria for bulimia nervosa declines as the duration of follow-up increases. Approximately 30 percent of the women, however, continued to engage in recurrent binge eating or purging behaviors. A history of substance use problems and a longer duration of the disorder at presentation predicted worse outcome (Keel et al., 1999).

■ ETIOLOGY

The etiology of bulimia nervosa has not been fully explicated, but as is the case with anorexia nervosa, may be best understood from a biopsychosocial perspective. Recently, there is emerging evidence supporting a genetic linkage with higher rates of both anorexia nervosa and bulimia nervosa in first-degree relatives of anorexia nervosa probands (Strober, Lampert, Morrell, Burroughs & Jacobs, 1990). The average concordance rate for bulimia nervosa in monozygotic twins is approximately 50 percent versus 15 percent for dizygotic twins (Bulik, Sullivan & Kendler, 1998). Genetic liability is expressed in a complex context with the final eating disorder symptoms representing an interaction of three broad classes of predisposing factors along with precipitating and perpetuating factors. The three classes of predisposing factors include cultural, individual (psychological and biological) and familial causal factors. The precipitating factors are less clearly delineated although there is substantial evidence that dieting is involved in the development of eating disorder behavior (Fairburn, 1985a). The cognitive behavioral model of disordered eating shows that people who develop bulimia nervosa become preoccupied with an idealized body weight and shape, which leads to dieting behaviors. This dieting behavior makes these people more susceptible to a loss of control over eating leading to binge eating. Binge eating leads to purging behaviors in order to compensate for the effects of the binge eating. Purging helps to maintain the bingeing by decreasing the anxiety related to potential weight gain, it also disrupts the learned satiety that normally regulates food intake. The bingeing and purging cause distress that serves to further lower self-esteem thereby perpetuating the cycle.

The serotonin system also plays a role in the development and maintenance of bulimia nervosa. There is substantial evidence for the existence of impaired central serotonin function in bulimia nervosa (Kaye et al., 1990; Goldbloom & Garfinkel, 1990; McBride, Anderson, Khalt, Sunday & Halmi, 1991; Jimerson, Lesem, Kaye & Brewerton, 1992; Brewerton, 1995). Bulimia nervosa is characterized by reduced post-synaptic hypothalamic serotonin receptor sensitivity that is independent of the presence of major depression or anorexia nervosa. Also, binge frequency has been shown to be inversely related to levels of CSF 5-HIAA (Jimerson et al., 1992). All of these findings are best accounted for by a dysregulation of the serotonin system that implies a relative failure of the neurotransmitter regulation rather than a simple decrease or increase in activity (Seiver & Davis, 1985).

■ MEDICAL COMORBIDITY

There are multiple effects of bulimia nervosa on the patient including medical, economic, vocational, legal, spiritual, and emotional sequelae. Patients with bulimia nervosa most often experience severe fluid and electrolyte imbalances due to purging behavior. Vomiting is the most common form of purging with 53–94 percent of people with bulimia nervosa reporting this behavior (Mitchell,

Hatzukami & Eckert, 1985a). Laxative abuse is also common with 20 percent of bulimia nervosa patients (Mitchell, Hatzukami, Eckert & Pyle, 1985b). The presence of metabolic acidosis should raise the suspicion of laxative abuse and the possibility of an underlying eating disorder. Up to 25 percent of bulimia nervosa patients report using diet pills and 10 percent use daily diuretics in order to achieve weight loss (Mitchell et al., 1985a). Caffeine is also used in large quantities because of its effect as an appetite suppressant, diuretic, and stimulant (Fahy & Treasure, 1991). Excessive exercise is less common in bulimia nervosa than in anorexia nervosa.

The medical consequences in bulimia nervosa are numerous and include, but are not limited to, parotidomegaly (enlarged parotid glands), Russell's sign (scars on the dorsum of the hand from self-induced gag and vomiting), dental decay, pharyngitis (inflammation of the pharynx), esophagitis (inflammation of the esophagus), gastritis (inflammation of the stomach), hiatal hernia, large bowel atony, gastric dilatation, hyperamylasemia, transient rebound edema, bradycardia, hypotension, and menstrual irregularities. As previously mentioned, there can be multiple fluid and electrolyte abnormalities secondary to purging including dehydration, hypochloremia, and hypokalemia. The physical symptoms associated with these abnormalities include muscle weakness, fatigue, cardiac arrhythmias, and seizures.

■ PSYCHOSOCIAL COMORBIDITY

Economical, financial and legal consequences are often related to the cost of foods required for binges, but also to the lack of productivity of these people. Patients often resort to stealing from family, friends or from stores in order to continue to support binges. Bingeing and purging behaviors are most often secretive and, when severe, can affect one's ability to hold a job or complete school. Family members are often more concerned about a bulimic's behavior than the patient themselves. Again, because of the secretive nature of this illness, these patients often lose touch with their family and friends becoming socially withdrawn and isolated.

■ ASSESSMENT

Because these people tend to be ashamed of their bingeing and purging behaviors, the assessment of bulimia nervosa may be difficult and is best done with an in-depth interview. A thorough assessment should include a physical examination to determine whether there are any medical consequences that need to be addressed. Again, there are several structured interviews and self-report measures that can be used. For more detail review the section on the assessment of anorexia nervosa. Remember that none of these structured interviews or self-report measures is a substitute for a thorough interview.

■ PSYCHIATRIC COMORBIDITY

Comorbidity with other psychiatric disorders is common. There is a high rate of depressive comorbidity and elevated rates of primary mood disorders in biological relatives. There are higher rates of affective and anxiety disorder diagnoses in first-degree relatives in bulimia nervosa probands. Bulimia nervosa occurs in persons at risk for substance-related disorders and a variety of personality disorders. Bulimia nervosa patients also have increased rates of anxiety disorders, bipolar type I disorder, dissociative disorders, and histories of sexual abuse. People with bulimia nervosa are at risk for developing substance abuse or dependence (Garfinkel et al., 1995). There are also higher rates of obsessive–compulsive personality disorder in first-degree relatives of bulimia nervosa probands (Lilenfeld et al., 1998).

■ TREATMENT

The treatment of bulimia nervosa consists of multiple modalities including individual psychotherapy, group therapy, family therapy, and pharmacotherapy. Most patients with uncomplicated bulimia nervosa do not require inpatient hospitalization. In some cases, inpatient hospitalization may be necessary. See Table 6-4 for criteria for inpatient treatment of bulimia nervosa. When in-

TABLE 6-4. CRITERIA FOR INPATIENT TREATMENT OF BULIMIA NERVOSA

When at least one of the following is present:

A. Bingeing and purging at least 4 times per day with severe impairment in life function which has failed to respond to at least 2 months of comprehensive outpatient treatment.

B. Interruption of the binge/purge cycle is required because medical complications threaten life or health. Possible complications include:

Pancreatitis

Uncontrolled diabetes

Esophagitis or esophageal tears

Severe electrolyte disturbance

Severe colitis

Gastric dilatation

Large bowel atony with obstruction

Renal impairment

Cardiac arrhythmia

C. Interruption of the binge/purge cycle is required because medication must be retained, as for treatment of a medical or psychiatric condition; or to maintain adequate nutritional status as during pregnancy.

D. If the patient is too depressed to be managed as an outpatient or there is a risk of suicide

patient hospitalization is necessary to address the bulimic symptoms, it is best accomplished in a subspecialized eating disorders unit that is highly structured. The goal of hospitalization is to stabilize the patient's eating patterns and to stop the cycle of bingeing and purging. These hospitalizations are generally brief and very symptom-focused. Inpatient programs typically use a behavioral management approach based on a cognitive behavioral model. There is typically a combination of group therapy, individual therapy, family education and therapy, nutrition education, and medications, if needed. Hospitalization to address other psychiatric symptoms often can be accomplished on a general inpatient psychiatric unit.

Outpatient treatment is usually indicated in the treatment of bulimia nervosa. There have been a number of randomized controlled trials that demonstrate the effectiveness of cognitive behavioral therapy in the treatment of bulimia nervosa. Cognitive behavior therapy is a semi-structured time limited (4–5 months) approach based on the cognitive behavioral model of disordered eating described above. There are manuals available (Fairburn, Jones, Peveler, Hope & O'Connor, 1993); however training in cognitive behavior therapy is desirable. There is considerable evidence that this therapy is useful in ameliorating symptoms of bulimia nervosa. In summary, these studies show that cognitive behavioral therapy is effective in decreasing the rates of bingeing and purging as well as dietary restraint (Agras, Schneider, Arnow, Raeburn & Telch, 1989; Agras et al., 1992; Fairburn et al., 1991; Garner, Rockert, Davis, Garner, Olmsted & Eagle, 1993; Wilson, Eldredge, Smith, Niles et al., 1991). Most patients improve substantially with this therapy and improvements are maintained for at least the first year after treatment (Agras et al., 1994; Fairburn et al., 1993; Wilson et al., 1991). The Oxford study looked at the long-term benefits of cognitive behavioral therapy and showed good maintenance of the benefits with abstinence rates of 48 percent at 5.8 years (Fairburn, Norman, Welch, O'Connor, Doll & Peveler, 1995). This therapy is based on the premise that chronic dieting in an effort to control weight promotes and maintains binge-eating behavior (Fairburn, 1985b; Fairburn, Marcus & Wilson, 1993). Treatment therefore focuses on decreasing dietary restraint, and on modifying maladaptive thoughts, beliefs, and values related to eating, shape, and weight. The treatment goal is the normalization of eating, not weight loss. Cognitive behavioral therapy has also been shown to have effects on associated psychopathology with improvement in depressive symptoms, self-esteem, social functioning and personality disorder symptoms (Fairburn, Kirk, O'Connor & Cooper, 1986; Fairburn, Agras & Wilson, 1992; Garner et al., 1993).

There is also evidence that interpersonal therapy is an efficacious treatment for bulimia nervosa. Interpersonal therapy like cognitive behavioral therapy was developed as a treatment for depression (Klerman, Weissman, Rounsaville & Chevron, 1984) and adapted for use in the treatment of bulimia nervosa (Fairburn, 1997). It is based on an assumption that problems in the interpersonal milieu maintain eating disorder symptoms. Interpersonal therapy was found to be somewhat less effective than cognitive behavior therapy immediately following treatment. However, patients who received interpersonal therapy continued to show improvement during follow-up. At one year, interpersonal therapy was equivalent to cognitive behavior therapy in terms of benefit (Fairburn et al., 1991, 1993).

There have been no controlled comparisons between long-term psychodynamic psychotherapy and other forms of treatment. There also have been no controlled studies of feminist therapies, which emphasize the importance of issues such as role conflicts, identity confusion, sexual abuse, and other forms of victimization in the development, maintenance, and treatment of eating disorders.

Pharmacotherapy in bulimia nervosa may be used as a supplement to education and psychotherapy. There are numerous studies looking at the efficacy of antidepressants in bulimia nervosa. Initial studies looked at antidepressants alone and fluoxetine showed the greatest benefits with the fewest side effects and lowest risk of lethality. Fluoxetine at 60 mg per day was superior to 20 mg per day in decreasing the frequency of bingeing and purging (Fluoxetine BN Collaborative Study Group, 1992; Goldstein et al., 1995). More recent studies have looked at the benefits of antidepressants, psychotherapy, and the combination. All of these studies demonstrate that cognitive behavior therapy is better than an antidepressant alone, but that the combination produces modest additional benefits (Mitchell, Pyle, Eckert, Hatsukami, Pomeroy & Zimmerman, 1990; Agras et al., 1992; Leitenberg, Rosen, Wolf, Vara, Detzer & Srebnik, 1994; Goldbloom, Olmsted, Davis, & Shaw, 1994; Walsh et al., 1995). Based on these data, antidepressants should be added if there is comorbid depression, anxiety disorder or if severe obsessionality is present or if the bulimia nervosa is severe or has had only a partial response to cognitive behavioral therapy alone. Antidepressants can also be used if psychotherapy for eating disorders are unavailable or if cost is a factor in the treatment of the patient. Mood stabilizers have been shown to have little benefit in the treatment of bulimia nervosa. There have been no studies of the use of benzodiazepines and they should be used with caution given the risk for developing substance abuse or dependence. There is no evidence of benefit with naltrexone (Mitchell et al., 1989; Alger, Schwalberg, Bigaouette, Michaelek & Howard, 1991) and fenfluramine has shown little effect with cognitive behavior therapy (Russel, Checkley, Feldman, & Eisler, 1988; Fahy, Eisler, & Russel, 1993).

Therefore, initial treatment recommendations for bulimia nervosa with limited comorbidity include systematic short-term psychotherapy. Cognitive behavior therapy is usually first recommended because there are more studies to support this type of therapy in bulimia nervosa. Also, it has more rapid onset of effects. Interpersonal therapy may be considered for patients with little or no response to cognitive behavior therapy or for patients who do not want a symptom-focused approach. For patients with very mild symptoms, psychoeducation alone may be adequate. There are also self-help or guided self-help therapies for use in mild cases or when other forms of therapy are not readily available. Antidepressant medication can be considered if there are significant comorbid symptoms or there is little or no improvement with psychotherapy.

For more severely ill patients or for those with significant comorbidity, there are various levels of care including inpatient hospitalization, partial hospitalization, and intensive outpatient. Refer to the section under anorexia nervosa for more details on these levels of treatment.

■ NUTRITION COUNSELING

Nutrition counseling is an extremely important part of treatment for the anorexic patient and a potentially useful treatment component for patients with bulimia nervosa. Often the easiest way to initially get a patient into treatment is to suggest nutrition consultation. It is important that the nutritionist have some experience with eating disorder patients or have access to a colleague who has eating disorders experience. These patients are frequently very knowledgeable about nutrition and will often attempt to manipulate the nutritionist. The nutritionist's role is to develop a meal plan, evaluate the patient's current food intake patterns, help normalize eating behaviors, estimate and determine an appropriate weight goal, and develop a meal plan to reach that goal. For bulimic patients, this does not include significant weight loss, at least initially. The role of the nutritionist is to help support the new eating behaviors and to inform other treatment team members of changes or reversals of progress. These goals can be accomplished through an initial assessment and regular follow-up. The nutritional assessment includes gathering information about height, weight, body mass index, body frame, highest weight, lowest weight, desired weight, average body weight, nutrition history, eating behaviors, food frequency, 24-hour food recall, percent body fat, daily caloric requirements, and reviewing laboratory values. Developing a meal plan is the next step. It is often difficult because of the patient's fear of gaining weight. The goal of developing a meal plan is to get the patient to eat commonly available foods in regularly scheduled meals.

It is often difficult to continue weight gain in the anorexic patient because of the need for high caloric intake, often greater than 65 cal/kg. When refeeding is started the metabolism begins to increase requiring continued calorie increases in order to continue weight gain. Weight gain typically begins with fluid weight gain with later tissue weight gain.

Sustaining calories, once a weight goal has been met, for an anorexic patient are approximately 34 cal/kg and for a bulimic patient approximately 28 cal/kg. These are typically higher for child and adolescent patients. The goal weight is the weight that will restore normal physiologic functioning, which can be determined by normalization of T_3, leutinizing hormone, estrogen/testosterone levels, and normal core body temperature. There are several different ways of determining goal weight. It is estimated a little differently in adult versus the still growing child and adolescent patients. Generally, ideal body weight is determined in adults using the 1959 Metropolitan Life charts (Metropolitan Life Insurance Company, 1959) and in adolescents using the pediatric growth charts. Premorbid weights are also taken into consideration, premorbid growth charts are important in determining goal weight in the child and adolescent patients. Body mass index (BMI) is being used more consistently in determining goal weight. The goal is to reach a BMI of 20.8 or more.

Eating Disorders Not Otherwise Specified

According to the DSM IV, eating disorders "not otherwise specified" (NOS) is a category for disorders of eating that do not fully meet the criteria for any specific eating disorder. The SDSM IV criteria for eating disorders NOS are shown in Table 6-5. This does not imply that these disorders are any less serious or that these individuals are any less in need of treatment. There are six examples given in the DSM IV (binge eating disorder will be discussed separately.) There is very little systematic information about eating disorder NOS despite the fact that this is the most common eating disorder diagnosis. Epidemiological studies are needed to learn more about the range of eating disorder behaviors. Also, treatment effectiveness studies that include patients with eating disorder NOS are needed to determine whether currently available treatments are of benefit. Until then, it makes sense to treat anorexia nervosa variants like anorexia nervosa itself and bulimia nervosa variants with interventions that work for bulimia nervosa.

TABLE 6-5. DIAGNOSTIC CRITERIA FOR EATING DISORDER NOT OTHERWISE SPECIFIED

The eating disorder NOS category is for disorders of eating that do not meet the criteria for any specific eating disorder. Examples include:

1. For females, all of the criteria for anorexia nervosa are met except the person has regular menses.
2. All of the criteria for anorexia nervosa are met except that, despite significant weight loss, the individual's current weight is in the normal range.
3. All of the criteria for bulimia nervosa are met except that the binge eating and inappropriate compensatory mechanisms occur at a frequency of less than twice a week or for a duration of less than 3 months.
4. The regular use of inappropriate compensatory behavior by a person of normal body weight after eating small amounts of food (e.g., self-induced vomiting after the consumption of two cookies).
5. Repeatedly chewing and spitting out, but not swallowing, large amounts of food.
6. Binge eating disorder: recurrent episodes of binge eating in the absence of the regular use of inappropriate compensatory behaviors characteristic of bulimia nervosa.

Binge Eating Disorder

Binge eating disorder (BED), recurrent episodes of binge eating in the absence of the inappropriate compensatory behaviors characteristic of bulimia nervosa, falls into the category for eating disorders NOS but, as mentioned previously, it has also been included in the appendix of the DSM IV. The DSM IV research criteria for binge eating disorder are shown in Table 6-6. Compensatory behaviors do occur among binge eating disorder patients but not with the regularity that is required for a diagnosis of bulimia nervosa. Most researchers feel that it is more accurate to report the number of days of binge eating rather than the number of episodes as is required for bulimia nervosa. Overall, these patients have an inability to regulate eating behaviors both within- and between-binge episodes. Most BED patients are overweight and seek treatment for obesity rather than for an eating disorder. Estimates are that about 2 percent of the general population has BED and 8 per-

---

TABLE 6-6. RESEARCH CRITERIA FOR BINGE EATING DISORDER

A. Recurrent episodes of binge eating. An episode of binge eating is characterized by both of the following:

    (1) Eating in a discrete period of time (e.g., within any 2 hour period), an amount of food that is definitely larger than most people would eat in a similar period of time under similar circumstances.

    (2) A sense of lack of control over eating during the episode (e.g., a feeling that one cannot stop eating or control what or how much one is eating).

B. The binge-eating episodes are associated with three (or more) of the following:

    (1) Eating much more rapidly than normal.

    (2) Eating until feeling uncomfortably full.

    (3) Eating large amounts of food when not feeling physically hungry.

    (4) Eating alone because of being embarrassed by how much one is eating.

    (5) Feeling disgusted with oneself, depressed, or very guilty after overeating.

C. Marked distress regarding binge eating is present.

D. The binge eating occurs, on average, at least 2 days a week for 6 months.

Note: The method of determining a frequency differs from that used for bulimia nervosa; future research should address whether the preferred method of setting a frequency threshold is counting the number of days on which binges occur or counting the number of episodes of binge eating.

E. The binge eating is not associated with the regular use of inappropriate compensatory behaviors (e.g., purging, fasting, excessive exercise) and does not occur exclusively during the course of anorexia nervosa or bulimia nervosa.

---

cent of the obese population (Bruce & Agras, 1992), but approximately 30 percent of people who receive obesity treatment at university-based clinics meet criteria for BED (Spitzer et al., 1992, 1993).

Obesity is associated with increased risks for cardiovascular disease, hypertension, diabetes, and certain cancers. The health risks associated with obesity are significant at a body mass index greater than 27 and increase with the severity of obesity (Pi-Sunyer, 1991).

Binge eating disorder is associated with significant psychiatric comorbidity, most importantly, depressive symptoms. Both binge eating and obesity can also contribute to shame and depressive symptoms.

Like bulimia nervosa, evidence is suggesting that cognitive behavioral therapy, interpersonal psychotherapy, and antidepressant treatment have a role in the treatment of binge eating disorder. However, cognitive behavioral therapy has been the best-studied treatment thus far. Cognitive behavioral therapy for binge eating disorder focuses on the moderation of food intake. Initially, the goal is to make a plan for regular eating and to minimize or eliminate binge episodes. The next goal is to moderate food intake and identify and modify thoughts and beliefs that perpetuate the eating problem. The final goal is to consolidate progress and teach relapse prevention. It should be emphasized that one of the goals is not weight loss; however, a weight loss program can be considered after treatment for the binge eating.

Interpersonal psychotherapy has been reported to be as effective as cognitive behavioral therapy in treating binge eating disorder (Wilfley et al., 1993). Dialectical behavior therapy is currently being adapted for use with binge eating disorder (Wiser and Telch, 1999).

Exercise should be a part of treatment for several reasons. Exercise is incompatible with binge eating. It can be an excellent way to manage stress and is an important part of any long-term weight management because of the energy expended.

Again, dietitians can work with the patient to become more aware of the amount of food that they consume, introduce basic principles of good nutrition, and give guidance for a reasonable caloric intake consisting of at least 1500 calories per day and up to 2500 calories per day.

There is some preliminary evidence that antidepressants (McCann & Agras, 1990; Alger et al., 1991; deZwaan, Nutzinger & Schoenbeck, 1992; Marcus, Wing, Ewing, Kern, McDermott & Gooding, 1990) and the opiate blocker naloxone (Drewnowski, Krahn, Demitrack, Nairn & Gosnell, 1995) may be useful in the treatment of binge eating disorder. However, there is very little research in this area. Antidepressants may be seen as helpful given the likelihood of co-occurring depression in binge eating disorder and the interaction between negative mood, binge eating, and weight gain.

Thus far there has been limited research in the treatment of binge eating disorder. The overall effects in these studies have been modest and there has been little long-term follow-up. More research is clearly needed in order to help better understand this illness and to develop effective treatment.

Conclusion

The aim of this chapter was to introduce the diagnosis and treatment of eating disorders. Although relatively rare, these illnesses are associated with a significant amount of morbidity and mortality. Milder variants of disordered eating also are associated with considerable morbidity and are seen commonly in clinical practice. The currently utilized treatments have proven to be moderately effective, but clearly more research is needed. This research should focus on the effectiveness of treatment modalities and also on epidemiology and the course of these illnesses. Additional research on the delineation and definition of the most common group of eating disorders, the eating disorders not otherwise specified, is also needed. As more is learned about the eating disorders the next area of focus may then be on primary prevention.

SUGGESTED READING

For the Clinician:

Handbook of treatment for eating disorders, 2nd ed., D.M. Garner & P.E
   Garfinkel (Eds.). Copyright 1997 by Guilford Publications, Inc., 72
   Spring Street, New York, NY 10012.

Medical issues and the eating disorders: The interface, A.S. Kaplan & P.E
   Garfinkel (Eds.). Copyright 1993 by Bruner/Mazel, Inc., 19 Union
   Square West, New York, NY 10003.

Anorexia nervosa and related eating disorders in childhood and adolescence, 2nd ed., B. Lask & R. Bryant-Waugh (Eds.). Copyright 1999
   by Lawrence Erlbaum, Hove, UK.

Overcoming binge eating by Christopher Fairburn, M.D. Copyright 1995
   by Guilford Publications, Inc., 72 Spring Street, New York, NY 10012.

Getting better bit(e) by bit(e) by U. Schmidt and J. Treasure. Copyright
   1993 by Lawrence Erlbaum, Hove, UK.

For Patients, Families and Friends:

Anorexia nervosa: A survival guide for families, friends, and sufferers, J.
   Treasure (Ed.). Copyright 1997 by Psychology Press.

The golden cage: The enigma of anorexia nervosa by Hilde Bruch.
   Copyright 1978 by the President and Fellows of Harvard College.

My sister's bones by Cathi Hanauer, 1996.

The best little girl in the world by Steven Levenkron, 1978.

Perk! The story of a teenager with bulimia by Liza F. Hall, 1997.

REFERENCES

Agras, W.S., Rossiter, E.M., Amow, B., Schneider, J.A., Telch, C.F.,
   Raeburn, S.D., Bruce, B., Perl, M., & Koran, L.M. (1992).
   Pharmacologic and cognitive-behavioral treatment for bulimia nervosa: A controlled comparison. American Journal of Psychiatry, 149,
   82–87.

Agras, W.S., Rossiter, E.M., Arnow, B., Telch, C.F., Raeburn, S.D.,
   Bruce, B., & Koran, L. (1994). One-year follow-up of psychosocial
   and pharmacologic treatments for bulimia nervosa. Journal of
   Clinical Psychiatry, 55, 179–183.

Agras, W.S., Schneider, J.A., Arnow, B., Raeburn, S.D., & Telch, C.F.
   (1989). Cognitive-behavioral treatment with and without exposure
   plus response prevention in the treatment of bulimia nervosa: A

reply to Leitenberg and Rosen. *Journal of Consulting and Clinical Psychology, 57*, 778–779.

Alger, S.A., Schwalberg, M.D., Bigaouette, J.M., Michaelek, A.V., & Howard, L.J. (1991). Effect of a tricyclic antidepressant and opiate antagonist on binge-eating in normal weight bulimic and obese, binge-eating subjects. *American Journal of Clinical Nutrition, 53*, 865–871.

American Psychiatric Association (APA) (1994). *Diagnostic and statistical manual of mental disorders*, 4th ed. (DSM IV). Washington, DC: American Psychiatric Association.

Anderson, A.E., Bowers, W., & Evans, K. (1997). Inpatient treatment of anorexia nervosa. In D.M. Garner & P.E. Garfinkel (Eds.), *Handbook of psychotherapy for anorexia nervosa and bulimia* (pp. 327–348). New York, NY: Guilford Press.

Brewerton, T.D. (1995). Toward a unified theory of serotonin dysregulation in eating and related disorders. *Psychoneuroendocrinology, 20*(6), 561–590.

Brewerton, T.D., & Jimerson, D.C. (1996). Studies of serotonin function in anorexia nervosa. *Psychiatry Research, 62*(1), 31–42.

Brewerton, T.D., Krahn, D.D., Hardin, T.A., Wehr, P.A., & Rosenthal, N.E. (1994). Findings from the seasonal pattern assessment questionnaire in patients with eating disorders and control subjects: effects of diagnosis and location. *Psychiatry Research, 52*(1), 71–84.

Bruce, B., & Agras, W.S. (1992). Binge eating in females: A population-based investigation. *International Journal of Eating Disorders, 12*, 65–373.

Bruch, H. (1962). Perceptual and conceptual disturbances in anorexia nervosa. *Psychosomatic Medicine, 24*, 187–194.

Bruch, H. (1973). *Eating disorders: Obesity, anorexia nervosa and the person within*. New York: Basic Books.

Bruch, H. (1978). *The golden cage*. Cambridge, MA: Harvard University Press.

Bryant-Waugh, R., Knibbs, J., Fosson, A., Kaminski, Z., & Lask, B. (1988). Long term follow up of patients with early onset anorexia nervosa. *Archives of Diseases of Childhood, 63*(1), 5–9.

Bulik, C.M., Sullivan, P.F., & Kendler, K.S. (1998). Heritability of binge-eating and broadly defined bulimia nervosa. *Biology of Psychiatry, 44*(12), 1210–1218.

Childress, A., Brewerton, T., Hodges, E., & Jarrell, M. (1993). The Kids Eating Disorder Survey (KEDS): a study of middle school students. *Journal of the American Academy of Child and Adolescent Psychiatry, 32*, 843–850.

Cooper, Z., & Fairburn, C.G. (1987). The Eating Disorder Examination: A semi-structured interview for the assessment of the specific psychopathology of eating disorders. *International Journal of Eating Disorders, 6*, 1–8.

Crisp, A.H. (1980). *Anorexia nevosa: Let me be*. London: Academic Press.

DaCosta, M., & Halmi, K.A. (1992). Classification of anorexia nervosa: Question of subtypes. *International Journal of Eating Disorders, 11*, 305–313.

DeZwaan, M., Nutzinger, D.O. & Schoenbeck, G. (1992). Binge eating in overweight women. *Comprehensive Psychiatry, 33*, 256–261.

Drewnowski, A., Krahn, D.D., Demitrack, M.A., Nairn, K., & Gosnell, B.A. (1995). Naloxone, an opiate blocker, reduces the consumption of sweet high-fat foods in obese and lean female binge eaters. *American Journal of Clinical Nutrition, 61*, 1206–1212.

Eisler, I., Dare, C., Russell, G.F., Szmukler, G., le Grange, D., & Dodge, E. (1997). Family and individual therapy in anorexia nervosa: A five-year follow-up. *Archives of General Psychiatry, 54*, 1025–1030.

Fahy, T., Eisler, I., & Russell, G.F.M. (1993). A placebo-controlled trial of d-fenfluramine in bulimia nervosa. *British Journal of Psychiatry, 162*, 597–603.

Fahy, T., & Treasure, J. (1991). Caffeine abuse in bulimia nervosa. *International Journal of Eating Disorders, 10*, 373–377.

Fairburn, C.G. (1985a). Cognitive-behavioral treatment for bulimia. In D.M. Garner & P.E. Garfinkel (Eds.), *Handbook of psychotherapy for anorexia nervosa and bulimia* (pp. 160–192). New York, NY: Guilford Press.

Fairburn, C.G. (1985b). The management of bulimia nervosa. *Journal of Psychiatric Research, 19*(2–3), 465–472.

Fairburn, C.G. (1997). Interpersonal psychotherapy for bulimia nervosa. In D.M. Garner & P.E. Garfinkel (Eds.), *Handbook of treatment for eating disorders*, 2nd ed. New York, NY: Guilford Press.

Fairburn, C.G., & Beglin, S.J. (1990). Studies of the epidemiology of bulimia nervosa. *American Journal of Psychiatry, 147*, 401–408.

Fairburn, C.G., & Cooper, Z. (1993). The Eating Disorder Examination (12th ed.). In C.G. Fairburn & G.T. Wilson (Eds.), *Binge eating: Nature, assessment, and treatment* (pp. 317–360). New York, NY: Guilford Press.

Fairburn, C.G., Agras, W.S., & Wilson, G.T. (1992). The research on the treatment of bulimia nervosa: Practical and theoretical implications. In G.H. Anderson & S.H. Kennedy (Eds.), *The biology of feast and famine: Relevance to eating disorders* (pp. 318–340). New York: Academic Press.

Fairburn, C.G., Jones, R., Peveler, R.C., Carr, S.J., Solomon, R.A., O'Connor, M.E., Burton, J., & Hope, R.A. (1991). Three psychological treatments for bulimia nervosa: A comparative trial. *Archives of General Psychiatry, 48*, 463–469.

Fairburn, C.G., Jones, R., Peveler, R.C., Hope, R.A., & O'Connor, M. (1993). Psychotherapy and bulimia nervosa: The longer-term effects of interpersonal psychotherapy, behavior therapy, and cognitive behavior therapy. *Archives of General Psychiatry, 50*, 419–428.

Fairburn, C.G., Kirk, J., O'Connor, M., & Cooper, P.J. (1986). A comparison of two psychological treatments for bulimia nervosa. *Behaviour Research and Therapy, 24*, 629–643.

Fairburn, C.G., Marcus, M.D., & Wilson, G.T. (1993). Cognitive behavioral therapy for binge eating and bulimia nervosa: a comprehensive treatment manual. In C.G. Fairburn & G.T. Wilson (Eds.), *Binge eating: Nature, assessment, and treatment* (pp. 361–404). New York; NY: Guilford Press.

Fairburn, C.G., Norman, P.A., Welch, S.L., O'Connor, M.E., Doll, H.A., & Peveler, R.C. (1995). A prospective study of outcome in bulimia nervosa and the long-term effects of three psychological treatments. *Archives of General Psychiatry, 52*, 304–312.

Ferguson, C.P., La Via, M.C., Crossan, P.J. & Kaye, W.H. (1999). Are serotonin selective reuptake inhibitors effective in underweight anorexia nervosa? *International Journal of Eating Disorders, 25*(1), 11–17.

Fichter, M.M., Elton, M., Engel, K., Meyer, A.E., Mall, H., & Poustka, F. (1991). Structured Interview for Anorexia and Bulimia (SIAB): Development of new instruments for the assessment of eating disorders. *International Journal of Eating Disorders, 10*, 571–592.

Fluoxetine Bulimia Nervosa Collaborative Study Group (1992). Fluoxetine in the treatment of bulimia nervosa. *Archives of General Psychiatry, 49*, 139–147.

Garfinkel, P.E., Lin, E., Goering, P., Spegg, C., Goldbloom, D., Kennedy, S., Kaplan, A., & Woodside D.B. (1995). Bulimia nervosa in a Canadian community sample: Prevalance and comorbidity. *American Journal of Psychiatry, 152,* 1052–1058.

Garfinkel, P.E., Lin, E., Goering, P., Spegg, C., Goldbloom, D.S., Kennedy, S., Kaplan, A.S., & Woodside, D.B. (1996). Should amenorrhoea be necessary for the diagnosis of anorexia nervosa. *British Journal of Psychiatry, 168,* 500–506.

Garner, D.M. (1991). *Eating Disorders Inventory—2.* Odessa, FL: Psychological Assessment Resources.

Garner, D.M., & Bemis, K.M. (1982). A cognitive-behavioral approach to anorexia nervosa. *Cognitive Therapy and Research, 6,* 123–150.

Garner, D.M., & Garfinkel, P.E. (1979). The Eating Attitudes Test: An index of the symptoms of anorexia nervosa. *Psychological Medicine, 9,* 273–279.

Garner, D.M., Olmsted, M.P., & Polivy, J. (1983). Development and validation of a multidimensional eating disorder inventory for anorexia nervosa and bulimia. *International Journal of Eating Disorders, 2,* 15–34.

Garner, D.M., Olmsted, M.P., Bohr, Y., & Garfinkel, P.E. (1982). The Eating Attitudes Test: Psychometric features and clinical correlates. *Psychological Medicine, 12,* 871–878.

Garner, D.M., Rockert, W., Davis, R., Garner, M.V., Olmsted, M.P., & Eagle, M. (1993). Comparison between cognitive-behavioral and supportive-expressive therapy for bulimia nervosa. *American Journal of Psychiatry, 150,* 37–46.

Garner, D.M., Vitousek, K.M., & Pike, K.M. (1997). Cognitive-behavioral therapy for anorexia nervosa. In D.M. Garner & P.E. Garfinkel (Eds.), *Handbook of treatment for eating disorders,* 2nd ed. New York, NY: Guilford Press.

Goldbloom, D.S., & Garfinkel, P.E. (1990). The serotonin hypothesis of bulimia nervosa theory and evidence. *Canadian Journal of Psychiatry, 35*(9), 741–744.

Goldbloom, D.S., Olmsted, M.P., Davis, R., & Shaw, B. (1994). A randomized control trial of fluoxetine and individual cognitive behavioral therapy for women with bulimia nervosa: Short-term outcome. *Behavioral Research Therapy, 35*(9), 803–811.

Goldstein, D.J., Wilson, M.G., Thompson, V.L., Polvin, J.H., Rampey, A.H., & the Fluoxetine Bulimia Nervosa Research Group (1995).

Long-term fluoxetine treatment of bulimia nevosa. *British Journal of Psychiatry, 166,* 660–665.

Hall, A. & Hay, P.J. (1991). Eating disorder patient referrals from a population region, 1977–1986. *Psychological Medicine, 21,* 697–701.

Halmi, K.A., Eckert, E., Marchi, P., Sampugnaro, V., Apple, R., & Cohen, J. (1991). Comorbidity of psychiatric diagnoses in anorexia nervosa. *Archives of General Psychiatry, 48,* 712–718.

Herzog, D.B., Keller, M.B., Sacks, N.R., Yeh, C.J., & Lavori, P.W. (1992). Psychiatric comorbodity in treatment-seeking anorexics and bulimics. *Journal of the American Academy of Child and Adolescent Psychiatry, 31,* 810–818.

Hetherton, T.E., & Polivy, J. (1992). Chronic dieting and eating disorders: A spiral model. In J.H. Crowther, D. Tennenbaum, S.E. Hobfall & M.A.P. Stephens (Eds.), *The etiology of bulimia nervosa: The individual and familial context* (pp. 133–135). Washington, DC: Hemisphere.

Hoek, H.W. (1991). The incidence and prevalence of anorexia nevosa and bulimia nervosa. *Psychological Medicine, 21,* 455–460.

Jimerson, D.C., Lesem, M.D., Kaye, W.H., & Brewerton, T.D. (1992). Low serotonin and dopamine metabolite concentrations in cerebrospinal fluid from bulimic patients with frequent binge episodes. *Archives of General Psychiatry, 49*(2), 132–138.

Johnson, C. (1987). Diagnostic Survey for Eating Disorders (DSED). In C. Johnson & M. Connors (Eds.), *The etiology and treatment of bulimia nervosa.* New York, NY: Basic Books.

Katzman, D.K., Zipursky, R.B., Lambe, E.K. & Mikulis, D.J. (1997). A longitudinal magnetic resonance imaging study of brain changes in adolescents with anorexia nervosa. *Archives of Pediatric and Adolescent Medicine, 151*(8), 793–797.

Kaye, W.H. (1997). Persistent alterations in behavior and serotonin activity after recovery from anorexia and bulimia nervosa. *Annals of the New York Academy of Science, 28*(817), 162–178.

Kaye, W.H., Ballenger, J.C., Lydiard, R.B., Stuart, G.W., Laraia, M.T., O'Neil, P., Fossey, M.D., Stevens, V., Lesser, S.R., & Hsu, G. (1990). CSF monoamine levels in normal-weight bulimia: Evidence for abnormal nonadrenergic activity. *American Journal of Psychiatry, 147*(2), 225–229.

Kaye, W.H., Gwirtsman, H.E., George, D.T. & Ebert, M.H. (1991). Altered serotonin activity in anorexia nervosa after long-term weight restoration. Does elevated cerebrospinal fluid 5-hydroxyindoleacetic acid level correlate with rigid and obsessive behavior? *Archives of General Psychiatry, 48*(6), 556–562.

Keel, P.K., Mitchell, J.E., Miller, K.B., Davis, T.L., & Crow, S.J. (1999). Long-term outcome of bulimia nervosa. *Archives of General Psychiatry, 56*(1), 63–69.

Klerman, G.L., Weissman, M.M., Rounsaville, B.J., & Chevron, E.S. (1984). *Interpersonal psychotherapy of depression.* New York, NY: Basic Books.

La Via, M.C., Gray, N., & Kaye, W. H. (2000). Case reports of olanzapine treatment of anorexia nervosa. *International Journal of Eating Disorders, 27*(3), 363–366.

Lacey, J.H., & Dolan, B.M. (1998). Bulimia in British blacks and Asians. A catchment area study. *British Journal of Psychiatry, 152,* 73–79.

Lambe, E.K., Katzman, D.K., Mikulis, D.J., Kennedy, S.H., & Zipursky, R.B. (1997). Cerebral gray matter volume deficits after weight recovery from anorexia nervosa. *Archives of General Psychiatry, 54*(6), 537–542.

Lask, B., & Bryant-Waugh, R. (1993). *Childhood onset anorexia nervosa and related eating disorders.* Hove, England: Erlbaum.

Leitenberg, H., Rosen, J.C., Wolf., J., Vara, L.S., Detzer, M.J. & Srebnik, D. (1994). Comparison of cognitive-behavioral therapy and desipramine in the treatment of bulimia nervosa. *Behavior Research and Therapy, 32,* 37–45.

Lilenfeld, L.R., Kaye, W.H., Greeno, C.G. Merikangas, K.R., Plotnicov, K., Pollice, C., Rao, R., Strober, M., Bulik, C.M. & Nagy, L. (1998). A controlled family study of anorexia nervosa and bulimia nervosa: psychiatric disorders in first-degree relatives and effects of proband comorbidity. *Archives of General Psychiatry, 55*(7), 603–610.

Lucas, A.R., Beard, C.M., O'Fallon, W.M., & Kurland, L.T. (1991). Fifty-year trends in the incidence of anorexia nervosa in Rochester, Minnesota: A population-based study. *American Journal of Psychiatry, 148,* 917–922.

Maloney, M.J., McGuire, J.B., & Daniels, S.R. (1988). Reliability testing of a children's version of the Eating Attitude Test. *Journal of the American Academy of Child and Adolescent Psychiatry, 27,* 541–543.

Marcus, M.D., Wing, R.R., Ewing, L., Kern, E., McDermott, M., & Gooding, W. (1990). A double-blind, placebo-controlled trial of fluoxetine plus behavior modification in the treatment of obese binge-eaters and non-binge-eaters. *American Journal of Psychiatry, 147,* 876–881.

Mazure, C.M., Halmi, K.A., Sunday, S.R., Romano, S.J., & Einhorn, A.M. (1994). The Yale–Brown–Cornell Eating Disorder Scale: development, use, reliability and validity. *Journal of Psychiatric Research, 28* (5), 425–445.

McBride, D.A., Anderson, G.M., Khalt, V.D., Sunday, S.R., & Halmi, K.A. (1991). Serotonergic responsivity in eating disorders. *Psychopharmacology Bulletin, 27*(3), 365–372.

McCann, V.D., & Agras, W.S. (1990). Successful treatment of non-purging bulimia nervosa with desipramine: A double-blind, placebo-controlled study. *American Journal of Psychiatry, 147,* 1509–1513.

Metropolitan Life Insurance Company (1959). *Metropolitan height and weight tables.* New York: MLIC.

Mitchell, J.E., Christensen, G., Jennings, J., Huber, M., Thomas, B., Pomeroy, C., & Morley, J. (1989). A placebo-controlled, double-blind crossover study of naltrexone hydrochloride in outpatients with normal-weight bulimia. *Journal of Clinical Psychopharmacology, 9,* 94–97.

Mitchell, J.E., Hatzukami, D., & Eckert, E. (1985a). Characteristics of 275 patients with bulimia. *American Journal of Psychiatry, 142,* 482–485.

Mitchell, J.E., Hatzukami, D., Eckert, E. & Pyle, R. (1985b), Eating Disorders Questionnaire. *Psychopharmacology Bulletin, 21,* 1025–1043.

Mitchell, J.E., Pyle, R.L., Eckert, E.D. Hatsukami, D., Pomeroy, C., & Zimmerman, R. (1990). A comparison study of antidepressants and structured intensive group psychotherapy in the treatment of bulimia nervosa. *Archives of General Psychiatry, 47,* 149–157.

Palla, B., & Litt, I. (1988). Medical complications of eating disorders in adolescents. *Pediatrics, 81,* 613–623.

Pi-Sunyer, F.X. (1991). Health implications of obesity. *American Journal of Clinical Nutrition, 53,* 1596–1603.

Polivy, J., & Herman, C.P. (1985). Dieting and bingeing: A causal analysis. *American Psychologist, 40,* 193–210.

Russell, G. (1979). Bulimia nervosa: an ominous variant of anorexia nervosa. *Psychological Medicine, 9,* 429–448.

Russell, G.F.M., Checkley, S.A., Feldman, J., & Eisler, I. (1988). A controlled trial of d-fenfluramine in bulimia nervosa. *Clinical Neuropharmacology, 22*(Suppl.), S146–S149.

Russell, G.F.M., Szmukler, G.I., Dare, C., & Eisler, I. (1987). An evaluation of family therapy in anorexia nervosa and bulimia nervosa. *Archives of General Psychiatry, 44*, 1047–1056.

Seiver, L.T. & Davis, K.L. (1985). Overview toward a dysregulation hypothesis of depression. *American Journal of Psychiatry, 142*(9).

Shore, R.A., & Porter, J.E. (1990). Normative and reliability data for 11 to 18 year olds on the Eating Disorder Inventory. *International Journal of Eating Disorders, 9*, 201–207.

Smith, M.C. & Thelan, M. H. (1984). Development and validation of a test for bulimia. *Journal of Consulting and Clinical Psychology, 52*, 863–872.

Spitzer, R.L., Devlin, M., Walsh, B.T., Hasin, D., Wing, R., Marcus, M.D., Stunkard, A., Wadden, T., Yanovski, S., Agras, S., Mitchell, J., & Nonas, C. (1992). Binge eating disorder: A multisite field trial of the diagnostic criteria. *International Journal of Eating Disorders, 11*, 191–203.

Spitzer, R.L., Yanovski, S., Wadden, T., Wing, R., Marcus, M.D., Stunkard, A., Devlin, M., Mitchell, J., Hasin, D., & Horne, R.L. (1993). Binge eating disorder: Its further validation in a multisite study. *International Journal of Eating Disorders, 13*, 137–153.

Strober, M., Freeman, R., & Morrell, W. (1997). The long-term course of severe anorexia nervosa in adolescents: survival analysis of recovery, relapse, and outcome predictors over 10–15 years in a prospective study. *International Journal of Eating Disorders, 22*(4), 339–360.

Strober, M., Lampert, C., Morrell, W., Burroughs, J., & Jacobs, C. (1990). A controlled family study of anorexia nervosa: Evidence of family aggregation and lack of shared transmission with affective disorders. *International Journal of Eating Disorders, 9*, 239–253.

Sullivan, P.F. (1995). Mortality in anorexia nervosa. *American Journal of Psychiatry, 152*, 1073–1074.

Sunday, S.R., Halmi, K.A., & Einhorn, A.N. (1995). The Yale–Brown–Cornell Eating Disorders Scale: A new scale to assess eating disorders symptomatology. *International Journal of Eating Disorders, 18*, 237–245.

Thelan, M.H., Farmer, J., Wonderlich, S., & Smith, M. (1991). A revision of the Bulimia Test: The BULIT-R. *Psychological Assessment: A Journal of Consulting and Clinical Psychology, 3*, 119–124.

Thelan, M.H., Mann, L. M., Pruitt, J., & Smith, M. (1987). Bulimia: Prevalence and component factors in college women. *Journal of Psychosomatic Research, 31*, 73–78.

Thelan, M.H., Powell, A.L., Lawrence, C., & Kuhnert, M.E. (1992). Eating and body image concerns among children. *Journal of Clinical Child Psychology, 21*, 41–47.

Vitousek, K.M., & Hollon, S.D. (1990). The investigation of schematic content and processing in eating disorders. *Cognitive Therapy and Research, 14*, 191–214.

Walsh, B.T., Wilson, G.T., Devlin, M.J., Pike, V.M., Roose, S.P., Fleiss, J., & Waternaux, C. (1997). Medication and psychotherapy in the treatment of bulimia nervosa. *American Journal of Psychiatry, 154*(4), 523–531.

Walters, E.E., & Kendler, K.S. (1995). Anorexia nervosa and anorexic-like syndromes in a population-based female twin sample. *American Journal of Psychiatry, 152*, 64–71.

Welch, G., Thompson, L., & Hall, A. (1993). The BULIT-R: Its reliability and clinical validity as a screening tool for DSM-III-R bulimia nervosa in a female tertiary education population. *International Journal of Eating Disorders, 14*, 95–105.

Wilfley, D.E., Agras, W.S., Telch, C.F., Rossiter, E.M., Schneider, J.A., Cole, A.G., Sifford, L., & Raeburn, S.D. (1993). Group cognitive behavioral therapy and group interpersonal psychotherapy for the non-purging bulimic individual: A controlled comparison. *Journal of Consulting and Clinical Psychology, 61*, 296–305.

Wilson, G.T., Eldredge, K.L., Smith, D., & Niles, B. (1991). Cognitive-behavioral treatment with and without responsive prevention for bulimia. *Behavior Research and Therapy, 29*, 575–583.

Wiser, S., & Telch, C.F. (1999). Dialectical behavior therapy for binge-eating disorder. *Journal of Clinical Psychology, 55*(6), 755–768.

Yager, J., et al. (Work Group on Eating Disorders) (2000). Practice guideline for the treatment of patients with eating disorders (Revision). *American Journal of Psychiatry, 157* (Suppl.), 1–39.

7

Chapter Seven

Diagnosis and Treatment of Borderline Personality Disorder and Antisocial Personality Disorder

Thomas M. Kelly ● Paul A. Pilkonis

Overview

The American Psychiatric Association DSM-IV multi-axial diagnostic system (APA, 1994) places the personality disorders on Axis II (see Chapter 1). This chapter will focus on the assessment and treatment of the two most severe types of the personality disorders, borderline personality disorder (BPD) and antisocial personality disorder (ASPD). The DSM-IV includes 13 personality disorders, 10 specific disorders and one nonspecific disorder referred to as personality disorders-not otherwise specified (PD-NOS). Two other disorders which are included as "exploratory" (i.e., requiring further study), are depressive personality disorder and passive-aggressive personality disorder. The DSM-IV also categorizes personality disorders into three general types, whereby disorders that share similar symptoms or traits are grouped into "clusters," referred to as Cluster A (the "odd" type), Cluster B (the "dramatic" type), and Cluster C (the "anxious" type) disorders. A detailed review of the DSM-IV system, these clusters, and their associated conditions is beyond the scope of this chapter. The reader is referred to the DSM-IV (APA, 1994) and Lively (1995) for an in-depth review of these topics.

The Cluster B personality disorders include: histrionic personality disorder, narcissistic personality disorder, borderline personality disorder, and antisocial personality disorder. The types of symptoms exhibited by patients diagnosed with Cluster B personality disorders include impulsivity, sensation seeking, severe mood swings, manipulative behavior, suicidal behavior and self-mutilation. The most severe of these disorders are the borderline and antisocial types, because the symptoms of these disorders are the most destructive to self and others. As a result of their functional level, motivation, and behavior in treatment, patients diagnosed with these disorders represent a substantial challenge to the clinician. Their "treatability" index is considered in the low to intermediate range (Sperry, 1995).

This chapter will address the prevalence, assessment, and treatment of these disorders. We will also discuss symptomatology from the patient's perspective, i.e., what is it like to have the traits associated with these disorders. Emphasis will be placed on the etiology and comorbidity of these disorders with other Axis-I conditions, such as the substance use disorders. How treatment and outcome is often complicated by comorbidity, or the co-occurrence of at least two separate disorders, will also be addressed. In the interest of space conservation, Borderline Personality Disorder will be referred to as BPD and Antisocial Personality Disorder will be referred to as ASPD.

Prevalence

Borderline Personality Disorder is fairly prevalent with approximately 2 percent of the general United States population exhibiting the disorder. The prevalence is higher in clinical populations with estimations that approximately 10 percent of outpatients in mental health clinics and 20 percent of psychiatric inpatients meet cri-

teria for BPD. Among patients with personality disorders it is estimated that 30–60 percent have a borderline personality (DSM-IV,
1994). There is some question about how gender differences for
comorbid Axis-I conditions may skew findings of gender differences in Axis-II conditions (Golomb, Fava, Abraham, &
Rosenbaum, 1995). However, most epidemiologic studies (e.g.,
Swartz, Blazer, George, & Winfield, 1990) find BPD more prevalent
among females. Estimates of ASPD vary. Using DSM-III criteria in
a large, multi-site epidemiologic study, Regier and others (1993)
found that only about one-half of 1 percent met criteria for ASPD.
Kessler et al. (1994) found 3.5 percent met criteria for ASPD and
the rate for males (5.8 percent) was almost 5 times that for
females (1.2 percent). The DSM-IV estimates that about 3 percent
of males have ASPD; only 1 percent of females are assumed to
have ASPD. Regier and others (1993) also found a similar gender
ratio with ASPD being 4 times as prevalent among males.
Prevalence estimates in clinical populations range from 3 to 30
percent, depending on the samples that have been studied and
there are very high rates of ASPD among substance users and in
prison populations (DSM-IV, 1994).

Assessment and Diagnosis of Borderline Personality Disorder

The DSM-IV defines Borderline Personality Disorder (BPD) as the
presence of at least 5 of the 9 possible symptoms (trait is actually
a better term since these symptoms are derived from enduring
constructs which begin in adolescence or early adulthood and are
likely to be present over many years). These symptoms include:
(1) frantic efforts to avoid real or imagined abandonment; (2) a
pattern of intense, unstable relationships that alternate between
idealization and devaluation of others; (3) identity disturbance,
i.e., a markedly and persistently unstable self-image or sense of
self; (4) impulsivity in at least two areas that are potentially self-

damaging, e.g., spending money, sex, reckless driving; (5) recurrent suicidal or self-mutilating behavior; (6) affective instability or marked changes in mood that last only a few hours or days; (7) chronic feelings of emptiness; (8) inappropriate, intense anger or difficulty controlling anger, and (9) transient, stress-related paranoid ideation or severe dissociative symptoms. This list includes a number of symptoms or traits that are shared with other Axis-I and Axis-II disorders, which often results in difficulty making a differential diagnosis. In addition, comorbidity further complicates the diagnostic process. However, several guidelines exist that provide some clarity for diagnosis of borderline personality disorder.

First, it is imperative to take a detailed psychiatric and developmental history. In addition, for those who have been treated before (as is often the case for ASPD and BPD patients), knowledge of previous treatment is very important. Personality traits establish patterns of behavior that begin in late adolescence and are enduring. Therefore, it is important to establish when the trait and any related behavior began. The course of the condition is also important, since any behavior that has not been observable at all times is more likely due to symptoms of an Axis-I condition. Second, the context of trait-related behaviors must be taken into account. While BPD traits cause behaviors that may be attributed to symptoms of other disorders, subtle differences can act as diagnostic guides. For example, both BPD and bipolar patients may engage in impulsive, uncontrolled spending sprees or promiscuous sexual behavior. However, BPD patients often evidence a pattern of these behaviors, which follow a real or perceived interpersonal loss. These impulsive behaviors therefore represent a defense against the depression associated with this loss. Such well-defined patterns will not be discernible in the histories of bipolar patients. Similarly, a differential diagnosis of BPD versus bipolar disorder must be based in part on the type of symptoms reported. BPD patients often have problems controlling such functions as temper, substance use, and sexual activity. Bipolar patients may also report such problems, but also report and/or display psychomotor symptoms such as thought racing, agitation, and distractibility. It is therefore important to not only record a detailed psychiatric history but to closely observe the patient during the interview for signs and behaviors that will assist in making a differential diagnosis. However, comorbidity with other disorders is almost a ubiquitous occurrence for the BPD patient and understanding how symptoms represent different disorders and different levels, i.e., acute versus chronic vulnerability is crucial to effective treatment planning. We will develop this theme as we discuss issues related to etiology and treatment.

■ SUBJECTIVE EXPERIENCE OF BPD

The psychoanalytic perspective of BPD is based on a psycho-developmental model, which centers on how developmental experiences affect relationships. This provides a good starting point for understanding the subjective experience of the BPD patient. Kernberg (1975) suggests failure to resolve psycho-developmental conflicts in childhood causes identity diffusion or problems with the "sense of self" that results in ego weakness in BPD patients. Psychologically, this prevents the BPD patient from perceiving him/herself as separate from significant others. Fear of separation and loss of these others therefore threatens the BPD patient's very existence. This drives BPD patients to maintain a feeling of closeness with people they consider necessary for their survival. Their frantic efforts to avoid abandonment and tendency to exhibit impulsive behaviors, which include physically and psychologically self-destructive behaviors, often follow their perception of being rejected. These dramatic behaviors can, of course, result in further withdrawal by people the BPD patient sought to draw closer.

Since it is critical for BPD patients to maintain closeness with others in order to feel "whole," they often become quickly involved in one self-destructive relationship after another. It is also common for BPD patients to describe long-term, intense, hostile-dependent relationships with others who evidence severe psychopathology, e.g., antisocial traits. These patients set up a pattern of intense, unstable, and self-destructive relationships which is easily discernible during history taking. The fear of separation in these relationships is reflective of conflicts in early childhood that have not been adequately resolved because BPD patients do not experience a "normal" rapprochment phase of childhood development (Mahler, Pine, & Bergman, 1975). During this phase, which begins around the age of 2, children learn that their separateness from others is not threatening and they successfully complete the individuation process. When individuation has not occurred, it is often observable during transitional phases in development. For example, the patterns of behavior described above may begin in early adolescence or when an older adolescent moves away from home. These transitions represent a reenactment of rapprochment and therefore reawaken many of the conflicts that remain unresolved. Hickey (1985) has creatively cited examples from literature to demonstrate the subjective experience of the BPD patient.

■ COMMON EFFECTS OF BPD

The histories of BPD patients often reveal very uneven patterns of functional abilities. This may be seen as a corollary to the "all-or-nothing" thinking, tendency to vacillate between idealization and devaluation, and the wide mood swings. BPD patients have the capacity for functioning at very high levels during periods of low stress and interpersonal tranquility, but they can quickly deteriorate to the point of requiring admission to an inpatient facility to save them from suicide. Gunderson, Kolb, and Austin (1981) included a section on "social adaptation" in the first version of the Diagnostic Interview for Borderline Patients (DIB), which systematically assesses this phenomenon. As indicated, this pattern is the result of ego-syntonic behaviors, which are based on an intense need for interpersonal closeness and the tendency to act out angrily or impulsively to achieve it. This often has devastating effects on the BPD patients' emotional well being, since they feel ashamed of their actions. Their self-esteem suffers and this can lead to a downward spiral of negative thinking, reinforcing like behavior. More severe BPD patients may deteriorate functionally and lose the capacity for working in the competitive labor force and socializing outside of a clinical population. Such behaviors may baffle families and friends, especially in the early stages of the disorder. Emotional support and psycho-educational intervention is often indicated to help them understand and cope with this behavior.

■ ETIOLOGY OF BPD

Developmental Formulations

The first widely accepted theories of the etiology of BPD were posited by psychoanalytic practitioners (Kernberg, 1975; Mahler, Pine & Bergman,1975; Masterson, 1976). Based on systematic interviews of mothers and children, Mahler and others (1975) concluded that there are three phases of early development, including: (1) symbiotic and differentiation during which the infant is, at first, not conscious of its separateness in the world and later becomes aware of its separateness; (2) practicing during which ambulation begins and the child "practices" his/her status as a separate being and; (3) rapprochment which occurs around the 2nd year and during which the child achieves his/her psychological status as a separate person from the mother. It is during this last phase that a "crisis" occurs due to the child's need to resolve the "ambitendency" to be both separate from the mother while still desiring to cling to her. This ambivalence is observable in alternating clinging and negativistic behaviors which, if not adequately resolved, results in the "all good" versus "all bad" and the splitting behavior often seen in adult BPD patients.

Rinsley (1982), citing his work with Masterson, emphasizes the interactional aspect of the resolution of the rapprochment phase. These authors suggest that often the mothers of BPD patients have BPD personalities and are struggling with the "loss" of the child during rapprochment. They present a detailed view of how withdrawal of maternal support for the child in his/her quest for separation–individuation during the rapprochment phase contributes to the development of a "split ego." This splitting causes the BPD patient to only feel "good" while perceiving those close to her as nurturing and, conversely, causes the BPD patient to feel inadequate, abandoned and depressed when perceiving those close to her as withdrawing. Masterson (1976) describes the major work of psychotherapy as the gradual integration of these good and bad split images of self and others so that the BPD patient can "mourn" the loss of the introjected mother.

Childhood Antecedents of BPD: Dysfunctional Parental Relationships, Separation and Loss and Sexual Abuse in Childhood

Although high rates of psychiatric symptoms and mental disorders are found in family studies of BPD, there is little evidence for the genetic transmission of BPD (Torgerson, 1994). However, sexual abuse, loss of caretakers, and alienation from family are common experiences for BPD patients and seem to be specific for the development of BPD (Soloff & Millward,1983; Young & Gunderson, 1995; Zanarini & Frankenburg, 1997). Zanarini, Gunderson, Marino, Schwartz, and Frankenburg (1989) found high rates of verbal and sexual abuse in childhood among BPD outpatients, and severity of childhood sexual abuse has also been found related to severity of BPD disorder, self-mutilation, and chronic suicidality (Dubo, Zanarini, Lewis, & Williams, 1997; Silk, Lee, Hill, & Lohr, 1995).

Parental incest was found to be predictive of worthlessness and intolerance of being alone in the study by Silk and colleagues. The authors conclude that repeated and severe sexual abuse represent early attachment failures that can distort interpersonal development in adulthood. A recent investigation found interpersonal sensitivity also predicted the BPD diagnosis and suggests that these experiences may interact, i.e., the more strongly childhood experiences reinforce interpersonal sensitivity, the less childhood trauma may be necessary to produce borderline psychopathology (Figueroa, Silk, Huth, & Lohr, 1997).

■ AXIS-I CONDITIONS COMORBID WITH BPD

Recent research on Axis-I conditions indicates that mood and anxiety disorders are most common among patients diagnosed with BPD. Zanarini et al. (1998) found that over 95 percent of a sample of severe BPD patients were diagnosed with an affective disorder, i.e. major depression (83 percent), dysthymia (39 percent) or bipolar II disorder (10 percent). Importantly, depression in BPD patients is qualitatively different than depression in non-BPD samples. BPD patients tend to experience more self-condemnation, emptiness, fears of abandonment, self-destructiveness, and hopelessness (Gunderson & Phillips, 1991; Rogers, Widiger, & Krupp, 1995).

Anxiety disorders in the Zanarini and colleagues (1998) study were almost as prevalent as affective disorders, with over 88 percent of BPD patients meeting DSM-III-R criteria for an anxiety disorder. Fifty-six percent met criteria for post-traumatic stress disorder, suggesting that a moderately high percentage of these patients may be suffering the results of childhood sexual abuse trauma. When compared to patients with other Axis-II conditions, including ASPD, more BPD patients were diagnosed with affective or anxiety disorders. A higher percentage of BPD patients were diagnosed with substance use disorders compared to those with other Axis-II conditions (64 percent versus 54 percent), but this was not a significant difference. Zanarini and colleagues noted that substance use disorders were more prevalent among males with BPD (82 percent versus 59 percent) and there were higher rates of eating disorders among females with BPD than among BPD males (62 percent versus 21 percent).

Oldham and others (1995) also found high rates of anxiety disorders among their BPD patients. Although they found that their BPD patients did not meet full criteria for mood disorders, they did find that patients with mood disorders in their sample had high rates of BPD traits. Similar to Zanarini and colleagues, these investigators found high rates of bulimia among BPD patients.

Antisocial Personality Disorder

Antisocial Personality Disorder (ASPD) is defined as the presence of at least three of the following traits after the age of 18: (1) failure to conform to social norms by repeatedly performing acts that are grounds for arrest; (2) deceitfulness, i.e. chronic lying, use of aliases, or conning others for personal profit or pleasure; (3) impulsivity or failure to plan for the future; (4) irritability or aggressiveness, as indicated by repeated physical fights or assaults; (5) a reckless disregard for the safety of self or others; (6) consistent irresponsibility, indicated by failure to sustain regular work behavior or to honor financial obligations; and (7) lack of remorse, as indicated by indifference to or rationalization of behavior which harms others. A further stipulation is that the above behaviors must be observable outside the course of schizophrenia or a manic episode.

In addition, ASPD can only be diagnosed if there is evidence of conduct disorder in childhood. Conduct disorder is diagnosed in children and adolescents when at least three, DSM defined symptoms related to the violation of other's rights or breaching of major societal norms is persistently evident for at least 12 months. Epidemiologic research suggests that even fewer of these childhood symptoms, i.e., 2 in males and 1 in females, may be predictive of adult ASPD (Robins & Price, 1991). Because the existence of a conduct disorder is a necessary criterion for the diagnosis of ASPD, obtaining a detailed history of the onset and course of antisocial behaviors is imperative. This is even more relevant to diagnosing ASPD because research exists which indicates that ASPD may be associated with other comorbid conditions, i.e., attention-deficit hyperactivity disorder (ADHD).

The most significant problem in diagnosing ASPD involves obtaining a valid history upon which to base the diagnosis. In general, diagnosing personality disorders is often more difficult than diagnosing many of the Axis-I conditions. Axis-I conditions are experienced as painful or distressing and are readily reported. Conversely, symptoms or traits of personality disorders are often "ego-syntonic," i.e., the patient does not feel distressed by what might be considered a "problem." For example, the life of the BPD patient is often replete with examples of manipulative behavior aimed at maintaining or re-establishing interpersonal stability. This may not be spontaneously reported since this is not perceived as a problem. Indeed it has become a mode of adapting to problems. Although the interviewer may need to direct the interview to elicit such information, most BPD patients do not attempt to conceal this.

This problem is intensified in the diagnosis of ASPD as a direct result of behavior related to the disorder itself, i.e., the penchant for lying or conning others. ASPD patients are often seen in health care settings where a "payoff" exists for conning behavior, e.g., drugs. Some settings may be more vulnerable than others, e.g., a private general practitioners office. However, practitioners must be alert to such behavior no matter where they may be practicing. As might be expected, ASPD patients with comorbid substance use disorders are particularly prone to this and may lie about symptoms related to other physical or psychiatric conditions, as well as conceal important information about their background, which may be important in recognizing the symptoms of ASPD. Meloy (1988) recommends a cyclical technique for history taking where ASPD is suspected. This technique assumes that antisocial patients will lie and tests this assumption by returning to the same material, in order to determine if it is recounted the same way each time. For this reason, it is most important to obtain information from corroborative sources whenever considering the presence of an Axis-II disorder. Zimmerman, Pfohl, Stangl, and Corenthal (1986) found that the presence/absence of any personality disorder was changed in almost 20 percent of the patients in their study, after considering information provided by an informant. In most cases informant data resulted in the patient receiving an additional personality disorder diagnosis.

■ SUBJECTIVE EXPERIENCE OF ASPD

Just as the traits of BPD revolve around interpersonal closeness, the primary motivation of the ASPD patient is dominance over others. Health care practitioners often enter their professions motivated by a desire to take care of and help others. As a result, they are often repulsed by patients who display behaviors that exploit or harm others. Here, it is critical for clinicians to detach themselves from the tendency to view the ASPD patient as "bad" and take an objective, clinical perspective.

Millon, Davis, and Associates (1996) provide a valuable synopsis of the ASPD patient's view of interpersonal relationships. These authors stress that ASPD patients' developmental experiences lead them to believe others will abuse or exploit them, if given the opportunity. Fear of exploitation becomes the ASPD patients' primary concern and they become constantly vigilant for signs of it. However, this fear must be masked because it is equated with weakness. As a reaction formation, fear is overcome by a drive to possess physical, psychological, and/or personal power over others. This guards against exploitation by effectively removing the means by which others can harm the ASPD patient.

■ COMMON EFFECTS OF ASPD

While the effects of BPD often take their greatest toll on the patient, it is likely that the effects of ASPD are at least as great on the patient's family and society. ASPD patients have a history of "acting out" behaviors, often beginning in early childhood (see Disorders of Childhood in ASPD) which include impulsivity, aggressiveness, and antisocial acts such as vandalism and theft. Millon and others (1996) suggest that milder forms of acting out represent rebelliousness to parental expectations or conflicts at one end of the spectrum, while more severe delinquent behaviors are likely to be fueled by parental indifference and hostility. Meloy (1988) indicates that parental abuse and neglect are common in the backgrounds of psychopaths and it is active abuse that appears to generate ASPD. Since uncaring parents do not react with affectation, most of the negative effects of this early behavior is foisted upon other family, e.g., siblings, peers and schoolmates. Typically, when the school can no longer tolerate problems, these children are referred to the criminal justice system. Often this is their introduction to a life of criminal activity, punctuated by periods of incarceration. Of course, the economic costs of ASPD, in terms of lost wages and productivity, as well as legal costs and costs of incarceration, are incalculable.

■ ETIOLOGY OF ASPD

Developmental Formulations

Kernberg (1975) considers the psychopath a severe type of the narcissistic personality. He suggests that, unlike the BPD patient who has not established adequate ego boundaries, the intrapsychic structure of the ASPD develops later, when self and object images have been differentiated. However, the images of the ideal self and ideal object have merged to protect the ASPD patient from a traumatizing interpersonal world. At the same time, intense anger, which develops during development due to abuse and exploitation by the child's caretakers is projected onto others. This masks the fear of abuse, which is responsible for the almost paranoid-like vigilance the ASPD patient keeps for signs of exploitation and his/her drive for dominance over others.

Millon and colleagues (1996) summarize the early life experiences of the person who develops ASPD, emphasizing that infancy for the ASPD personality is one replete with parental indifference, neglect and even hostility. Having never experienced parental warmth and affection they do not desire gratification from relationships and, subsequently, have no interest in forming relationships later in life. The neglect and hostility that marks infancy and early childhood for these children continues through middle childhood and adolescence. This essentially forces ASPD children to fend for themselves with the primary damage being to their intrapsychic structure. ASPD patients form their own value system, which is based on their early childhood experiences of neglect and hostility from others. This is reflected in their drive to dominate others so as to disarm them, as discussed above. If they hold allegiance to others, it is only to their peer group. Even then however, the ASPD patient uses others as a means to an end and is loyal to no one.

Disorders of Childhood in ASPD

Externalizing disorders that generally onset in childhood, i.e. those that include impulsivity, motoric hyperactivity and even substance abuse, may be critical to the etiology of ASPD. Studies suggest that Oppositional Defiant Disorder precedes the onset of conduct disorder (Loeber, Keenan, Lahey, Green, & Thomas, 1993), and may be an independent risk for the later development of ASPD (Langbehn, Cadoret, Yates, Troughton, & Stewart, 1998). Similarly, Weiss, Hechtman, Milroy, and Perlman (1985) and Mannuzza, Klein, Bessler, Malloy, and LaPadula (1993) found ASPD more prevalent in the backgrounds of adult males who had been diagnosed with ADHD as children. It is not clear how childhood disorders interact in contributing to ASPD (Pilkonis & Klein, 1999) but these conditions should be considered in the differential diagnosis of adult ASPD.

■ AXIS-I CONDITIONS COMORBID WITH ASPD

There have been very few investigations of co-occurrence of Axis-I disorders in ASPD. The research that has been done indicates that ASPD patients are at some risk for developing mood and substance use disorders. However, some qualifications exist with regard to these comorbidities. Carter, Joyce, Mulder, Sullivan, and Luty (1999) found higher rates of ASPD only among depressed males. Oldham et al. (1995) did not find ASPD associated with any of the major Axis-I disorders but found patients with substance use disorders had more comorbid antisocial traits, compared to non-substance abusing patients. Similarly, data from the Epidemiologic Catchment Area study indicate that the prevalence of ASPD among alcoholics is over 14 percent and those diagnosed with an alcohol use disorder were 21 times more likely to have a comorbid ASPD, an odds ratio higher than any other mental disorder; the prevalence of ASPD among those with any other drug disorder was 18 percent and again, the odds of having a comorbid ASPD was higher than that for any other disorder (Regier et al., 1993).

Millon and colleagues (1996) state that ASPD patients tend to act out against feelings of anxiety or tension, thereby externalizing their discomfort. The tendency for ASPD patients to develop substance use disorders is likely related to their desire to quickly rid themselves of intrapsychic pain and/or to their involvement with criminal activity associated with drug trafficking. Therefore, while they may have relatively brief feelings of anxiety or depression, they rarely develop major Axis-I mood or anxiety disorders because of the length of time and intensity associated with meeting criteria for these disorders. However, Cleckley (1976) suggests that psychopaths can be categorized as primary or secondary, based on the development of their moral conscience and capacity for feeling guilt. Research indicates that some ASPD patients do meet criteria for mood and anxiety disorders, and it is likely that these are Cleckley's secondary psychopaths.

■ NEUROLOGICAL DYSFUNCTION COMMON TO BPD AND ASPD

One area which has been found potentially etiological for both BPD and ASPD symptoms is that associated with neurochemical deficiencies, specifically serotonin dysregulation. Serotonin is a neurotransmitter involved in the regulation of mood and affect. Serotonin inhibits impulsivity and aggression and Brown and colleagues (1979, 1982) reported decreased levels of serotonin metabolites in convicted criminals who were found to be higher on a measure of aggression. Roy and Linnoila (1989) summarized the literature on other personality correlates of decreased serotonergic function, indicating that studies show increased levels of monotony avoidance and nonconformity in those low in serotonergic activity. Behaviorally, subjects with low serotonin levels have more contact with police, arguments with others, hostility at the time of research interviews, and arguments on the job. Low levels of serotonin have been found associated with the violent, impulsive suicidal acts often displayed by ASPD and BPD patients (Mann, 1987) and with nonsuicidal, self-aggressive behaviors common in BPD, e.g., self-mutilation (New et al., 1997). This biologic substrate has also been found genetically related to ASPD. Constantino, Morris, and Murphy (1997) found decreased serotonergic function in newborns of parents whom had reported high rates of ASPD in their biological relatives. Fortunately, antidepressants known as "SSRIs" (selective serotonin reuptake inhibitors) are effective in increasing serotonergic activity.

■ SELF-REPORT MEASURES OF ASPD AND BPD

Self-report measures can be very useful in diagnosing personality disorders because they are easily administered. In addition, when found to be valid indicators of the relevant constructs, they also save time and resources in making diagnoses that otherwise require additional interviewing or record reviews to corroborate information and sophistication with making a differential diagnosis. Unfortunately, while they may add to an informational base, there are no self-report measures of BPD and ASPD that can be used as the sole basis of the diagnosis.

No self-report measures of ASPD have been developed but measures of psychopathy have been used extensively. There is debate about the utility of the psychopathic personality diagnosis and self-report measures of it have been found not to correlate with its core features (Lilienfeld, 1998). Furthermore, to reiterate, theorists generally consider psychopathy to encompass a broader dimension of personality than what is captured by the categorical diagnostic entity of ASPD. Our purpose is not to join in this debate but to present methods, which may assist in the diagnosis of ASPD. Therefore, we will confine ourselves to discussion of one of these self-report instruments, the Minnesota Multiphasic Personality Inventory Psychopathic Deviate Scale (MMPI-Pd) (McKinley & Hathaway, 1944).

This scale includes 50 items, which were developed in testing older adolescents and young adults involved in legal proceedings and with groups of prisoners and psychiatric inpatients. The Pd scale has been found to identify at least one-half of subjects considered to be psychopathic personalities. Raw scores are converted to "T-scores," which are related to the mean of normative groups and interpretation of results requires knowledge specific to the use of the MMPI. However, the scale has been found fairly stable in test–retest reliability trials, suggesting consistency in results across time (Greene, 1980).

There is little research on the utility of self-report instruments for the diagnosis of BPD. Similar to the situation with ASPD, one has been developed which appears to provide assistance in diagnosing BPD, the Borderline Syndrome Index (BSI) (Conte, Plutchik, Karasu, & Jerrett, 1980). This is a 52-item self-report, which demonstrated high internal consistency and discriminative validity in a four-group sample composed of patients with BPD, major depression, schizophrenia, and volunteers who had no history of psychiatric illness. The BSI has not been widely used in studies to determine its utility in discriminating between BPD and Axis-I disorders, e.g., bipolar disorders or other personality disorders. Marlowe, O'Neill-Byrne, Lowe-Ponsford, and Watson (1996) found the constructs measured by the BSI more closely identified features associated with dependent personality disorders. Skodol and Oldham (1991) reviewed instruments for diagnosing BPD and found that no single instrument has been found clearly superior and that instrument driven assessments may be helpful in clinical settings but are not necessary, if accurate information is gathered in clinical interviews.

■ DIAGNOSTIC INTERVIEWS FOR ASPD AND BPD

The most widely used interviews for the diagnosis of ASPD and BPD are the International Personality Disorder Examination (IPDE) (Loranger, Janca, & Sartorius, 1997) and the Structured Clinical Interview for DSM-III-R Personality Disorders (SCID-II) (First et al., 1995). Both of these interviews are based on DSM-defined criteria and assess the full range of DSM-defined personality disorders.

The IPDE is a 157-item, semi-structured instrument that provides diagnoses for the Axis-II personality disorders contained in the DSM-IV, as well as items for diagnosis of personality disorders according to the *International Classification of Diseases—Tenth Edition*. The IPDE items are designed to tap information relevant to the criteria which comprise each disorder and are scored on a three-point scale of absent, sub-threshold, and present. The IPDE is not designed to be used with individuals under 18 (this is in line with the DSM stipulation that personality disorders are not to be diagnosed in individuals under the age of 18), although modifications have been used with subjects as young as age 15. The interview can generally be completed within 90 minutes and sessions should not run longer than this to avoid subject and interviewer fatigue (Loranger et al., 1997). The IPDE has been widely field tested on over 700 patients and has achieved reliability ratings similar to those associated with other diagnostic instruments. There has been little validity testing of the IPDE but clinicians who have used it generally consider it a good indicator of DSM-IV personality disorders. However, as with all diagnostic instruments based on self-report, its validity cannot be separated from the interviewer's clinical acumen (Loranger, 1997).

The SCID-II (First, Spitzer, Gibbon, & Williams, 1995) is a semi-structured interview designed for the diagnosis of 11 of the DSM-III-R personality disorders and the one nonspecific disorder, Personality Disorder-Not Otherwise Specified (PD-NOS). The SCID-II bases questions on the criteria for each diagnosis, which unlike the IPDE, are grouped together under a general description of the disorder. This provides the clinician with a better overall sense of what constitutes the diagnosis but may contribute to a "halo effect" for over-diagnosing the disorder (First et al., 1995).

The SCID-II includes a self-report questionnaire which contains items associated with DSM-defined disorders and the subject endorses or denies criteria associated with each disorder. This self-report should be administered prior to the interview and can be quickly scored to determine disorders that can be deleted, thereby reducing interview time (the interview should take 35–40 minutes). The assumption is that patients who respond negatively to items related to particular disorders on the self-report will also respond negatively to questioning related to these disorders during the interview. However, the interviewer can choose to include these items (questions) in the interview, if their clinical judgment suggests that the patient should be assessed for any and all DSM defined Axis-II personality disorders (First et al., 1995). The SCID-II has demonstrated reliability ratings similar to other instruments designed to assess DSM-defined personality disorders and preliminary evidence suggests that patients diagnosed with a personality disorder on the SCID-II score lower on global functioning. This suggests that the constructs measured by the SCID-II are valid indicators of constructs associated with DSM-defined Axis-II disorders (First et al., 1995).

Two other instruments that measure full-spectrum DSM-defined Axis-II conditions deserve mention. The Structured Interview for the DSM-III Personality disorders (SID-P) (Stangl, Pfohl, Zimmerman, Bowers, & Corenthal, 1985) and the Diagnostic Interview for Personality Disorders (DIPD) (Zanarini, Frankenburg, Chauncey, & Gunderson, 1987). The SID-P was the first instrument developed for diagnosing the full range of DSM-defined Axis-II disorders. It consists of a 60–90 minute patient interview, using 160 questions based on DSM-III criteria and incorporates information from a 30-minute interview with a knowledgeable informant. Scoring is based on a three-point system, which emphasizes increasing severity in meeting the criteria for the disorder. Initial testing suggested moderate to high reliability with some of the DSM-III Axis-II disorders. However, reliability with other Axis-II conditions could not be determined due to low base rates in the testing sample (Stangl et al., 1985).

The DIPD is a semi-structured interview consisting of 252 questions which can be administered in 60–90 minutes, and which is also designed to assess DSM-III Axis-II disorders. Like the SCID-II, its items conform to the criteria sets of the DSM-defined disorders and, therefore, administering criteria for selected disorders is easily accomplished. Separate interrater and test–retest reliability studies indicate moderate to high reliability of the DIPD in determining DSM-defined Axis-II diagnoses among inpatients (Zanarini et al., 1987).

The Diagnostic Interview for Borderline Patients (DIB) (Gunderson et al., 1981) is a widely used instrument for determining the diagnosis of BPD. It includes measurements of social adaptation, impulse actions, intense affects, psychotic thinking, and behaviors associated with interpersonal relationships. Scores on each of these sections are summed and scaled scores of 0, 1 or 2 are derived to produce a total score ranging from 0 to 11. Scores of 7 and above are considered indicative of "definite" borderline pathology. Some changes have been made in the most recent version of this instrument, the DIB-R (revised). For example, the social adaptation scale has been removed because it was found to poorly discriminate BPD from other disorders. The DIB-R has been found reliable in distinguishing clinically diagnosed BPD patients from patients diagnosed with other Axis-II disorders (Zanarini, Gunderson, Frankenburg, & Chauncey, 1990).

It should be noted that all of the above interviews should be administered only after determining the absence of pervasive Axis-I psychopathology. The presence of mental disorders as disabling as schizophrenia or the active phase of a manic disorder precludes any valid personality disorder testing. Accordingly, testing for Axis-II disorders should only follow determination of other Axis-I pathology by clinical interview or research testing. Should the patient be diagnosed with a serious Axis-I disorder from which they are expected to recover, Axis-II testing should be conducted following recovery. These instruments (the SCID-II being a possible exception) were designed for use in research settings and by interviewers who are very conversant with the mental disorders defined by the Diagnostic and Statistical Manuals. The validity of these diagnostic instruments relies heavily on the interviewer's ability to differentiate symptoms of Axis-II disorders within a multi-axial taxonomic system.

■ SUMMARY

BPD and ASPD patients are likely to report dysfunctional family backgrounds but ASPD patients are more likely to experience neglect and hostility while BPD patients may have been over-involved with their parents, especially their mothers. These disorders are likely to share a common biologic substrate, which fuels a propensity for impulsivity and aggressiveness. However, such behavior for BPD patients appears associated with desperate attempts to maintain closeness with significant others, while the behaviors of ASPD patients are as likely to be toward unknown others. Differences also exist in terms of family psychopathology and childhood experiences. There are high rates of diagnosable childhood disorders among ASPD patients and a clearer link to antisocial behaviors in the families of ASPD patients. Comorbid substance use problems are found in both BPD and ASPD patients and BPD patients are likely to develop affective and anxiety-related disorders. Research often finds that both ASPD and BPD patients have been exposed to physical and sexual abuse, but sexual abuse is a better predictor of BPD. This is particularly traumatic when the perpetrator is a family member. Parental incest has been found linked to feelings of worthlessness and intolerance of being alone in adult BPD patients. Further, there may be an interaction effect between sexual abuse and interpersonal sensitivity. Childhood experiences that intensify interpersonal sensitivity, e.g., feelings that others do not understand or are unsympathetic, reduce the amount of sexual trauma necessary to produce BPD in adulthood. These findings appear to support psychodynamic theories that self and object boundaries never become established in BPD, which intensifies intolerance of being alone and regressive experiences at the time of real or perceived abandonment.

Treatment of BPD and ASPD

■ OVERVIEW

As indicated by our review, comorbidity of Axis-I and Axis-II disorders is common and, therefore, the treatment of BPD cannot be separated from treatment associated with the symptoms of other conditions. In fact, due to the emphasis the patient often places on their Axis-I, "ego-dystonic" symptoms, therapists often consider the maladaptive traits associated with personality disorders to be complications for first-line treatments of symptoms related to these more acute Axis-I symptoms. As such Axis-II traits produce a slower response, a less complete response, or both in the treatment of Axis-I conditions (Pilkonis & Frank, 1988; Shea, Widiger, & Klein, 1992).

We believe that principles of treatment must be guided by a formulation of how Axis-I and Axis-II disorders are linked. Tyrer,

Gunderson, Lyons, and Tohen (1997) have outlined one view, suggesting that the presence of an Axis-II personality disorder implies greater vulnerability to Axis-I conditions. In essence, traits such as impulsivity and risk-taking result in a greater propensity for developing Axis-I conditions such as depression or substance use disorders. Accordingly, we have adopted a longitudinal perspective, i.e., a chronic (rather than an acute or "infectious") disease model in which the Axis-I symptoms occur in the context of the Axis-II condition (Pilkonis, 1999). We have attempted to present this in our review of the etiology and comorbidity of BPD and ASPD. Consistent with this is recognizing the potential value of thinking in developmental terms. While it is important to bring acute symptom relief as soon as possible, one's approach should also reflect attention to normative issues in adult development in order to address the chronic vulnerability set up by the Axis-II condition. Implied in this perspective is the setting of mid- to long-term treatment goals that include improvement in the areas that represent difficulties which have evolved over time, e.g., problems in attachment and interpersonal relationships, self-sufficiency, accomplishment, self-image, and generativity on behalf of others.

In general, given the mechanisms in this paradigm, it can be assumed that pharmacotherapy will bring relief more quickly for the acute symptoms of BPD and ASPD. Such acute symptoms are related to the serotonergic imbalance we have already discussed. Interestingly, however, research suggests that psychotherapy can produce the same effect on the serotonergic system as pharmacotherapy with SSRI medication (Saxena, Brody, Schwartz, & Baxter, 1998). This notwithstanding, psychotherapeutic intervention is necessary to address the chronic Axis-II traits that make the patient vulnerable to their acute symptoms. Exceptions to this might include hopelessness that treatment can be helpful at all. It is imperative to address such hopelessness directly and rapidly in the therapeutic relationship with patients who have a long history of treatment failures in order to decrease the potential for premature termination of treatment. We will now turn our attention to treatment models.

■ MODIFIED PSYCHOANALYTIC PSYCHOTHERAPY

Kernberg delineated his modified psychoanalytic treatment of BPD over the past three decades. His early recommendations regarding treatment of borderline conditions are couched in psychoanalytic terms that many clinicians find technical and difficult to grasp (e.g., Kernberg, 1975). However, he and his colleagues have recently published a very readable manual of psychotherapy of borderline personality organization (Clarkin, Yeomans, & Kernberg, 1999).

Clarkin and colleagues (1999) refer to their model as transference focused psychotherapy (TFP). This model is based on patient deficiencies in ego functioning, which result from distorted self and object relationships. The term is descriptive because most of the work in psychotherapy is conducted through analysis of emotions and behavior associated with the therapeutic relationship. Indeed TFP includes developing a highly structured therapeutic contract in order to control acting-out outside the psychotherapy sessions, in order to encourage the focusing of intrapsychic conflicts on the therapist-patient relationship. This structuring includes, for example, explicit guidelines as to how emergencies and contacts such as telephone calls outside of treatment are to be handled. Generally, the early stage of treatment includes dealing with breaches of this contract and limit setting.

Effective TFP assumes that acting out and regressive behaviors will occur throughout therapy. However, these should decrease sufficiently within the first 6 months so that treatment will then primarily consist of analysis of the patient's intrapsychic conflicts as they are revealed in the therapeutic relationship. Clarkin and colleagues (1999) emphasize that the process is important in that it includes the therapist's ability to recognize three levels of communication: (1) the patient's verbal content, (2) the behavior they exhibit, and (3) the countertransference or emotions evoked in the therapist during this exchange. The therapist must understand and synthesize these channels of communication in order to decide on a therapeutic priority, which is then pursued in treatment. These priorities are based on behaviors that include threats to self or other destructive behaviors (most important) to pursuit of affect-laden material not associated with the therapeutic relationship (least important).

TFP assumes that the behaviors exhibited in treatment are reflective of intrapsychic conflicts based on the BPD patient's distorted early caretaker attachments and repeated in the therapeutic relationship. Psychotherapy involves first eliciting information in order to clarify the nature of these conflicts. During this process the patient is tactfully confronted with discrepancies in their reports or between the verbal and non-verbal aspects of their behavior. These conflicts usually represent distortions of the therapeutic relationship so that the therapist is seen as an "all-bad" persecutor or and "all-good" caretaker. At the same time the patient may see themselves as a completely innocent victim or a total failure, deserving of the therapist's disdain. As these themes are revealed the therapist must interpret them for the patient. As this process continues the BPD patient develops integrated images of self and others, which include both positive and negative qualities. The psychotherapy process, which focuses on the interpersonal relationship with the therapist, reinforces tolerance of anxiety related to simultaneous recognition of these qualities.

Clarkin and colleagues (1999) suggest a number of transference themes that predominate in psychotherapy, e.g., antisocial, narcissistic, and depressive. Antisocial themes are the most severe and, consistent with the views of others, these authors believe antisocial patients often bring hidden agendas to treatment. In addition, the superegos of ASPD patients are severely damaged and do not allow for internalization of control or psychotherapeutic intervention. Clarkin and colleagues (1999) make some distinction between violent and non-violent psychopaths. They indicate that the ability to remain non-violent suggests some limited potential to benefit from treatment, while violent psychopaths generally benefit from nothing short of external societal control. Narcissistic presentations reflect a higher order of personality organization and, although grandiosity and envy are dominate themes, these patients can identify with the therapist and are therefore open to therapeutic intervention. The highest order of transference is the depressive position. At this point the patient has integrated self and object images but now must mourn the loss of idealized images. Importantly however, patients at this stage experience a full range of affect and a capacity for feeling guilt appropriate to interpersonal situations, resulting in increased abilities for restoration of relationships.

This is consistent with Masterson (1976), who believes psychotherapy for the BPD patient involves structuring a situation whereby the patient can work through the abandonment depression set up by his/her failure to attain individuation from the mother. He suggests that early phases of treatment for some BPD patients may involve primarily supportive treatment. In general however, Masterson (1976) describes three general phases of treatment: (1) the testing phase, (2) the working through phase, and (3) the separation phase. The testing phase is the first during which the patient is determining whether the therapist can be trusted. During this phase the patient offers much resistance to the therapist's pointing out his/her self-destructive patterns because, as we discussed earlier, these are the ways the patient has learned to cope while denying their self-destructive quality.

Most of the work in therapy is done by confronting the patient with how his/her coping mechanisms are self-destructive. As BPD patients learn the therapist can be trusted, they begin to give up their defensive, self-destructive behavior, and become more depressed. This begins the working-through phase during which these patients attempt to deal with their abandonment depression but act out their anger toward their mother/father in the relationship with the therapist. Masterson (1976) sees this as the most common resistance to treatment offered by BPD patients. The separation stage begins when BPD patients indicate significant resolution of their depression, even though they may still report anxiety over terminating therapy. Ideally, the decision to terminate therapy should come from the patient, but the therapist should remain available for future contacts as needed.

■ DIALECTICAL BEHAVIOR THERAPY (DBT)

DBT is based on the principle of the dialectic. Treatment necessarily involves the interaction of a thesis with its (or an) antithesis, which produces a new outcome or synthesis. Linehan (1993) points out that this tension is a continuous process by which change occurs and it is this "process" that is the essential nature of life. While it is beyond our objective to detail the development of DBT, Linehan (1993) describes the development of the therapy and her discovery of its dialectical underpinnings, as she struggled to apply cognitive-behavioral therapy (CBT) (see p. 33), in the treatment of BPD patients. It is essential reading for a comprehensive understanding of how these techniques operate in clinical practice. Our objective is to delineate the principles and structure of DBT.

First, the practice of DBT involves use of cognitive-behavioral techniques but with close attention to the development and influence of the therapeutic relationship. Linehan (1993) points out that cognitive-behavioral components may be primarily responsible for the effectiveness of DBT but the therapeutic process differs from CBT. CBT has been presented as a "technology of change," which does not stress accepting the validity of the behaviors displayed by the patient and has not historically emphasized the patient/therapist collaboration. Conversely, an empathic understanding of patient experiences and the patient's reaction to these experiences are necessary for establishing a close patient/therapist collaboration, which is critical to conducting DBT.

This relates closely to the second principle of DBT, which emphasizes patient validation. Linehan (1993) points out that, by not emphasizing patient validation throughout treatment, many psychotherapists effectively blame the patient. She stresses that therapists are often quite tolerant with the BPD patient at the outset of therapy. Early on they will even increase their efforts to help but eventually become exasperated with the lack of improvement and soon begin to see the patient as either causing his/her own problems or being manipulative or resistant. This recapitulates the invalidating environment BPD patients have previously experi-

enced. Worse, due to their vulnerable self-image and their invest-
ment in the relationship with their therapist, BPD patients may
accept the therapist's view of them as the root of their own problems, thereby reinforcing some the negative self-image that psychotherapy is designed to combat. The longitudinal perspective
on treatment we propose is consistent with Linehan's recognition
of the deleterious effects of the invalidating environments BPD
patients have experienced throughout their lives. She stresses
that much of psychotherapy for these patients involves reversing
this trend through the therapeutic relationship.

With patient acceptance and validation as a backdrop, DBT is
based on the therapist and patient closely collaborating on analyz-
ing maladaptive behaviors and considering alternatives to them.
Linehan (1993) proposes three dialectical behavioral dimensions
that BPD patients experience: (1) emotional vulnerability/self-
invalidation; (2) unrelenting crisis/inhibited grieving; and (3)
active passivity/apparent competence. These dimensions are
experienced as polar opposites between which the BPD patient
vacillates. The therapist must be able to recognize these dimensions and, while not invalidating the patient through suggesting
that the patient's behaviors could be improved (this would imply
that the expectations of the invalidating environment were correct
and the patient wrong), teach the patient how to change. The tension between acceptance and change is the central dialectic of
DBT. The primary objective of DBT is to promote the dialectical
process whereby the patient can find more balanced, integrated
alternatives to their extreme responses.

Dialectical-behavior therapy is a system of therapy, which
includes, at a minimum, weekly psychotherapy with an individual
therapist and a skills training group session in which the patient
participates for the first year of therapy. Individual psychotherapy
sessions are generally 1 hour long. However, provisions are made
for lengthening them as needed. Skills training sessions are generally 2 to $2\frac{1}{2}$ hours long, in groups consisting of 2–10 patients and
are conducted in a psychoeducational format. Linehan (1993) discusses a hierarchy of the types of behaviors that are targeted in
individual treatment. There are seven primary targets of DBT:

(1) decreasing suicidal behaviors; (2) decreasing behaviors that threaten the therapy; (3) decreasing behaviors that reduce the quality of life; (4) increasing behavioral skills; (5) decreasing post-traumatic stress; (6) increasing self-respect; and (7) achieving individual goals. In the individual therapy, behaviors are examined, as are responses to life situations with an emphasis on problem-solving and increasing the use of adaptive behaviors. The skills training group involves practicing and role play of interpersonal skills and adaptive behaviors. As in all group therapy, modeling is considered a significant aspect of skill training and Linehan emphasizes the importance of therapist recognition and reinforcement of newly acquired skills and adaptive behaviors.

Linehan (1993) points out that the decision to separate therapy into individual psychotherapy and skills training was a practical one. Both are necessary components of treatment but the nature of each generally precludes the other. Individual therapists must focus on emphasizing the inhibition of typical borderline thinking and behaviors and their replacement with more adaptive responses and do not have the time nor the structure necessary for teaching the "nuts and bolts" of behavioral and interpersonal skills. Similarly, training in interpersonal effectiveness, emotion regulation, and distress tolerance are important aspects of treatment for patients who lack these skills but are best presented as learned behaviors.

The most important factor in recommending DBT with BPD patients is preliminary evidence of its effectiveness. Linehan and her colleagues have conducted several longitudinal studies and have demonstrated that patients treated in DBT engage in fewer and less damaging suicidal behaviors, have fewer days spent on inpatient units, and drop out of treatment less frequently, compared to BPD patients enrolled in treatments otherwise offered in the community (Linehan, Armstrong, Suarez, Allmon, & Heard, 1991; Linehan, Heard, & Armstrong, 1993; Shearin & Linehan, 1994). In addition to these behavioral improvements there is evidence that DBT was more effective in reducing anger and promoting social adjustment, compared to other treatments. These studies had small sample sizes and some improvements associated with DBT appear to fade after the first year of therapy (Linehan et al., 1993; Shearin & Linehan, 1994). However, DBT is the first psychosocial treatment of BPD that has been systematically researched and these results are encouraging. Linehan and colleagues have called for research of DBT effectiveness outside of that conducted in their clinic (Shearin & Linehan, 1994).

■ INTERPERSONAL THERAPY OF BPD AND ASPD

Benjamin (1996) describes an interpersonal approach to psychotherapy of BPD and ASPD, emphasizing assessment and treatment using structural analysis of social behavior (SASB). In her view most symptoms of Axis-II disorders included in the DSM can be translated into interpersonal themes represented by continuums from "attack" to "active love" and "control" to "emancipation." Theoretically, these continuums intersect, allowing for placement of the patient's behavior in a particular quadrant of the graph based on complementary pairings of the patient's actions and reactions to others. Developmental experiences, e.g., having been sexually abused, are used to understand current interpersonal themes. These themes are used in treatment to help the patient recognize and block associated patterns of maladaptive behaviors and learn new, more adaptive ones. Benjamin (1996) suggests facilitating collaboration early in treatment by stressing an exploratory approach whereby the patient and therapist work together against "it," i.e., the patient's disorder. As the patient's identification with the therapist deepens, it is important for the therapist to strengthen the patient's will to give up maladaptive patterns by showing enthusiasm for apparent improvement.

■ COGNITIVE BEHAVIORAL THERAPY OF BPD

Originally developed for use with depressed patients, cognitive behavioral therapy (CBT) has been adapted for use with BPD patients (Beck, Freeman, & Associates, 1990; Ryle, 1995; Young, 1994). Although the approaches we will discuss differ somewhat in their conceptualizations of the disorder and interventions to be used, these systems all assume a cognitive-behavioral theoretical base. This theory espouses that perception of a stimulus begins the process whereby cognitive schemas, e.g., the perception of danger triggers affective schemas which include anxiety, followed by motivational schemas, e.g., flight, to cope with the situation (Beck et al., 1990). CBT proposes to alter the cognitive schemas and thereby impact the affective and behavioral responses that follow.

Similar to Kernberg (1975) and Linehan (1993), Beck and colleagues emphasize the need for structure in psychotherapy with BPD patients. Testing of the therapist's resolve and concern often arises in treatment of BPD patients and setting limits is a necessary backdrop for the patient's successfully working through this. For example, Beck and colleagues suggest limiting the duration of telephone contacts outside of therapy and setting up subsequent face-to-face contacts as soon as possible to deal with the issue. However flexibility is also emphasized. Beck and colleagues recommend focusing on the patient's collaboration in treatment planning and suggest that patients be given some control over seating arrangements and topics to be discussed.

Cognitive behavioral therapy with less severely disordered patients follows a rather systematic delineation and confrontation of problems. It may be necessary to allow for a more crisis-oriented approach, addressing issues as they arise in treatment of BPD. Still, Beck and colleagues recommend that some priority be given to consistency of focus by possibly splitting the sessions to permit discussing current problems, while allowing for a shift to ongoing goals.

The primary target of treatment is dichotomous thinking. This is similar to the concept of "all-or-nothing" or "black and white" thinking and parallels the concept of emotional "splitting," whereby incongruent affects cannot be simultaneously recognized and drives the BPD patient to idealize or devalue others. Beck and colleagues (1990) suggest that this can best be addressed early in treatment by eliciting the patients perceptions about others and clarifying whether these people are, for example, completely untrusting or completely trusting. This type of questioning often results in the patient's admitting to times when they viewed the same people differently. Then, by the use of an "all-or-nothing" continuum, the concept of people being rated at different levels of trustworthiness can be introduced. As dichotomous thinking is reduced, increasing control over moods and emotions is established. The therapeutic relationship should be used to work on emotional control in vivo, i.e., the therapist should be attuned to emotional changes in the BPD patient and encourage expression of feelings in therapy. This allows patients to experiment with "opening up" without the fear that this may have devastating consequences.

Impulse control is also a target of treatment. However, Beck and colleagues (1990) indicate that this goal should be approached as a necessary part of helping the patient simply decide whether they want to control their impulses, so that they have a choice in situations where they may want to exercise greater control. This approach emphasizes the therapist's recognition that the patient may want to give in to their impulses and implies the patient's right to choose. In this way it is similar to Linehan's (1993) admonition that patient reactions are legitimate and failure to recognize this in therapy produces an invalidating experience.

Strengthening the patient's sense of identity is one of the more remote goals of CBT and is accomplished as the patient identifies accomplishments and positive characteristics and by the therapist consistently recognizing when the patient makes good decisions and copes effectively. Honesty is imperative here and it can be counterproductive for the therapist to be ingenuine about his/her evaluation of the patient's functioning. It is important however, to remember that even the patient's willingness to be honest about their improper or ineffective behavior should be regularly reinforced as indicative of growth in challenging their perceptions of risking rejection or abandonment.

Beck and colleagues (1990) discuss the importance of the therapeutic relationship in their approach to BPD patients. They take care to point out that, due to basic assumptions of a dangerous, malevolent world, the patient's powerlessness and vulner-

abilities and their perception that they are inherently unacceptable, BPD patients are often not capable of moving with the speed
that other patients may exhibit in addressing their dysfunctional
thinking. Beck and colleagues (1990) stress that it is not uncommon for CBT therapists to help non-BPD patients change rather
quickly, i.e., 15–20 sessions. However, for BPD patients who
have not had extensive treatment, it is possible that cognitive-
behavioral therapy may take 18–30 months of weekly sessions to
produce significant change.

Young (1994) has developed a cognitive approach specifically designed for use with patients who have personality disorders. His conceptualization is that cognitive and affective
schemas result during early developmental experiences, which
are played out in every day life for patients with personality disorders and during the course of psychotherapy. These schemas are
very rigid and dictate how these patients view the world and react
to it. This inflexibility around cognition, affect, and behavior make
personality disordered patients poor candidates for short-term
cognitive therapy. These schemas occur automatically in these
patients' lives when they experience situations that involve autonomy, connectedness with others, worthiness, and expectations
and limits. In essence, these schemas represent defenses, and
patients will attempt to maintain and avoid discussing them and
adopt behaviors that compensate for them. Young (1994) has
identified 18 of these early maladaptive schemas, and the work in
therapy involves recognizing them and demonstrating the connection between triggering events, the patients' emotions, and the
schemas. A "Schema Questionnaire" has been developed which
the patient fills out during the assessment period to help in focusing
on significant problem schemas. CBT with less severely disordered patients often involves guided discovery whereby the
patient and therapist collaborate more effectively in uncovering
dysfunctional thinking and develop ways of challenging it. Young
(1994) indicates that more confrontation by the therapist is
needed to challenge the validity of the early maladaptive schemas
in personality disordered patients. However, this schema-focused
approach shares much with Beck and colleagues (1990) cogni-

tive-behavioral therapy of BPD, including a long-term approach, emphasis on use of the therapeutic relationship, as well as homework and standard behavioral techniques used by the patient to challenge these schemas.

Cognitive analytic therapy (CAT) (Ryle, 1995) is a form of psychotherapy that combines concepts and techniques used in modified psychoanalytic psychotherapy with CBT. In CAT the first objective is to construct a reformulation of what brought the patient to therapy. Considerable time is spent in interviewing patients and reviewing self-reports to construct this reformulation. Like Young's Schema Questionnire (1994), a self-report called The Psychotherapy File is completed by CAT patients to help in the identification of "traps," "dilemmas," and other difficulties these patients routinely encounter. The reformulation specifies and validates the pains in life the patient has experienced, the procedures they use to cope and target problems and target problem procedures to be addressed in therapy. Target problem procedures involve the maladaptive behaviors patients use to cope. Again, there is some parallel with Young's schemas in that these target problem procedures are routine methods of coping.

Like CBT, Ryle (1995) advocates the use of rating scales and other paper and pencil therapy adjuncts such as diagrams to clearly define patient problem states and how these are continued and reinforced through the patient's target problem procedures. The point of therapy is to reformulate, recognize, and revise the reformulated patterns. As in CBT and Young's schema-based approach, Ryle (1995) emphasizes that more of the therapeutic work with personality disordered patients will be done in the therapy sessions by confronting patients with their target problem procedures and how these procedures operate through the therapeutic relationship. Similar to psychoanalytic psychotherapy, Ryle (1995) suggests that the therapist be alert for signs of transference and countertransference as guides to structuring the sessions. In the sessions the CAT therapist and patient collaborate on rating improvement in revising the target problem procedures. Outside the sessions CAT stresses the use of diaries to record significant events and circumstances related to target problem procedures.

■ PHARMACOTHERAPY OF BPD

Pharmacotherapy of BPD is complicated because symptoms that are typically the targets of pharmacologic intervention are diverse. As a result, research into medication efficacy in BPD have included investigations of the full spectrum of psychoactive medications, i.e., antidepressants, neuroleptics, minor tranquilizers, anticonvulsants, and lithium carbonate. Soloff (1990) summarized this literature and reported overall findings that low-dose neuroleptics (e.g., Haldol, Mellaril) are effective against anger, hostility, impulsivity, and transient cognitive and perceptual distortions. Interestingly, these medicines were also effective against depressive symptoms in BPD. Conversely, one tricyclic antidepressant (amitriptyline; Elavil) seemed to increase referential thinking, impulsivity, suicidal threats, and assaults in some patients who participated in one study of BPD patients (Soloff, George, Nathan, Shulz, & Perel 1986), and alprazolam (Xanax) appeared to contribute to self-destructive behavior and assaults in females who participated in another pharmacotherapy trial of BPD (Cowdry & Gardner, 1988).

In general, specialists agree tricyclic antidepressants appear to be effective against endogenous pattern depressions, i.e., depressions that do not have an observable external stressor, and in which melancholic symptoms such as loss of pleasure in life and guilt are prominent symptoms. Monoamine oxidase inhibitors (MAOI), antidepressants such as Parnate and Nardil, appear to be most effective against atypical depressive symptoms such as intolerance of being alone and the chronic emptiness/boredom of which BPD patients often complain (Coccaro & Kavoussi, 1991; Soloff, 1990).

While tricyclic and MAOI antidepressants may be indicated for some patients, they carry great medical risk (cardio-toxicity) and may be lethal in overdose. Therefore, they should never be prescribed for outpatients who may be actively suicidal unless it is possible to enlist the aid of a responsible person, e.g., family member or residence counselor, to oversee the use of these medicines. Anticonvulsant medications such as Tegretol and lithium carbonate are of more limited utility, appearing to be effective primarily against impulsivity and aggressiveness and also represent relatively high medical risk (Links, Steiner, Boiago, & Irwin, 1990; Soloff, 1990). Clinicians must be continuously aware of the risk–benefit ratio of providing potentially harmful medications to BPD patients given their tendency to "create" emergencies. Further, some potentially beneficial medications can cause problematic side effects, e.g., long-term use neuroleptic medications can cause irreversible involuntary movements of the mouth and/ or extremities (tardive dyskinesia).

The class of antidepressants known as selective serotonin reuptake inhibitors (SSRIs, e.g. Prozac) appear to offer enhanced efficacy against more of the symptoms often seen in BPD. These medicines have few deleterious risks associated with long-term use and are relatively safe in overdose (Soloff, 1998). Coccaro et al. (1989) found inverse relationships between sertonergic function and depressive symptoms in patients who had both affective and personality disorders, compared to control subjects. These investigators also found an inverse relationship between serotonergic function and impulsive aggression but only in those diagnosed with Axis-II personality disorders, suggesting that a similar biologic mechanism underlies the depression and the impulsive, self-destructive behaviors seen in BPD. This is consistent with findings cited in the etiology of BPD and ASPD and suggests the treatment with SSRIs may be of benefit in treating both depressive and impulsive symptoms.

Soloff (1998) reviewed the literature and has proposed psychopharmologic algorithms for use with personality disordered patients based on the empirical evidence. He suggests a decision tree approach in choosing lines of medication treatment for patients presenting with different symptom profiles. Patients presenting with primarily cognitive-perceptual symptoms should first be treated with antipsychotic medicines with changes in dosage or medication types made only following adequate trials of the preceding medications. Similarly, for patients who present with primarily depressed, angry, anxious, and labile moods and patients with aggressive, impulsive, or self-destructive symptoms should be started first on SSRIs, with use of additional medications or changes to more novel medications made only at prescribed intervals. In general, pharmacotherapy of BPD produces a mild to moderate response in the symptoms BPD patients complain about most. Algorithms such as those outlined by Soloff (1998) are likely to maximize medication efficacy. However, the underlying character structure of BPD will remain and will require treatment, as suggested by our vulnerability paradigm.

■ PSYCHOTHERAPY OF ASPD

Unlike BPD, no one psychosocial therapy has been developed specifically for the treatment of ASPD. In fact, most descriptions of psychotherapy with ASPD patients are generally very pessimistic about the efficacy of such treatment. Gabbard (1990) suggests that outpatient psychotherapy of ASPD patients is "doomed" to failure due to the lack of structure associated with such treatment. He stresses that truly psychopathic patients will act on their impulses outside of treatment and routinely lie to their therapist in session, thereby sabotaging any potential benefit. Gabbard and Coyne (1987) found that the presence of anxiety and major depression were positive predictors of treatment completion in ASPD inpatients. While comorbidity often complicates treatment, it may be that the capacity to feel anxiety and depression is indicative of the ASPD patient's potential to benefit from psychotherapy.

Meloy (1988) provides guidelines as to the types of patients who represent the most severe of ASPD types and recommends strongly against offering them treatment due to the potential danger for the treating clinician. These include: (1) patients who have a sadistic, aggressive history; (2) those who offer no remorse or rationalizations for previous antisocial behavior; (3) patients who are either of high intelligence or low intellect; (4) patients who have demonstrated no capacity for establishing bonds or attachments, and (5) patients who trigger an unshakable fear of being preyed upon in the clinician, in the absence of any current behavior that would provoke such a reaction.

Given this, experts agree that treatment of the ASPD patient is best conducted in a highly structured environment, i.e., prison or secure inpatient facilities (Lion & Leaff, 1973; Vailliant, 1975). While inpatient treatment is a reasonable alternative this should be preceded by a risk-benefit analysis on a case-by-case basis, given the limited benefit that is likely and the potential for problems associated with hospitalizing such patients in a general psychiatric facility (Gabbard, 1990). General psychiatric units are structured environments but lack the high level of security necessary to deal with ASPD patients. It is important to remember that, although ASPD is a psychiatric disorder, ASPD patients routinely commit crimes against others, e.g., assaults and robberies. Further most modern psychiatric units are based on a community model and encourage interaction among patients because such activities are therapeutic for most patients who are severely depressed or are not grounded in reality. Yet, severely ill patients can be easily preyed upon by those inclined to criminality. Finally, the staff of inpatient psychiatric units are often not trained and equipped to deal with criminal behavior. These elements combine to represent very real threats to both patients and staff when ASPD patients are admitted to general psychiatric units.

For ASPD patients who are taken into psychotherapy, Frosch (1983) suggests that the major problems in the treatment of all severe personality disorders emanate from patient resistance and therapist countertransference. For the ASPD patient resistance to treatment is associated with two factors, an incapacity for interpersonal closeness and objectives that are incompatible with goals of ethical treatment. Due to abuse and hostility from others during development, many ASPD patients do not have the capacity for establishing meaningful interpersonal attachments, which is a necessary component for psychotherapy. This usually results in the ASPD patient's disinterest in any form of outpatient psychotherapy. Therapists however may be viewed as a means to an end. ASPD patients may get involved in outpatient treatment, but often with ulterior motives, e.g., seeking attention or gaining access to drugs or resources from entitlement programs. Again, it should be emphasized that for the ASPD patient lying and conning others has become a natural part of their behavioral repertoire in adapting to a deep-seated fear of exploitation.

The problem of countertransference, i.e., the feelings and emotional reactions therapists have for their patients, is as significant a problem as patient resistance. Most health-care workers enter their professions in order to help or care for others. As such, their care-taking sensitivities are offended when confronted with patients whose backgrounds are replete with examples of harm or exploitation of others. This often results in clinicians choosing not to work with ASPD patients or, worse, being unaware of how their feelings are negatively impacting any potentially therapeutic interventions they might otherwise make in treatment with the ASPD patient. Meloy (1988) discusses the common effect of "therapeutic nihilism," i.e., the clinician's adopting the attitude that all psychopaths are not amenable to treatment simply by virtue of their status as psychopaths. Frosch (1983) suggests that clinicians can become better therapists for ASPD patients by recognizing and using their emotional reactions to guide their responses to ASPD patients.

■ COGNITIVE BEHAVIORAL THERAPY OF ASPD

Beck and colleagues (1990) suggest that CBT of ASPD patients is possible but emphasize that therapists must maintain control of their feelings and behaviors and approach these patients differently than patients with only Axis-I conditions. First, the ASPD patient has not learned to think beyond the stage of concrete operations and, therefore, focuses on a personal, rather than an interpersonal, view of the world. ASPD patients assume that they are always right and, however they choose to behave to meet their needs is acceptable because they have the right to do so. Beck and colleagues suggest that the cognitive therapist's role is to convince ASPD patients of the possibility that their perceptions are incorrect and that this can keep them from getting what they want (or as much as they can) out of life. In this way, the CBT therapist avoids moralizing or focusing on making the ASPD patient a better person. On the other hand, ASPD patients may be able to learn to do things with others in mind, even if it is for their own ultimate gain. Beck and colleagues (1990) recommend using techniques such as the "Choice Review Exercise," which allows the ASPD patients to review the advantages and disadvantages of alternative behaviors in getting what they want. This exercise can show ASPD patients how, restraining themselves from giving in to their impulses or considering the feelings of others can be helpful in getting their own needs met.

Beck and colleagues stress that the therapist should stay out of control struggles, pointing out that the ASPD patient is often in control and can "win" them. Therapists should, in fact, discuss this with patients in therapy because doing so can remove the incentive the ASPD patient may have for engaging the therapist in such struggles. This is similar to Kernberg's (1975) admonition that therapists remain "neutral" in their dealings with BPD patients and Masterson's (1976) suggestion that therapists pay close attention to their countertransference and focus on being the "good enough therapist," so as to avoid doing too much or too little in working with BPD patients.

According to Beck and colleagues (1990), the CBT therapist needs to display self-assurance and a reliable (but not infallible) demeanor, along with a non-defensive interpersonal style and a sense of humor. Understanding one's limits in dealing with ASPD patients is crucial since ASPD patients rarely follow through properly in treatment and often drop out prematurely. Beck and colleagues point out that ASPD patients who are court committed or otherwise coerced into treatment will often participate grudgingly. Continuing an ineffective therapy with such patients effectively keeps the patient from being responsible for their antisocial behavior, which is countertherapeutic. They suggest the therapist have a realistic discussion with their ASPD patients about commitment to therapy, if they are not following through after the fourth session. As with BPD patients, CBT with this population is lengthier (at least 50 sessions) and symptoms of comorbid Axis-I conditions should be addressed first, e.g., substance abuse or suicidality.

■ PHARMACOTHERAPY OF ASPD

As above, the most acute symptoms of ASPD are impulsivity and aggressiveness. Like BPD patients, medications with significant side effects are not well tolerated by ASPD patients. Further, treatment of ASPD should be approached similarly to treatment of BPD, i.e., acute symptoms can be treated pharmacologically but the long-term issues related to problems in attachments, self-absorption in achieving one's own ends, require psychotherapeutic intervention. The similarity in the biological substrate of ASPD and BPD supports the use of similar medications in treatment of their symptomatology. The potential efficacy of lithium carbonate and anticonvulsants against these symptoms has already been noted.

There have been comparatively fewer studies of pharmacotherapy of ASPD. Impulsive aggression and irritability in personality disordered patients has been found to decrease with increased serotonergic function (Coccaro et al., 1989), and Kavoussi, Liu, and Coccaro (1994) found that SSRI antidepressants such as Prozac and Zoloft are effective against impulsive-aggressive symptoms in a sample that included ASPD patients. Soloff's (1998) algorithm therapy also applies to treatment of ASPD. Conversely, the antidepressant Desipramine has not demonstrated efficacy in ASPD patients addicted to cocaine (Arndt, McLellan, Dorozynsky, Woody, & Obrien, 1994; Leal, Ziedonis, & Kosten, 1994). Furthermore, medicines with addictive properties such as benzodiazepines (e.g., Valium) should be avoided due to the tendency for ASPD patients to develop substance use disorders. It is especially important to avoid use of such medicines for those with a history of substance abuse, whether or not the patient has recovered.

■ FAMILY TREATMENT

The family histories of BPD indicate these patients experience significant family disorganization. Recent research has found the families of BPD patients to be characterized as conflict ridden and controlling (Weaver & Clum, 1993) and patient's ratings of their relationships with their parents were more negative than parental ratings of the parent/child relationship (Gunderson & Lyoo, 1997). Studies have found high rates of psychopathology and low functioning among parents of BPD patients during their development (Shachnow, Clarkin, Smith-DiPalma, Thurston, Hull, & Shearin, 1997). This study found that low functional abilities and high rates of symptoms in their own lives resulted in the parents of BPD patients feeling ill-prepared for raising children.

Family intervention should be routinely considered as part of treatment planning for BPD patients, especially in the treatment of young patients. Research argues strongly for the need to interview as many family members or friends as may be available to obtain an "objective" view of family functioning as part of comprehensive treatment planning. While different family problems necessitate different treatment plans, most research finds families of BPD patients describe poor communication as a problem and this is likely to be a target early of intervention early in any family therapy. Often attempting to "normalize" family relationships is also important.

Finding ways of creating distance between over-involved parents and BPD patients or, conversely, engendering togetherness in a family where the parental union has excluded the BPD patient may promote significant movement in recovery. Creative problem-solving in promoting these changes is critical, as is the need to do so without suggesting any particular person is to blame for family problems. Defensiveness promotes "scapegoating" in BPD families. Allowing the continuation of such "scapegoating" not only hinders communication but can deepen schisms which family therapy should help resolve. One principle of family therapy is not to align oneself continuously with particular family members but to encourage all members to assert their own past concerns and to support overall improvement in family functioning. This is especially critical in conducting family therapy with BPD patients.

Generally, there is less opportunity to conduct family treatment with ASPD patients because families of these patients are often less involved with them and/or the patient is resistant. However, when feasible, the sooner family treatment is initiated the more likely it is to have a therapeutic impact, especially with juvenile delinquents or younger ASPD patients. Sperry (1995) notes that a major goal of family treatment with ASPD patients is for parents and spouses to set and maintain consistent limits around acceptable behavior. While it is a formidable undertaking, reversing this process can be critical to recovery for the ASPD patient and should be implemented to the degree that the patient will permit. Millon and colleagues (1996) suggest that supportive therapies may be indicated for family members who do not understand the patient's antisocial behavior, while attempts at family system change should be the focus with family members who may be knowingly or unknowingly promoting antisocial behaviors.

■ GROUP THERAPY

Group therapies, whether they be self-help groups or professionally led, can be effective adjunctive treatments for BPD and ASPD. Linehan's (1993) inclusion of skills training groups as an integral part of DBT has already been noted. Group treatments for BPD patients outside of more traditional individual psychotherapies have been recognized as effective in several other ways. Gunderson (1984) notes that one of the explicit goals of group psychotherapy is a striving for independence, which is an ongoing issue in treatment with BPD patients. In addition, confrontation with the maladaptive nature of regressive behaviors by groups of peers validates and reinforces that which is brought out in individual psychotherapy. Group participation also diffuses what may be an otherwise intense emotional transference to an individual therapist and provides additional structure to the patient's life (Kernberg, 1975; Clarkin et al., 1999).

The general resistance of ASPD patients to psychotherapy has already been noted and BPD patients may be resistant to group therapy due to their attachment to individual caregivers. Group treatment can be made a contingency of individual psychotherapy and this may allow time for BPD patients to see the benefits of the experience, thereby increasing the chances of their following through (Gunderson, 1984). It should be noted that Kernberg and colleagues (1989) advise against group treatment during individual therapy and admonish individual therapists not to function in the dual capacity as a group therapist for their patients. This treatment strategy decreases the potential for acting out in psychotherapy. Outside of self-help groups, with which the individual therapist should have no contact, the therapy contract in individual therapy should stipulate whether contacts with group therapists will take place and under what circumstances this might occur. This is absolutely essential for therapies such as DBT, where therapists perform different roles in treating the same patients.

■ OTHER REHABILITATIVE EFFORTS

Gunderson (1984) has recognized the importance of other rehabilitative efforts, e.g., vocational rehabilitation in the lives of BPD patients. He points out that longitudinal studies find one-half or more BPD patients are unemployed and suggests that therapists should take this into consideration in assessing treatment needs. Routine activities such as work offers additional structure to patient lives and the potential for relationships outside of those formed in clinical settings. In addition, the value such activity has for building self-esteem should not be minimized. Clarkin and colleagues (1999) point out that personality disordered patients can, at the least, perform volunteer jobs or attend day hospitals and recommend that they be involved in some productive activity outside of psychotherapy.

Most BPD and ASPD patients are capable of arranging for such services but more severely disabled patients may benefit from referrals and/or consultations with rehabilitation counselors. Some settings may employ case managers for this purpose. However, while therapeutic "neutrality" is important, there is little validity to the argument that individual therapists should not advocate for their patients in this regard, when clinical judgment suggests that it is appropriate.

■ RELAPSE ISSUES

The concept of relapse for BPD and ASPD patients is not as relevant as that of stability or rate of improvement during the course of these relatively long-term disorders. After reviewing the major follow-up studies to date, Mehlum and colleagues (1991) concluded that BPD patients rarely develop other, severe forms of psychopathology such as schizophrenia. Approximately two-thirds follow a course similar to patients with major affective disorders and improve functionally by the time they reach their forties. About one-third could be considered severely impaired. Stone (1990) was able to follow-up over 190 BPD patients approximately 20 years following inpatient treatment at the New York State Psychiatric Institute. He found that 3 out of 4 were functioning in the "fair" to "good" range. The other 25 percent had either completed suicide, were incapacitated, or were functioning poorly. He characterized outcome based on improvement trajectories in this sample and found that those who recovered quickly, slowly, or had atypical patterns had the best long-term outcomes. BPD patients whose course was linear or had a "wavy," rather erratic quality, did not fare well long term.

Borderline patients in this study were originally diagnosed using Kernberg's criteria for Borderline Personality Organization. Stone rediagnosed them using DSM criteria for BPD and found patients who met DSM criteria generally had the worst outcomes, the highest rates of suicide gestures and suicide. Thirty-eight percent of females in this study who were diagnosed with BPD, an affective disorder, and alcohol abuse completed suicide. Among those with the worst outcomes were patients who were substance abusers who had both borderline and antisocial traits. This group had a death rate six times that of non-antisocial borderline patients.

Follow-up studies that have reassessed patients for the presence of BPD find a rather wide range of patients continue to meet criteria for the diagnosis, i.e., 25–78 percent (McDavid and Pilkonis, 1996). While this may indicate that the diagnosis is unreliable, patients who no longer meet criteria for BPD often do not have other major Axis-I or Axis II symptomatology (Links, Heselgrave, & Van Reekum, 1999). Links and colleagues (1999) analyzed the core symptoms of BPD 7 years after initial assessment and found that impulsivity was the best predictor of persistence of the disorder. They suggest that this is in line with neurochemical research which demonstrates a negative correlation between serotonergic functioning and impulsivity (e.g., Coccaro et al., 1989), and that this should be a priority in treatment of BPD.

These findings indicate that most BPD patients do not deteriorate psychologically over time, but most improve only moderately. Comorbidity of mental disorders is associated with negative outcomes and BPD patients with affective, antisocial, and substance use disorders are at greatest risk for premature death. However, time spent in treatment has been found to correlate positively with improvement (Waldinger & Gunderson, 1984) and rapid control of anger and impulsivity within the first 6 weeks of outpatient therapy is important to retention of BPD patients in treatment (Kelly, Soloff, Cornelius, George, Lis, & Ulrich, 1992). Initiation of effective psychotherapy and use of SSRI antidepressants may permit faster and more effective control of core traits, i.e., traits that constitute a significant vulnerability to acute symptoms in BPD and ASPD patients.

Conclusion

Diagnosis and treatment cannot be separated in applying an infectious versus chronic disease model to treatment of ASPD and BPD. This review suggests that acute symptoms, those indicative of "infection," should be the first targets of treatment. Often this will involve treatment of cognitive/perceptual distortions or impulsivity, which are indications for pharmacotherapy. However, assessment may reveal other acute symptoms, e.g., a lack of hope that symptoms will improve, which can only be addressed by competent intervention from the outset of treatment.

Assessments of ASPD and BPD patients should include an understanding of what treatments have been applied and, importantly, the circumstances under which they may have failed. Simply introducing more structure into psychotherapy or use of a different technique which emphasizes new constructs, e.g., DBT, can be useful in instilling hope that things may be different this time.

When acute symptoms such as impulsivity have been addressed in treatment, it is more likely that BPD and ASPD patients will benefit from psychotherapy geared toward understanding their second-order symptoms. These generally consist of maladaptive behaviors that have been learned in the context of more basic symptomatology, e.g., the BPD patient's impulse to act out in order gain attention from significant others or the ASPD patient's failure to plan ahead. Just as acute symptoms must be considered in the context of the chronic disease, the value the therapeutic relationship holds for the patient is enhanced by the therapist's capacity for understanding this symptom hierarchy. Therapy becomes a cyclical process whereby therapeutic accuracy of how to intervene leads to patient improvement and trust, which enhances the therapeutic relationship. Continuing cooperation in treatment based on this history increases openness in the patient and the probability of accurate therapeutic interventions.

As treatment unfolds there is a third order of symptoms that are the interactive products of developmental experiences, temperament, and learning—the traits that underlie behaviors. ASPD patients may lack remorse, while BPD patients may be intolerant of being alone. These are among the most "deep-seated" traits and ones that often are never approached in psychotherapy because patients drop out when confronted with them. It may be that confrontation with these traits occurs too soon for many ASPD and BPD patients. Psychoanalysts emphasize the importance of exercising clinical judgment and timing in applying interpretive statements during treatment. Similarly, understanding how comorbidities of Axis-I disorders interact with ASPD and BPD is crucial for constructing the hierarchy of symptoms to be used in individual treatment planning.

SUGGESTED READINGS

Beck, A.T., Freeman, A., & Associates (1990). *Cognitive therapy of personality disorders.* New York, NY: Guilford Press.

Benjamin, L.S. (1996). *Interpersonal diagnosis and treatment of personality disorders.* New York, NY: Guilford Press.

Clarkin, J.F., Yeomans, F.E., & Kernberg, O.F. (1999). *Psychotherapy for borderline personality.* New York, NY: John Wiley & Sons, Inc.

Gabbard, G.O. (1990). *Psychodynamic psychiatry in clinical practice.* Washington, DC: American Psychiatric Press.

Kernberg, O.F., Selzer, M.A., Koenigsberg, H.W., Carr, A.C., & Appelbaum, A.H. (1989). *Psychodynamic psychotherapy of borderline patients.* New York, NY: Basic Books.

Meloy, J.R. (1988). *The psychopathic mind.* Northdale, NJ: Jason Aronson.

Stone, M. (1990). *The fate of borderline patients: Successful outcome and psychiatric practice.* New York, NY: Guilford Press.

REFERENCES

American Psychiatric Association (APA) (1994). *Diagnostic and statistical manual of mental disorders,* 4th ed. Washington, DC: American Psychiatric Association.

Arndt, I.O., McLellan, A.T., Dorozynsky, L., Woody, G.E., & Obrien, C.P. (1994). Desipramine treatment for cocaine dependence role of Antisocial Personality Disorder. *Journal of Nervous and Mental Disease, 182,* 151–156.

Beck, A.T., Freeman, A., & Associates (1990). *Cognitive therapy of personality disorders.* New York, NY: Guilford Press.

Benjamin, L.S. (1996). *Interpersonal diagnosis and treatment of personality disorders.* New York, NY: Guilford Press.

Brown, G., Ebert, M., Goyer, P., Jimerson, D., Klein, W., Bunney, W., & Goodwin, F. (1982). Aggression, suicide and serotonin: Relationships to CSF amine metabolites. *American Journal of Psychiatry, 139,* 741–746.

Brown, G., Goodwin, F., Ballenger, J., Goyer, P., & Major, L. (1979). Aggression in humans correlates with cerebrospinal fluid metabolites. *Psychiatric Research, 1,* 131.

Carter, J.D., Joyce, P.R., Mulder, R.T., Sullivan, P.F., & Luty, S.E. (1999). Gender differences in the frequency of personality disorders in depressed outpatients. *Journal of Personality Disorders, 13,* 67–74.

Clarkin, J.F., Yeomans, F.E., & Kernberg, O.F. (1999). *Psychotherapy for borderline personality.* New York, NY: John Wiley & Sons, Inc.

Cleckley, H. (1976). *The mask of sanity,* 5th ed. St. Louis: C.V. Mosby.

Coccaro, E.F., & Kavoussi, R.J. (1991). Biological and pharmacological aspects of Borderline Personality Disorder. *Hospital and Community Psychiatry, 42,* 1029–1033.

Coccaro, E.F., Siever, L.J., Klar, H.M., Maurer, G., Cochrane, K., Cooper, T.B., Mohs, R.C., & Davis, K.L. (1989). Serotonergic studies in patients with affective and personality disorders. *Archives of General Psychiatry, 46,* 587–599.

Constantino, J.N., Morris, J.A., & Murphy, D.L. (1997). CSF-5HIAA and family history of antisocial personality disorder in newborns. *American Journal of Psychiatry, 154,* 1771–1773.

Conte, H.R., Plutchik, R., Karasu, T.B., & Jerrett, I. (1980). A self-report borderline scale discriminative validity and preliminary norms. *Journal of Nervous and Mental Disease, 168,* 428–435.

Cowdry, R.W., & Gardner, D.L. (1988). Pharmacotherapy of borderline personality disorder: Alprazolam, carbamezapine, trifluoperazine and trancyclopromine. *Archives of General Psychiatry, 45,* 111–119.

Dubo, E.D., Zanarini, M.C., Lewis, R.E., & Williams, A.A. (1997). Childhood antecedents of self-destructiveness in Borderline Personality Disorder. *Canadian Journal of Psychiatry, 42,* 63–69.

Figueroa, E.F., Silk, K.R., Huth, A., & Lohr, N.E. (1997). History of childhood sexual abuse and general psychopathology. *Comprehensive Psychiatry, 38,* 23–30.

First, M.B., Spitzer, R.L., Gibbon, M., & Williams, J.B.W. (1995). The structured clinical interview for DSM-III-R personality disorders (SCID-II). Part I: Description. *Journal of Personality Disorders, 9,* 83–91.

First, M.B., Spitzer, R.L., Gibbon, M., Williams, J.B.W., Davies, M., Borus, J., Howes, M.J., Kane, J., Pope, H.G., & Rounsaville, B. (1995). The Structured Clinical Interview for DSM-III-R Personality Disorders (SCID-II). Part II: Multi-site test-retest reliability study. *Journal of Personality Disorders, 9,* 92–104.

Frosch, J.P. (1983). The treatment of antisocial and borderline personality disorders. *Hospital and Community Psychiatry, 34,* 243–248.

Gabbard, G.O. (1990). *Psychodynamic psychiatry in clinical practice.* Washington, DC: American Psychiatric Press.

Gabbard, G.O., & Coyne, L. (1987). Predictors of response of antisocial patients to hospital treatment. *Hospital and Community Psychiatry, 38,* 1181–1185.

Golomb, M., Fava, M., Abraham, M., & Rosenbaum (1995). Gender differences in personality disorders. *American Journal of Psychiatry, 152,* 579–582.

Greene, R.L. (1980). *The MMPI: An interpretive manual.* New York, NY: Grune and Stratton.

Gunderson, J.G. (1984). *Borderline personality disorder.* Washington, DC: American Psychiatric Press.

Gunderson, J.G., Kolb, J.E., & Austin, V. (1981). The diagnostic interview for borderlines. *American Journal of Psychiatry, 138,* 869–903.

Gunderson, J.G., & Lyoo, I.K. (1997). Family problems and relationships for adults with Borderline Personality Disorder. *Harvard Review of Psychiatry, 4,* 272–278.

Gunderson, J.G., & Phillips, K.A. (1991). A current view of the interface between borderline personality disorder and depression. *American Journal of Psychiatry, 148,* 967–975.

Hickey, B.A. (1985). The borderline experience subjective impression. *Journal of Psychosocial Nursing, 23,* 24–29.

Kavoussi, R.J., Liu, J., & Coccaro, E.F. (1994). An open trial of sertraline in personality disordered patients with impulsive aggression. *Journal of Clinical Psychiatry, 55,* 137–141.

Kelly, T.M., Soloff, P.H., Cornelius, J., George, A., Lis, J.A., & Ulrich, R. (1992). Can we study (treat) borderline patients? Attrition from research and open treatment. *Journal of Personality Disorders, 6,* 417–433.

Kernberg, O.F. (1975). *Borderline conditions and pathological narcissism.* New York, NY: Jason Aronson.

Kernberg, O.F., Selzer, M.A., Koenigsberg, H.W., Carr, A.C., & Appelbaum, A.H. (1989). *Psychodynamic psychotherapy of borderline patients.* New York, NY: Basic Books.

Kessler, R.C., McGonagle, K.A., Zhao, S., Nelson, C.B., Hughes, M., Eshelman, S., Wittchen, H., & Kendler, K.S. (1994). Lifetime and 12-month prevalence of DSM-III-R psychiatric disorders in the United States. *Archives of General Psychiatry, 51,* 8–19.

Langbehn, D.R., Cadoret, R.J., Yates, W.R., Troughton, E.P., & Stewart, M.A. (1998). Distinct contributions of conduct and oppositional defiant symptoms to adult antisocial behavior: Evidence from an adoption study. *Archives of General Psychiatry, 55*, 821–829.

Leal, J., Ziedonis, D., & Kosten, T. (1994). Antisocial personality disorder as a prognostic factor for pharmacotherapy of cocaine dependence. *Drug and Alcohol Dependence, 35*, 31–35.

Lilienfeld, S.O. (1998). Methodological advances and developments in the assessment of psychopathy. *Behaviour Research and Therapy, 36*, 99–125.

Linehan, M.M. (1993). *Cognitive-behavioral treatment of borderline personality disorder*. New York, NY: Guilford Press.

Linehan, M.M., Armstrong, H.E., Suarez, A., Allmon, D., & Heard, H. (1991). Cognitive-behavioral treatment of chronically parasuicidal borderline patients. *Archives of General Psychiatry, 48*, 1060–1064.

Linehan, M.M., Heard, H.L., & Armstrong, H.E. (1993). Naturalistic follow-up of a behavioral treatment for chronically parasuicidal borderline patients. *Archives of General Psychiatry, 50*, 971–974.

Links, P.S., Heselgrave, R., & Van Reekum, R. (1999). Impulsivity: Core aspect of borderline personality disorder. *Journal of Personality Disorders, 13*, 1–9.

Links, P.S., Steiner, M., Boiago, L., & Irwin, D. (1990). Lithium therapy for borderline patients: Preliminary findings. *Journal of Personality Disorders, 4*, 173–181.

Lion, J.R., & Leaff, L.A. (1973). On the hazards of assessing character pathology in an outpatient setting. *Psychiatric Quarterly, 47*, 104–109.

Livesly, W.J. (1995). *The DSM-IV Personality Disorders*. New York, NY: Guilford Press.

Loeber, R., Keenan, K., Lahey, B.B., Green, S.M., & Thomas, C. (1993). Evidence for developmentally based diagnoses of oppositional defiant disorder and conduct disorder. *Journal of Abnormal Child Psychology, 21*, 377–410.

Loranger, A.W. (1997). International personality disorder examination (IPDE). In A.W. Loranger, A. Janca, & Sartorius, N. (Eds.), *Assessment and diagnosis of personality disorders: The ICD-10 international personality disorder examination (IPDE)* (pp. 43–51). Cambridge: Cambridge University Press.

Loranger, A.W., Janca, A., & Sartorius, N. (1997). *Assessment and diagnosis of personality disorders: The ICD-10 international personality disorder examination (IPDE) manual* (pp. 114–129). Cambridge: University Press.

Mahler, M.S., Pine, F., & Bergman, A. (1975). *The psychological birth of the human infant.* New York, NY: Basic Books.

Mann, J.J. (1987). Psychobiologic predictors of suicide. *Journal of Clinical Psychiatry, 48*, 39–43.

Mannuzza, S., Klein, R.G., Bessler, A., Malloy, P., & LaPadula M. (1993). Adult outcome of hyperactive boys. *Archives of General Psychiatry, 50*, 565–576.

Marlowe, M.J., O'Neill-Byrne, K., Lowe-Ponsford, F.L., & Watson, J.P. (1996). The Borderline Syndrome Index: A validation study using the Personality Assessment Schedule. *British Journal of Psychiatry, 168*, 72–75.

Masterson, J.F. (1976). *Psychotherapy of the borderline adult.* New York, NY: Bruner/Mazel.

McDavid, J.D., & Pilkonis, P.A.(1996). The stability of personality disorder diagnoses. *Journal of Personality Disorders, 10*, 1–15.

McKinley, J.C., & Hathaway, S.R. (1944). The MMPI: V. Hysteria, hypomania and psychopathic deviate. *Journal of Applied Psychology, 28*, 153–174.

Mehlum, L., Friis, S., Irion, T., Johns, S., Karterud, S., Vaglum, P., & Vaglum, S. (1991). Personality disorders 2–5 years after treatment: A prospective follow-up study. *Acta Psychiatrica Scandanavica, 84*, 72–77.

Meloy, J.R. (1988). *The psychopathic mind.* Northdale, NJ: Jason Aronson.

Millon, T., Davis, R.D., & Associates (1996). *Disorders of personality DSM-IV and beyond.* New York, NY: John Wiley and Sons.

New, A.S., Trestman, R.L., Mitropolulou, V., Benishay, D., Coccaro, E., & Siever, L.J. (1997). Serotonergic function and self-injurious behavior in personality disorder patients. *Psychiatry Research, 69*, 17–26.

Oldham, J.M., Skodol, A.E., Kellman, H.D., Hyler, S.E., Doidge, N., Rosnick, L., & Gallaher, P.E. (1995). Comorbidity of Axis I and Axis II disorders. *American Journal of Psychiatry, 152*, 571–578.

Pilkonis, P.A. (1999). Treatment of personality disorders in association with symptom disorders. In W.J. Lively (Ed.), *Handbook of personality disorders.* New York, NY: Guilford Press.

Pilkonis, P.A., & Frank, E. (1988). Personality pathology in recurrent depression: Nature, prevalence, and relationship to treatment response. *American Journal of Psychiatry, 145,* 435–441.

Pilkonis, P.A., & Klein, K.R. (1999). Commentary on the assessment and diagnosis of antisocial behavior and personality. In D. Stoff, J. Brieling, & J.D. Masur (Eds.), *Handbook of antisocial behavior.* New York, NY: John Wiley and Sons.

Regier, D.A., Farmer, M.E., Rae, D.S., Myers, J.K., Kramer, M., Robins, L.N., George, L.K., Karno, M., & Locke, B.Z. (1993). One-month prevalence of mental disorders in the United states and sociodemographic characteristics: The Epidemiologic Catchment Area study. *Acta Psychiatrica Scandanavica, 88,* 35–47.

Rinsley, D.B. (1982). *Borderline and other self disorders. A developmental and object-relations perspective.* New York and London: Jason Aronson.

Robins, L.N., & Price, R.K. (1991). Adult disorders predicted by childhood conduct problems: Results from the NIMH Epidemiologic Catchment Area project. *Psychiatry, 54,* 116–132.

Rogers, J.H., Widiger, T.A., & Krupp, A. (1995). Aspects of depression associated with borderline personality disorder. *American Journal of Psychiatry, 152,* 268–270.

Roy, A., & Linnoila, M. (1989). CSF studies on alcoholism and related behaviours. *Progress in Neuro-Psychopharmacology and Biological Psychiatry, 13,* 505–511.

Ryle, A. (1995). The practice of CAT. In A. Ryle (Ed.), *Cognitive analytic therapy developments in theory and practice* (pp. 23–53). New York, NY: John Wiley & Sons.

Saxena, S., Brody, A.L., Schwartz, J.M., & Baxter, L.R. (1998). Neuroimaging and frontal-subcortical circuitry in obsessive-compulsive disorder. *British Journal of Psychiatry, 173* (Suppl. 35), 26–37.

Shachnow, J., Clarkin, J., Smith-DiPalma, Thurston, F., Hull, J., & Shearin, E. (1997). Biparental psychopathology and Borderline Personality Disorder. *Psychiatry, 60,* 171–181.

Shea, M.T., Widiger, T.A., & Klein, M.H. (1992). Comorbidity of personality disorders and depression: Implications for treatment. *Journal of Consulting and Clinical Psychology, 60,* 857–868.

Shearin, E.N., & Linehan, M.M. (1994). Dialectical behavior therapy for borderline personality disorder: Theoretical and empirical foundations. *Acta Psychiatrica Scandanavica, 89* (Suppl. 379), 61–68.

Silk, K., Lee, S., Hill, E., & Lohr, N.E. (1995). Borderline Personality Disorder symptoms and severity of sexual abuse. *American Journal of Psychiatry, 152,* 1059–1064.

Skodol, A.E., & Oldham, J.M. (1991). Assessment and diagnosis of Borderline Personality Disorder. *Hospital and Community Psychiatry, 42,* 1021–1028.

Soloff, P.H. (1990). Psychopharmacologic therapies in borderline personality disorder. In A. Tasman, E. Hales, & A.J. Frances (Eds.), *Review of psychiatry,* Vol. 8 (pp. 65–83). Washington, DC: American Psychiatric Press.

Soloff, P.H. (1998). Algorithms for pharmacological treatment of personality dimensions: Symptom-specific treatments for cognitive-perceptual, affective, and impulsive-behavioral dysregulation. *Bulletin of the Menninger Clinic, 62,* 195–213.

Soloff, P.H., George, A., Nathan, R.S., Shulz, P.M., & Perel, J.M. (1986). Paradoxical effects of amitriptyline in borderline patients. *American Journal of Psychiatry, 143,* 1603–1605.

Soloff, P.H., & Millward, J.W. (1983). Developmental histories of borderline patients. *Comprehensive Psychiatry, 24,* 574–588.

Sperry, L. (1995). *Handbook of diagnosis and treatment of DSM-IV personality disorders.* New York, NY: Bruner/Mazel.

Stangl, D., Pfohl, B., Zimmerman, M., Bowers, W., & Corenthal, C. (1985). A structured interview for the DSM-III personality disorders, a preliminary report. *Archives of General Psychiatry, 42,* 591–596.

Stone, M. (1990). *The fate of borderline patients: Successful outcome and psychiatric practice.* New York, NY: Guilford Press.

Swartz, M., Blazer, D., George, L., & Winfield, I. (1990). Estimating the prevalence of borderline personality disorder in the community. *Journal of Personality Disorders, 4,* 257–272.

Torgerson, S. (1994). Genetics in borderline conditions. *Acta Psychiatrica Scandanavica, 89* (Suppl. 379), 19–25.

Tyrer, P., Gunderson, J.G., Lyons, M., & Tohen, M. (1997). Special feature: Extent of comorbidity between mental state and personality disorders. *Journal of Personality Disorders, 11,* 242–259.

Vailliant, G.E. (1975). Sociopathy as a human process: A viewpoint. *Archives of General Psychiatry, 32,* 178–183.

Waldinger, R.J., & Gunderson, J.G. (1984). Completed psychotherapies with borderline patients. *American Journal of Psychotherapy*,
38, 190–202.

Weaver, T.L., & Clum, G.A. (1993). Early family environments and traumatic experiences associated with Borderline Personality Disorder.
Journal of Consulting and Clinical Psychology, *61*, 1068–1075.

Weiss, G., Hechtman, L., Milroy, T., & Perlman, T. (1985). Psychiatric
status of hyperactives as adults: A controlled prospective 15-year
follow-up of 63 hyperactive children. *Journal of the American
Academy of Child and Adolescent Psychiatry*, *24*, 211–220.

Young, D.W., & Gunderson, J.G. (1995). Family images of borderline
adolescents. *Psychiatry*, *58*, 164–172.

Young, J.E. (1994). *Cognitive therapy for personality disorders: A
schema-focused approach*. Sarasota, FL: Professional Resource Press.

Zanarini, M.C., & Frankenburg, F.R. (1997). Pathways to the development of borderline personality disorder. *Journal of Personality
Disorders*, *11*, 93–104.

Zanarini, M.C., Frankenburg, F.R., Chauncey, D.L., & Gunderson, J.G.
(1987). The diagnostic interview for personality disorders: Interrater
and test-retest reliability. *Comprehensive Psychiatry*, *28*, 467–480.

Zanarini, M.C., Frankenburg, F.R., Dubo, E.D., Sickel, M.A., Trikha, A.,
Levin, A., & Reynolds, M.A. (1998). Axis I comorbidity of borderline
personality disorder. *American Journal of Psychiatry*, *155*, 1733–
1739.

Zanarini, M.C., Gunderson, J.G., Frankenburg, F.R., & Chauncey, D.L.
(1990). Discriminating Borderline Personality Disorder from other
Axis II disorders. *American Journal of Psychiatry*, *147*, 161–167

Zanarini, M.C., Gunderson, J.G., Marino, M.F., Schwartz, E.O., &
Frankenburg, F.R. (1989). Childhood experiences of borderline
patients. *Comprehensive Psychiatry*, *30*, 18–25.

Zimmerman, M., Pfohl, B., Stangl, D., & Corenthal, C. (1986).
Assessment of DSM-III personality disorders: The importance of interviewing an informant. *Journal of Clinical Psychiatry*, *47*, 261–263.

Index

ISBN 0-07-134716-X